Z SCORE NEUROFEEDBACK

Z SCORE NEUROFEEDBACK

Clinical Applications

Edited by

ROBERT W. THATCHER
JOEL F. LUBAR

AMSTERDAM • BOSTON • HEIDELBERG • LONDON
NEW YORK • OXFORD • PARIS • SAN DIEGO
SAN FRANCISCO • SINGAPORE • SYDNEY • TOKYO

Academic Press is an imprint of Elsevier

Academic Press is an imprint of Elsevier
32 Jamestown Road, London NW1 7BY, UK
225 Wyman Street, Waltham, MA 02451, USA
525 B Street, Suite 1800, San Diego, CA 92101-4495, USA
The Boulevard, Langford Lane, Kidlington, Oxford OX5 1GB, UK

ISBN: 978-0-12-801291-8

British Library Cataloguing-in-Publication Data
A catalogue record for this book is available from the British Library

Library of Congress Cataloging-in-Publication Data
A catalog record for this book is available from the Library of Congress

For information on all Academic Press publications
visit our website at http://store.elsevier.com/

Typeset by MPS Limited, Chennai, India
www.adi-mps.com

Printed and bound in United States of America

Contents

Preface

EEG biofeedback also called neurofeedback has a 60-year history in the scientific literature. However, a problem with human neurofeedback methods was inefficiency because improved clinical outcome and changes in the EEG occurred only after many sessions, e.g., 40–80 sessions. A large number of sessions are expensive with reduced patient compliance and the need for good clinical outcome in fewer sessions is a pressing need. The first indication that more efficient biofeedback is related to increased specificity of the physiological event was proven in the 1960s when scientist's operant conditioned single neurons, groups of neurons, and evoked potentials in only a few sessions. The lack of specificity in human neurofeedback studies was evident by the use of one or two scalp electrodes arbitrarily placed on the scalp in which each electrode was influenced by widespread electrical sources inside the brain and therefore was nonspecific as to the Brodmann areas and networks inside the brain. Also, researchers and clinicians had no standards by which to select thresholds to determine if a feedback signal was to be delivered or not. For example, clinicians would argue for different protocols in which the threshold for alpha rhythms may be 20 μV for one clinician or 15 or 25 μV for others, etc. Arbitrary thresholds to inhibit rhythms like theta (4–8 Hz) also occurred, e.g., is the threshold 5 or 10 or 15 μV, etc. Still worse was that different clinicians would use different metrics. Some would use relative power, which is a percentage, others would use absolute amplitude in microvolts, others would use ratios of power, others would use ratios of relative power, and others would use arbitrary measures of coherence at different scalp locations and different ages.

In the late 1990s, it became obvious that the lack of specificity and uniform standards resulted in inefficient clinical applications of neurofeedback. As a consequence, the idea of using real-time Z scores to simplify and standardize neurofeedback was suggested by Robert Thatcher in the 1990s and implemented in 2006 with almost an immediate improvement in the efficiency of neurofeedback. That is, good clinical outcome was noticed in <20 sessions and often in <10 sessions soon after the first application of Z-score EEG biofeedback. The reason for the improved clinical efficacy was that different and multiple metrics were reduced to a single common metric, i.e., the metric of a Z score that ranges from ±2 or 3 standard deviations no matter what the original metric may be. Further, the

Z score removes arbitrary guessing about thresholds because the goal is to reinforce any given EEG measure in the direction of $Z = 0$ which is the center of a reference healthy age-matched normal population that has no psychological problems nor a history of clinical disorders. Reinforcing toward $Z = 0$ is also reinforcing toward greater stability and efficiency in networks of the brain. Dr. Joel Lubar was one of the first to embrace and adopt the Z-score EEG neurofeedback method and immediately reported improved clinical outcome in fewer sessions than had been his history prior to the introduction of Z-score biofeedback.

It was also noticed in the 1990s that clinicians were not linking a patient's symptoms to the patient's brain. Instead a "one size fits all" approach dominated the field of EEG neurofeedback for decades in which electrodes were placed, for example, at bilateral temporal locations (T3/T4) or midline line central locations (e.g., Cz) for all patients independent of their symptoms and clinical history. As a consequence, the concept of seamless integration of a "Symptom Check List" was introduced by which hypotheses can be formed to confirm or disconfirm which networks of the brain were likely linked to the patient's symptoms. This introduced another major increase in specificity since it has long been known that dysregulation in parts of a network called the "weak" system results in compensatory activity by the stronger or healthier networks. Not separating the "weak" network most likely responsible for the patient's symptoms from the compensatory networks is inefficient and results in more sessions before clinical improvement is noticed.

The next innovation was the 2010 introduction of Z scores to real-time three-dimensional EEG source localization integrated with symptom checklists. This advancement further increased specificity in which one begins with the patient's symptoms and hypothesis formation followed by QEEG assessment to confirm or reject hypotheses followed by low-resolution electromagnetic tomography (LORETA) Z-score neurofeedback that targets Brodmann areas (network nodes) and connections between nodes linked to the patient's symptoms. This not only increased specificity but also clinician efficiency by seamless integration of QEEG assessment treatment in a single 40-min session. The goal was to reinforce increased stability and efficiency of information processing in dysregulated network nodes and connections linked to the patient's symptoms. As evidenced in this book, the seamless integration and linking of symptoms to dysregulated networks in patient's brains resulted in improved clinical outcome in fewer sessions, which is the ultimate goal of EEG biofeedback.

Biofeedback of functional connectivity in three-dimensional neural networks linked to symptoms by real-time LORETA coherence, phase difference, phase lock, and phase shift referenced to an age-matched referenced normal population is one of the main topics in this book. Functional connectivity coupled with LORETA current density of neural networks linked to symptoms has become a standard method of EEG biofeedback now used by hundreds of clinicians and we expect that these scientific advancements will continue into the future. For example, reinforcement of effective connectivity also called "directional connectivity" is currently under development.

Another recent scientific advancement of EEG biofeedback is the introduction of Brain–computer interface (BCI) methods as described in the chapter on BrainSurfer. BCI involves the same neuromodulators and reinforcement toward increased stability in neural networks linked to symptoms as with EEG biofeedback but differs by involving continuous feedback with real-time visualization of the patient's brain network nodes and connections. No discrete feedback by a DVD or video or signal is used with BCI, instead patients employ cognitive and emotional strategies to change networks in their brains by viewing changes in nodes and connections in real time. The use of *Z* scores to simplify and guide toward the center of an age-matched normal reference is again a central concept designed to reinforce increased stability in networks linked to the patient's symptoms.

Important feedbacks regarding clinical efficacy and good clinical outcome by Dr. Lubar and others were major factors in the design and development of *Z*-score biofeedback technology. This new technology required step-by-step improvements in implementation and adherence to the basic scientific principles of EEG operant conditioning as discovered in the 1940s and extensively explored in the 1960s. Given the successes of the past as evidenced in this book, we anticipate further developments and implementation of similar technologies in the near future. We see a bright and maturing future of the field of EEG neurofeedback and see this book as one example of a growing scientific literature going forward.

Robert W. Thatcher and Joel F. Lubar

List of Contributors

Richard D. Abbey Abbey Neuropsychology Clinic, Palo Alto, CA, USA

Brianna H. Bendixsen Abbey Neuropsychology Clinic, Palo Alto, CA, USA

Carl J. Biver Applied Neuroscience Research Institute, Seminole, FL, USA; NeuroImaging Laboratory, Applied Neuroscience, Inc., Seminole, FL, USA

Wesley D. Center Liberty University, Lynchburg, VA, USA; Focus for Living, PLLC, Burleson, TX, USA

Scott L. Decker University of South Carolina, Barnwell College, Columbia, SC, USA

Dale S. Foster Memphis Integral Neurofeedback Institute (MINI), Cordova, TN; Applied Neuroscience Research Institute, Seminole, FL, USA

Gerald Gluck Center for Family Counseling and Biofeedback, Coral Springs, FL, USA

Jessica J. Green University of South Carolina, Barnwell College, Columbia, SC, USA

J. Lucas Koberda Tallahassee NeuroBalance Center, Tallahassee, FL, USA

William A. Lambos ABF Behavioral Health, Tampa, FL, USA

Rachael M. Little Abbey Neuropsychology Clinic, Palo Alto, CA, USA

Joel F. Lubar Southeastern Neurofeedback Institute, Pompano Beach, FL, USA

Duane M. North Applied Neuroscience Research Institute, Seminole, FL, USA; NeuroImaging Laboratory, Applied Neuroscience, Inc., Seminole, FL, USA

Andrea Reid-Chung ADD Centre & Biofeedback Institute of Toronto, Mississauga, ON, Canada

Alycia M. Roberts University of South Carolina, Barnwell College, Columbia, SC, USA

Robert W. Thatcher Memphis Integral Neurofeedback Institute (MINI), Cordova, TN, USA; Applied Neuroscience Research Institute, Seminole, FL, USA

Lynda Thompson ADD Centre & Biofeedback Institute of Toronto, Mississauga, ON, Canada

Michael Thompson ADD Centre & Biofeedback Institute of Toronto, Mississauga, ON, Canada

Paul Wand Private Practice, Coral Springs, FL, USA

Rebecca A. Williams ABF Behavioral Health, Tampa, FL, USA

CHAPTER

1

History and Technical Foundations of Z Score EEG Biofeedback

Robert W. Thatcher, Carl J. Biver and Duane M. North

NeuroImaging Laboratory, Applied Neuroscience, Inc., Seminole, FL, USA

INTRODUCTION

The statistical foundations of Z score electroencephalogram (EEG) biofeedback are based on the fact that after the appropriate transform, all EEG variables are Gaussian distributed with sample sizes equal to or greater than about 20 subjects per age group. A review of the statistical foundations is in the paper "History of the Scientific Standards of QEEG Normative Databases" (Thatcher & Lubar, 2008). The Z score is a statistic of distance from the mean adjusted for variance or Z = mean−measure divided by the standard deviation where at infinity with a random sampling the ideal Gaussian mean = 0 and the standard deviation = 1. This is a powerful statistic that also has a multivariate expression called the Mahalanobis distance (Cooley & Lohnes, 1971). The interpretation of a Z score depends on the assumptions of (1) a Gaussian distribution (>0.95) after transform of the raw digital data, (2) a $N > 20$ of a representative sample of the measure of interest, (3) the measures to compute the mean must be the same variables used to compute a Z score (e.g., FFT means cannot be used to compute joint time−frequency analysis (JTFA) Z scores or vice versa). The reason there is a violation of statistical sampling theory if one uses the FFT to compute a JTFA Z scores is because the FFT multiplies sine/cosine waves over a discrete interval of time (e.g., 1−2 s) as well as windowing

Z Score Neurofeedback.
DOI: http://dx.doi.org/10.1016/B978-0-12-801291-8.00001-7

to approximate infinity, whereas JTFA methods like Wavelets or Complex Demodulation do not use windowing or the convolution of sine waves over a discrete window of time. Although the FFT and digital filters can converge at infinity, the fact is that the same group of subjects produce different means when comparing the FFT to JTFA and therefore, standard #3 is violated. It is easy to show that the FFT produces different means than the JTFA on the same data samples, e.g., we find over 14% differences and Brainmaster 8% difference in means between the FFT and filter means which is a significant error and is in violation of statistical sampling theory.

The remainder of this chapter will review and integrate the statistical and technical methods used and described in various forums. In the sections to follow, steps are taken to adhere to the basic statistical foundations in which there is no violation of statistical sampling theory because only complex demodulation means are used to compute complex demodulation Z scores in all Neuroguide analyses of Z score biofeedback measures presented in this chapter.

FIRST USE OF GAUSSIAN PROBABILITIES TO IDENTIFY "DYSREGULATION" IN THE BRAIN

The fundamental design concepts of Z score biofeedback were first introduced by Thatcher (1998, 1999, 2000a,b,c). The central idea of the instantaneous Z score is the application of the mathematical Gaussian curve or "bell-shaped" curve by which probabilities can be estimated using the auto- and cross-spectrum of the EEG in order to identify brain regions that are deregulated and depart from expected values. Linkage of symptoms and complaints to functional localization in the brain is best achieved by the use of a minimum of 19 channel EEG evaluation so that current source density and LORETA source localization can be computed. Once the linkage is made, then an individualized Z score protocol can be devised. However, in order to make a linkage to symptoms, an accurate statistical inference must be made using the Gaussian distribution. The Gaussian distribution is a fundamental distribution that is used throughout science, e.g., the Schrodinger wave equation in Quantum mechanics uses the Gaussian distribution as basis functions (Robinett, 1997). The application of the EEG to the concept of the Gaussian distribution requires the use of standard mathematical transforms by which all statistical distributions can be transformed to a Gaussian distribution (Box & Cox, 1964). In the case of the EEG, transforms such as the square root, cube root, $\log_{10}$, Box-Cox, and hyperbolic sine are applied to the power spectrum of the digital time series in order to approximate a normal distribution (Duffy, Hughes, Miranda, Bernad, & Cook, 1994; Gasser, Jennen-Steinmetz, Sroka, Verleger, & Mocks, 1988; John, Prichep, & Easton, 1987; John, Prichep, Fridman, & Easton, 1988; Thatcher, North, & Biver, 2005a,b; Thatcher, Walker, Biver, North, & Curtin, 2003). The choice of the exact transform depends on the accuracy of the approximate match to a Gaussian distribution. The fact that accuracies of 95–99% match to a Gaussian are commonly published in the EEG literature encouraged by Thatcher and colleagues to develop and test the Z score biofeedback program.

The majority of cortical pyramidal neurons resonate at specific center frequencies depending on the membrane potential and ionic conductances and behave like "band pass" filters that gate action potentials. The pyramidal neuron resonances wax and wane and exhibit rhythmic bursts and periods of asynchrony in a non-Gaussian distribution as a function of time. It is necessary to mathematically transform EEG digital data to approximate a Gaussian in shape and then the EEG normative database can be cross-validated and estimates of error can be made. Z score biofeedback using the target of reinforcing toward $Z = 0$ with respect to the center of an age matched group of healthy individuals is designed to reinforce increased information processing in networks of the brain. The real-time EEG Z score utilizes a representative sample of normal and healthy subjects with no history of neurological psychological disorders with normal performance on neuropsychological tests measured while the first author (Thatcher) was the principal investigator and professor at the University of Maryland. Initially a sample of 625 "normal" subjects constituted the reference normal database and then the number was expanded to today with a total of 860 subjects. Standard equilibration of the amplifier frequency and gain characteristics was used to exactly match the amplifiers used to measure EEG from a patient to the frequency characteristics of the normative database amplifiers. The normative database includes clinical selection criteria, age range (2 months to 82 years), cross-validation tests, demographics, and other details of the Z score normative database have been published and are recommended reading for those interested in deeper details than is briefly reviewed in this document (see Thatcher, 1998, 1999, 2000a; Thatcher & Lubar, 2008; Thatcher et al., 2003).

In 2009, a method to aid in reinforcing extreme Z scores or outliers to move toward $Z = 0$ was called "Z Tunes." This real-time Z score biofeedback method was implemented in recognition of the neurophysiological linkage to resonant cortical pyramidal neurons that operate by reinforcing outliers over a 10 s history if the slope of the time history of the outliers is in the direction of $Z = 0$. That is, not reinforce outliers if they are diverging or becoming more extreme and only reinforce outliers if they are moving in the direction of increased stability in the direction of $Z = 0$.

APPLICATION OF GAUSSIAN PROBABILITY DISTRIBUTIONS TO INSTANTANEOUS Z SCORE BIOFEEDBACK AND WHY JTFA Z SCORES ARE SMALLER THAN FFT Z SCORES

The second design concept is the application of the Gaussian distribution to averaged "instantaneous" time domain spectral measures from groups of normal subjects and then to cross-validate the means and standard deviations for each subject for each instant of time (Thatcher, 1998, 1999, 2000a,b). The cross-validation is directly related to the variance of the distribution (Thatcher et al., 2003, 2005a,b). However, in order to achieve a representative Gaussian distribution, it is necessary to include two major categories of statistical variance: (1) the moment-to-moment variance or within session variance and (2) between subject variance across an age group. In the case of the fast Fourier transform (FFT), there is a single "integral" of the power spectrum for each subject and each frequency and, therefore, there is only between subject variance in normative databases that use noninstantaneous analyses such as the FFT. Thus, there is a fundamental and important difference between an instantaneous Z score and an integrated FFT Z score with the former having two sources of variance, while the latter has only one source of variance. Figure 1.1 illustrates the relationship between an FFT-based normative database versus an "instantaneous" or JTFA database such as used for the computation of instantaneous Z scores.

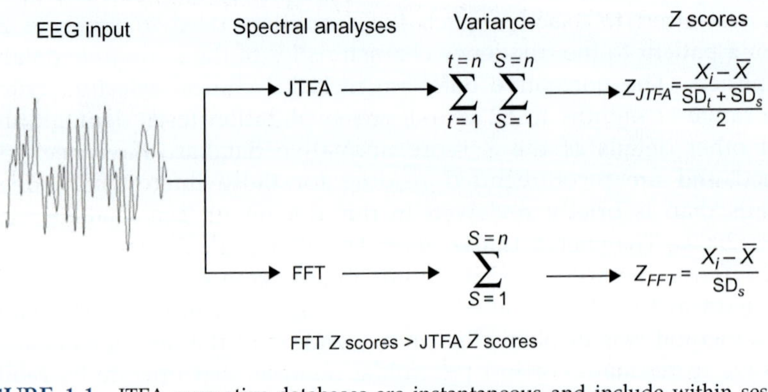

FIGURE 1.1 JTFA normative databases are instantaneous and include within session variance plus between subject variance. In contrast, FFT normative data only contains between subject variance. t = time, s = subjects, and SD_t = standard deviation for the within session and SD_s = standard deviation between subjects. Thus, FFT Z scores are larger than JTFA Z scores and a ratio of 2:1 is not uncommon.

SIMPLIFICATION AND STANDARDIZATION

Another design concept is simplification and standardization of EEG biofeedback by the application of basic science. Simplification is achieved by the use of a single metric, namely, the metric of the "Z score" for widely diverse measures such as power, coherence, and phase delays. Standardization is also achieved by EEG amplifier matching of the frequency response of the normative database amplifiers to the frequency characteristics of the EEG amplifiers used to acquire a comparison subject's EEG time series.

Once a quantitative (QEEG) normative database analysis is completed, then one can use a Z score biofeedback program to train patient's to move their instantaneous Z scores toward zero or the center of the age matched normal population. The absolute value and range of the instantaneous Z scores while smaller than those obtained using the offline QEEG normative database are nonetheless valid and capable of being minimized toward zero. An advantage of a Z score biofeedback program is simplification by reducing diverse measures to a single metric, i.e., the metric of a Z score. Thus, there is greater standardization and less guess work about whether to reinforce or suppress coherence or phase differences or power, etc., at a particular location and particular frequency band. The difference between standard and conventional EEG biofeedback versus Z score biofeedback is shown in Figure 1.2.

INDIVIDUALIZED EEG BIOFEEDBACK PROTOCOLS

An intertwined clinical concept in the design of Z score biofeedback is "individualized" EEG biofeedback and nonprotocol-driven EEG biofeedback based on a symptom checklist. The idea of linking patient symptoms and complaints to functional localization in the brain and resonant frequencies of the EEG as evidenced by "dysregulation" of neural populations is fundamental to individualized biofeedback. For example, dysregulation is recognized by significantly elevated or reduced power or network measures such as coherence and phase within regions of the brain that subserve particular functions that can be linked to the patient's symptoms and complaints. The use of Z scores for biofeedback is designed to "re-regulate" or "optimize" the homeostasis, neural excitability, and network connectivity in particular regions of the brain. The functional localization and linkage to symptoms is based on modern knowledge of brain function as measured by fMRI, PET, penetrating head wounds, strokes, and other neurological evidence acquired over the last two centuries (see Brazis et al., 2007; Heilman & Valenstein, 1993; Thatcher, 2011a,b, 2012). Thus, the false concern that Z

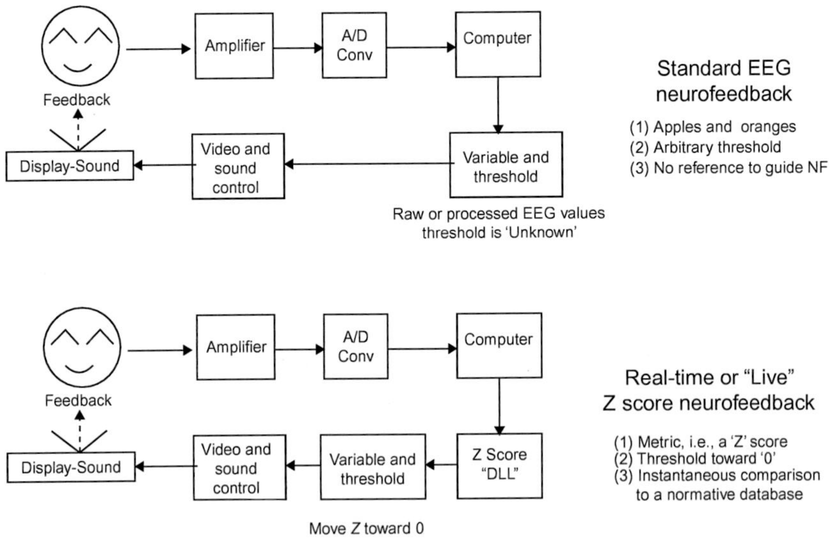

FIGURE 1.2 Top row is conventional or standard EEG biofeedback in which different units of measurement are used in an EEG analysis (e.g., μV for amplitude, theta/beta ratios, relative power 0–100%, coherence 0–1, phase in degrees or radians) and the clinician must "guess" at a threshold for a particular electrode location and frequency and age as to when to reinforce or inhibit a give measure. The bottom row is Z score biofeedback in which different metrics are represented by a single and common metric, i.e., the metric of a Z score and the guess work is removed because all measures are reinforced to move Z scores toward Z = 0 which is the approximate center of an average healthy brain state based on a reference age matched normative database in real time.

score biofeedback will make exceptional people dull and an average individual a genius is misplaced. The concept is to reinforce stability and not periods of "chaos" in networks linked to symptoms and complaints and then monitor improvement or symptom reduction during the course of treatment using a single metric for all measures, i.e., the Z score. For peak performance applications, a careful inventory of the client's personality style, self-assessment of weaknesses and strengths, and identification of the client's specific areas that he/she wishes to improve must be obtained before application of Z score biofeedback. Then, the practitioner attempts to link the client's identification of areas of weakness that he/she wants to improve to functional localization as expressed by "deregulation" of deviant neural activity that may be subject to change.

As mentioned previously, the instantaneous Z scores are much smaller than the FFT Z scores in Neuroguide™ which uses the same subjects for the normative database. Smaller Z scores when using the instantaneous Z scores is expected because of the necessary inclusion of the moment-to-moment within session variance. One should not be surprised by a 50% reduction in JTFA Z scores in comparison to FFT Z scores and this is why it is best to first use 19 channel EEG measures and the highly stable FFT Z scores to link symptoms to functional localization in the brain to the extent possible. Then use the Z score program inside of Neuroguide™ to evaluate the patient's instantaneous Z scores in preparation before the biofeedback procedure begins. This will allow one to obtain a unique picture of the EEG instantaneous Z scores of each unique patient prior to beginning Z score biofeedback. The clinician must be trained to select which Z scores best match the patient's symptoms and complaints. A general rule is the choice of Z scores to use for biofeedback depends on two factors obtained using a full 19 channel EEG analysis: (1) scalp location(s) and (2) magnitude of the Z scores. Dysregulation by hyperpolarization produces slowing in the EEG and deregulation due to reduced inhibition produces deviations at higher frequencies. The direction of the Z score is much less important than the location(s) of the deviant Z scores and the linkage to the patient's symptoms and complaints.

IMPLEMENTATION OF THE Z SCORE BIOFEEDBACK

Step one is to compute means and standard deviations of instantaneous absolute power, relative power, power ratios, coherence, phase differences and amplitude asymmetries, phase reset, etc., on selected age groups of normal subjects from the 19 channel 10/20 electrode locations using the within session and between session variance as described previously. The inclusion/exclusion criteria, number of subjects, number of subjects per age group, cross-validation procedures, and other details of the means and standard deviation computations have been published (Thatcher et al., 2003; Thatcher, Walker, & Guidice, 1987). Step two is to develop a Dynamic Link Library or DLL that can be distributed to EEG biofeedback manufacturers such as BrainMaster, EEG Spectrum, Thought Technology, Mind Media BV (NeXus), EEG Spectrum, and Deymed which allows the manufacturers to integrate the instantaneous Z scores inside of their already existing software environments. The DLL involves only four command lines of code and is designed for software developers to easily implement the instantaneous Z scores by passing raw digital data to the DLL and then organizing the Z scores that are returned in less than 1 μs. This rapid analysis and return of Z scores is essential for timely feedback when specific EEG features are measured by the Complex Demodulation JTFA operating inside of the DLL.

JTFA COMPLEX DEMODULATION COMPUTATIONS

The mathematical details of complex demodulation used to compute the instantaneous Z scores as contained in the Applied Neuroscience, Inc. "DLL" are provided in the Appendix section and are described in Otnes and Enochson (1977), Bloomfield (2000), Granger and Hatanka (1964), and Thatcher, North, and Biver (2009). Complex demodulation is a time/frequency domain digital method of spectral analysis, whereas the FFT is a frequency domain method. These two methods are related by the fact that they both involve sines and cosines and both operate in the complex domain and in this way represent the same mathematical descriptions of the power spectrum. The advantage of complex demodulation is that it is a time/frequency domain method and is less sensitive to artifact and does not require windowing nor even integers of the power of 2 as does the FFT. The FFT integrates power in a frequency band over the entire epoch length and requires windowing functions which can dramatically affect the power values whereas, as mentioned previously, complex demodulation does not require windowing (Otnes & Enochson, 1972). Complex demodulation was computed for the linked ears and eyes open and eyes closed conditions for all 625 subjects in the normative database.

Table 1.1 gives the center frequencies and bandwidths used by the Neuroguide DLL as well as the temporal equivalent of frequency in the right column.

Figure 1.3 is an illustration of the method of complex demodulation for the computation of power, coherence, and phase. The mathematical details are given in the Appendix.

Z SCORES AND QEEG NORMATIVE DATABASES

Matousek and Petersen (1973) computed means and standard deviations in 1 year age groups and were the first to use Z scores to compare an individual to the normative database means and standard deviations. The Z score is an excellent statistic defined as the difference between the value from an individual and the mean of the population divided by the standard deviation of the population or

$$Z = \frac{x_i - \overline{X}}{\mathrm{SD}}$$

John and colleagues expanded on the use of the Z score for clinical evaluation including the use of multivariate measures such as the Mahalanobis distance metric. A direct normalization of the Gaussian

TABLE 1.1 Time Domain Conversion of Frequencies to Time of the Z Score Biofeedback DLL and Neuroguide

	Center Frequency (Hz)	Bandwidth (Hz)	Time Domain (ms)
Delta	2.5	1–4	1,000–250
Theta	6.0	4–8	250–125
Alpha	8.0	8–12	125–83
Beta	18.5	12–25	83–40
Hi-Beta	27.5	25–30	40–33
Beta 1	13.5	12–15	83–67
Beta 2	16.5	15–18	67–56
Beta 3	21.5	18–25	56–40
Alpha 1	9.0	8–10	125–100
Alpha 2	11.0	10–12	100–83
Gamma 1*	FFT only	30–35	33–29
Gamma 2*	FFT only	35–40	29–25
Gamma 3*	FFT only	40–50	25–20

*, Neuroguide only.

distribution using Z scores is useful in comparing individuals to a QEEG normative database. That is, the standard-score form of the Gaussian is where the mean = 0 and standard deviation = 1 or, by substitution into the Gaussian equation for a bell-shaped curve, then

$$Y = \frac{1}{\sqrt{2\pi}} e^{-z^2/2}$$

where Y = Gaussian distribution and the Z score is a deviation in standard deviation units measured along the baseline of the Gaussian curve from a mean of 0 and a standard deviation = 1 and deviations to the right of the mean being positive and those to the left negative. By substituting different values of Z, then different values of Y can be calculated. For example, when $Z = 0$, $Y = 0.3989$ or, in other words, the height of the curve at the mean of the normal distribution in standard-score form is given by the number 0.3989. For purposes of assessing deviation from normal, the values of Z above and below the mean, which include 95% of the area of the Gaussian, is often used as a level of confidence necessary to minimize Type I and Type II errors. The standard-score equation is also used to cross-validate a normative database which again emphasizes the importance of approximation to a Gaussian for any normative QEEG database.

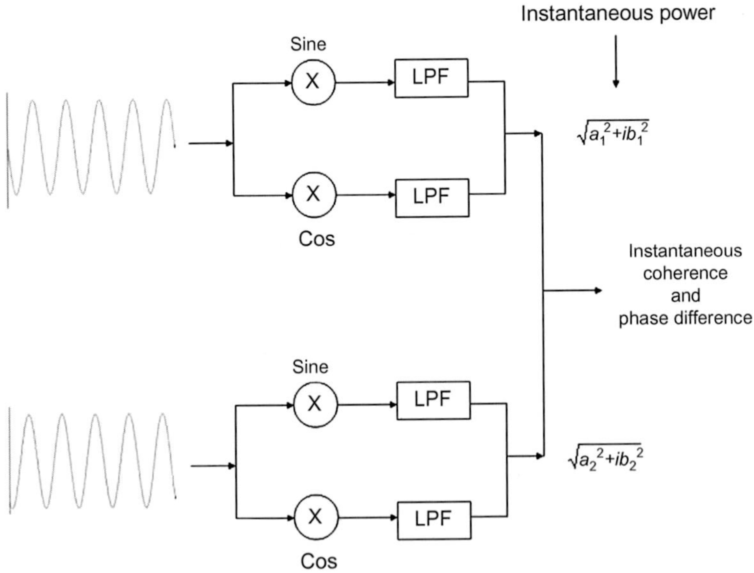

FIGURE 1.3 Diagram of complex demodulation. Left is a sine wave as input which is multiplied by the sine and cosine waves at the center frequency of a given frequency band as described in Table 1.1 which transforms the digital time series to the complex plane. A sixth-order Butterworth low-pass filter is used to shift the frequency to zero where power at the center frequency is then calculated using the Pythagorean theorem. Complex numbers are then used to compute coherence and phase as described in the Appendix.

STANDARDIZATION BY AMPLIFIER MATCHING AND QEEG NORMATIVE DATABASES

Surprisingly, matching of amplifier frequency characteristics as a standard was largely neglected during much of the history of QEEG normative databases. E. Roy John and colleagues (1982–1988) formed a consortium of universities and medical schools that were using QEEG who met several times over a few years and this consortium was one of the supporters of the edited volume by John titled "Machinery of the Mind" (John, 1990). One of the important issues consistently raised at the consortium meetings was the need for "standardization." In the 1980s, it was technically difficult to match different EEG systems because of the infantile development of analysis software. This history forced most QEEG users to use relative power because absolute power was not comparable between different EEG machines. There was no frequency response standardization between different EEG machines and thus there was no cross-platform standardization of QEEG. It was not until the mid-1990s that computer speed and software development

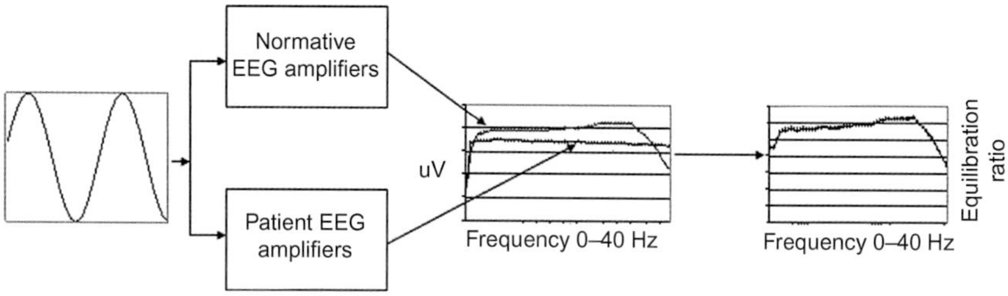

FIGURE 1.4 Flow chart of the amplifier standardization procedure. Microvolt sine waves are injected into the input of amplifiers and the frequency responses are calculated. The frequency response of the normative database amplifiers and the frequency response of other EEG amplifier systems are then equated and the spectral analysis is adjusted so that there is a standardized import and matching of amplifier systems with the common unit being microvolts (μV).

made amplifier matching and normative database amplifier equilibration a possibility. The first use of standardized matching of amplifiers was to the University of Maryland (UM) database (Thatcher et al., 2003). The procedure involved injecting microvolt calibration sine waves into the input of amplifiers of different EEG machines and then injecting the same microvolt signals into the normative database amplifiers thus obtaining two frequency response curves. The equilibration of a normative QEEG database to different EEG amplifiers is the ratio of the frequency response curves of the two amplifiers that are then used as coefficients in the power spectral analysis. This was an important step because suddenly absolute power Z scores and normative database comparisons became possible. The frequencies in absolute power are independent of each other and are not distorted. It is always best to use absolute values whenever possible and not relative values or even ratios. A ratio can change due to the denominator or the numerator and one cannot determine which has changed without evaluating the absolute values used to compute the ratios.

As illustrated in Figure 1.4, a simple method of amplifier equilibration to exactly match the frequency characteristics of different amplifiers is to calibrate the amplifiers using microvolt sine waves at discrete frequencies from 1 to 40 Hz and injecting the sine waves into the inputs of the EEG amplifiers. Then take the ratio of the microvolt values at each frequency and use the ratios to exactly equate the spectral output values at different frequencies for different amplifiers. This method creates a universal equilibration process so that microvolts in a given amplifier are equal to microvolts in all other amplifiers including the normative database amplifiers. By equilibrating amplifiers, direct comparisons between a given patient's EEG and the normative database means and standard deviations are valid and meaningful.

AGE GROUPINGS OF THE INSTANTANEOUS Z SCORE NORMATIVE POPULATION

The selected normal subjects are grouped by age with sufficiently large sample size and the means and standard deviations of the EEG time series and/or frequency domain analyses are computed for each age group. Transforms are applied to approximate a Gaussian distribution of the EEG measures that comprise the means. Once approximation to Gaussian is completed, then Z scores are computed for each subject in the database and leave one out Gaussian cross-validation is computed in order to arrive at an optimum Gaussian cross-validation sensitivity. Finally the Gaussian validated norms are subjected to content and predictive validation procedures such as correlation with neuropsychological test scores and intelligence, etc., and also discriminant analyses and neural networks and outcome statistics, etc. The content validations are with respect to clinical measures such as intelligence, neuropsychological test scores, school achievement, and clinical outcomes. The predictive validations are with respect to the discriminative, statistical, or neural network clinical classification accuracy. Both parametric and nonparametric statistics are used to determine the content and predictive validity of a normative EEG database.

Figure 1.5 shows the number of subjects per year in the normative EEG life span database. It can be seen that the largest number of subjects are in the younger ages (e.g., 1–14 years, $N = 470$) when the EEG is changing most rapidly. As mentioned previously, a proportionately smaller number of subjects represents the adult age range from 14 to 82 years ($N = 155$). The Z score normative database includes a total of 727 carefully screened individual subjects ranging in age from 2 months to 82 years. In order to increase the time resolution of age, sliding averages were used for the stratification in Neuroguide and for instantaneous Z scores (Thatcher et al., 2003). Two-year means were computed using a sliding average with 6-month overlap of subjects. This produced a more stable and higher age resolution normative database and a total of 21 different age groups. The 21 age groups and age ranges and number of subjects per age group are shown in the bar graph in Figure 1.5.

Figure 1.6 is an illustration of a step-by-step procedure by which the Z instantaneous score normative EEG database was validated and sensitivities calculated. The left side of the figure is the edited and artifact clean and reliable digital EEG time series which may be re-referenced or re-montaged, which is then analyzed in either the time domain or the frequency domain.

Figure 1.7 is an example of how the distribution of a raw or nontransformed EEG variable approximates a Gaussian distribution after a Box-Cox transform. Different transforms were selected to produce the best fit possible to a Gaussian distribution and the fit varied from about 97% to 99% accuracy.

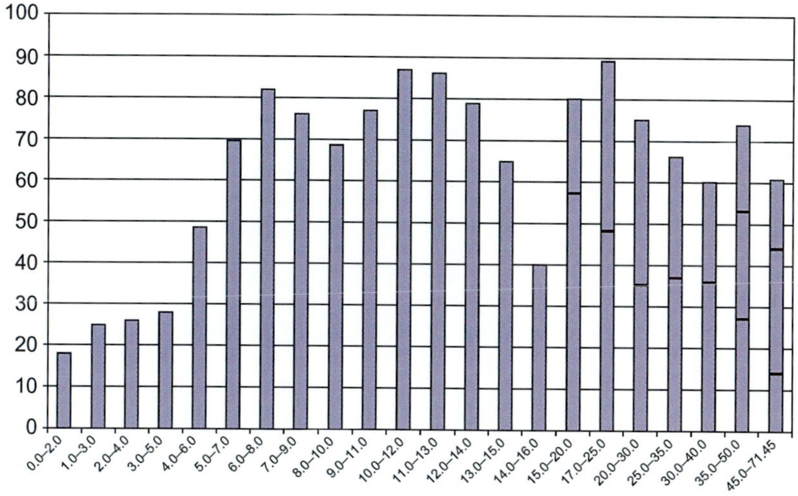

FIGURE 1.5 The number of subjects per age group in the *Z* score life span EEG reference normative database. The database is a "life span" database with 2 months of age being the youngest subject and 82.3 years of age being the oldest subject. Two year means were computed using a sliding average with 6-month overlap of subjects. This produced a more stable and higher age resolution normative database and a total of 21 different age groups. The 21 age groups and age ranges and number of subjects per age group are shown in the bar graph.

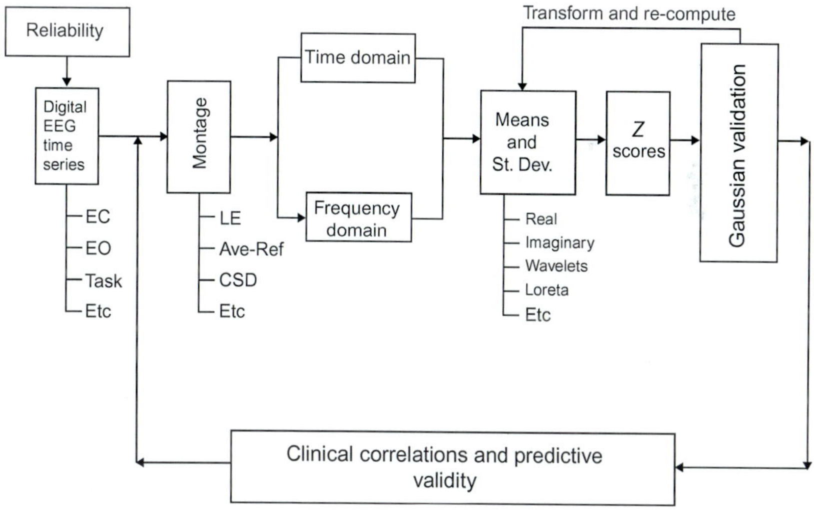

FIGURE 1.6 Illustration of the step-by-step procedure to Gaussian cross-validate and then validate by correlations with clinical measures in order to estimate the predictive and content validity of any EEG normative database. The feedback connections between Gaussian cross-validation and the means and standard deviations refer to transforms to approximate Gaussian if the nontransformed data is less Gaussian. The clinical correlation and validation arrow to the montage stage represents repetition of clinical validation to a different montage or reference or condition, such as eyes-open, active tasks, eyes-closed, etc., to the adjustments and understanding of the experimental design(s). *From Thatcher et al. (2003).*

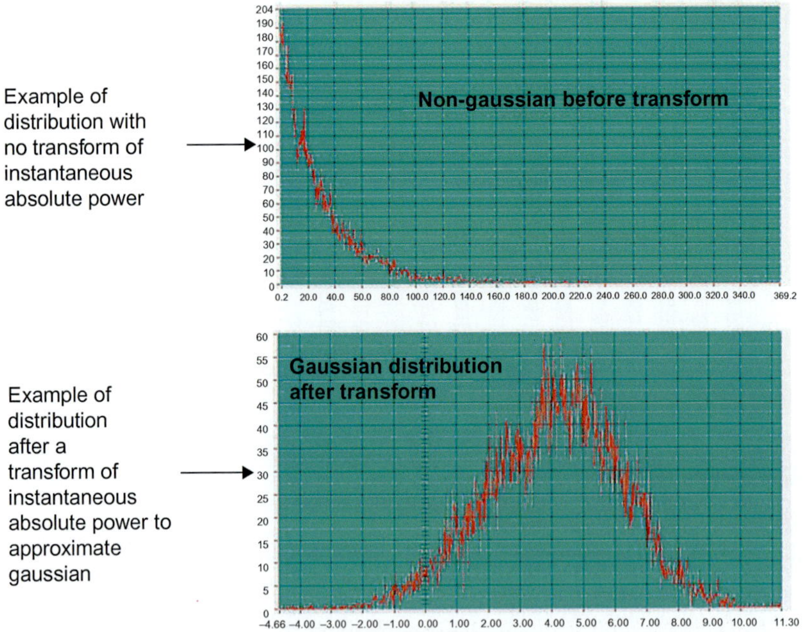

FIGURE 1.7 Example of the distribution of instantaneous absolute values before and after a transform is applied to approximate Gaussian. If no transform is used, then the instantaneous Z scores are totally invalid and should not be used.

SAMPLING FROM THE SAME POPULATION OF MEASURES OF THE HUMAN BRAIN

As mentioned, an important design concept is the application of the Gaussian distribution to averaged "instantaneous" time domain spectral measures from groups of normal subjects and then to cross-validate the means and standard deviations for each subject for each instant of time with respect to the measurement (Thatcher, 1998, 1999, 2000a,c). The cross-validation is directly related to the mean and variance of the distribution from which the same samples are obtained (Thatcher et al., 2003, 2005a,b). This includes the physiological basis for the measures, which must be the same because spatial and temporal localization validation is sufficient to prove validity. However, in order to achieve a representative sample of Z scores, the variables must be drawn from the same physiological population and be in agreement with respect to frequency and location. Over the last 25 years, the NYU and ANI normative databases have been repeatedly and independently cross-validated and are used worldwide in many institutions and serve as a historical reference in the history of QEEG normative databases (see Thatcher & Lubar, 2008). Because of the 25-year history of high cross-validation, the NYU and ANI databases in the "static" FFT domain then when used in the instantaneous domain, they must also cross-validate between ANI and NYU. Testing the foundations and examining the statistics is a crucial part of this process, and full disclosure of equations and procedures allows for independent replication and validation in the future.

In the case of the FFT, there is a single spectral value for each subject and power at each frequency is computed over a one to several minute period and, therefore, there is only between subject variance in "static" QEEG normative databases that use noninstantaneous analyses such as the FFT "static" norms, i.e., the average of subjects over an age range. Instantaneous or JTFA raw digital values differ from the FFT by being measures of the "instantaneous" state of the brain as defined by the center frequency and bandwidth of the JTFA time/frequency transform without windowing. In contrast, the FFT is a frequency domain transform that uses windowing and estimates the average spectral value over an extended period of time (e.g., 1–2 min) to produce a single average value that is then added across subjects in a given age range. The sample size is usually around 20–70 subjects in an age group and not tens of thousands of instantaneous JTFA values with variance as a function of age.

The FFT and JTFA measure the same physiological processes in a statistically and computationally different manner and these two methods are essentially identical to each other when using large sample sizes and no FFT windowing. Nonetheless, an important difference is that the average spectral values produced by an FFT involve different mathematical procedures and require windowing. Therefore, the means of the FFT and JTFA are different when computed using the same group of subjects and the same EEG data samples. Also, the variance is larger with the instantaneous JTFA than the distribution over age as with the FFT. For example, the FFT is calculated over an entire epoch of time (e.g., 1 or 2 s) and must use windowing to prevent discontinuities in the computation and is noisy with low degrees of freedom. In contrast, JTFA methods compute spectral values at each instant of time, do not involve windowing, have higher degrees of freedom, and a different non-Gaussian distribution than the FFT average over an age range.

Figure 1.8 is an example of the large and dramatic differences between the FFT and the JTFA instantaneous spectrum over a 2 s period of time. The mismatch occurs in all frequencies. Also, the FFT requires windowing in order to eliminate discontinuities at the boundary of the epoch which produces ringing and false frequencies. Figure 1.3 top is the FFT computed over the first 2 s of the Neuroguide demo. Note the low degrees of freedom and noisy nature of the FFT. Figure 1.4 bottom

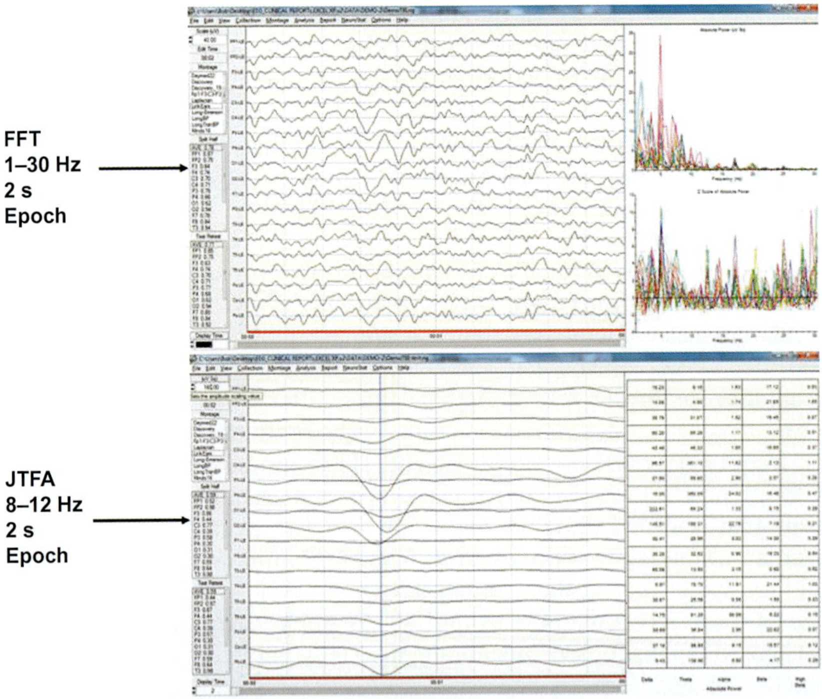

FIGURE 1.8 Top is the FFT absolute power spectrum over the first 2 s of EEG and the bottom is the JTFA absolute power spectrum in the theta frequency band (4–8 Hz) over the same 2 s of EEG data. This figure shows the dramatic difference between the FFT and the JTFA at low degrees of freedom. The FFT requires windowing, whereas the JTFA does not require windowing which results in slight differences in the total power measurements. Nonetheless, at high degrees of freedom, the JTFA and FFT converge to very similar values, but not identical values. The use of the FFT mean to calculate instantaneous Z scores is not optimal and presents scaling problems because of different mean values. The simple computation is JTFA means to calculate JTFA Z scores and FFT means to calculate FFT Z scores. As shown in Figures 1.5 and 1.6, there are slight differences between the FFT and JTFA when testing with mathematically ideal sine waves.

is the JTFA over the same 2 s epoch of time and demonstrates a different measure set. Nonetheless, if one sums over the entire epoch, then the statistical degrees of freedom between the FFT and JTFA more closely match and both methods produce approximately the same, but not identical values due to the FFT windowing.

Figures 1.9 and 1.10 illustrate the relationship between the mean of an FFT-based normative database versus the mean of an "instantaneous" or JTFA database.

This shows a convergence or cross-validation of the same exact underlying EEG linearly scaled differently. However, in the statistics of sampling theory, if a scaling factor is used to equate the JTFA and FFT

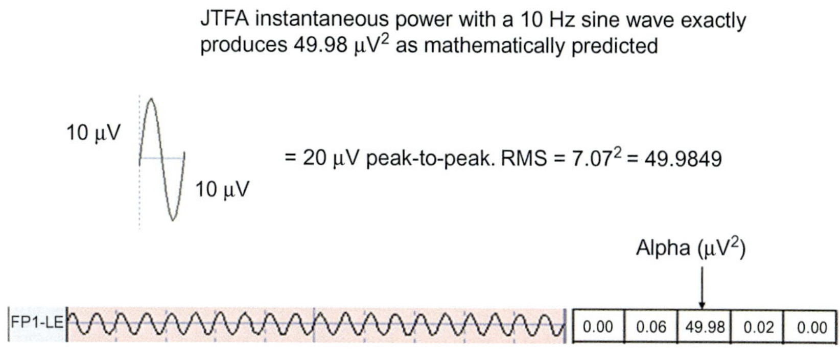

FIGURE 1.9 Top illustrates a 10 Hz and 10 μV sine wave. The expected power is the RMS value of the sine wave which $= 7.07^2 = 49.9849$ μV². The middle trace is a 10 Hz, 10 μV sine wave produced by the Neuroguide signal generator. With the free Neuroguide demo click View > JTFA > Absolute Power and select average of Absolute Values which produces 49.98 μV² which is exactly as mathematically predicted.

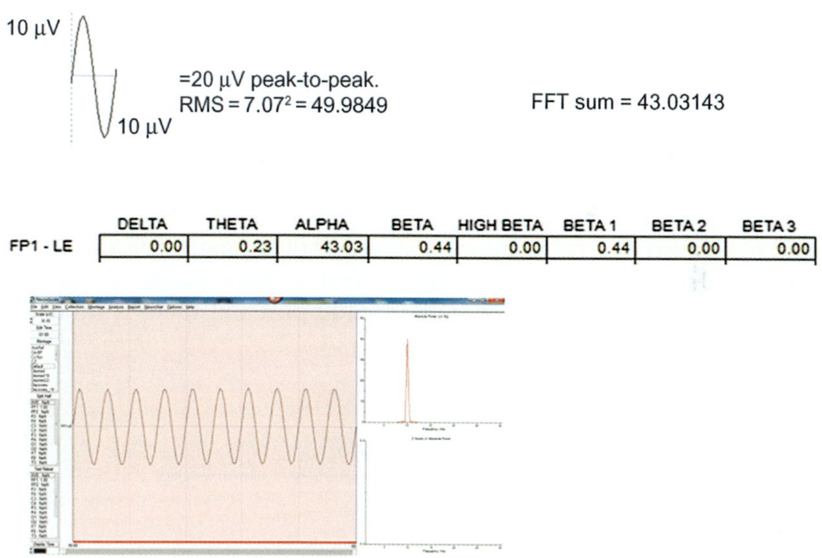

FIGURE 1.10 Top illustrates a 10 Hz and 10 μV sine wave. The expected power is the RMS value of the sine wave which $= 7.07^2 = 49.9849$ μV². The middle trace is the FFT power spectrum showing 43.03143 μV² or 6.953 μV² less power than the mathematical ideal and the JTFA. The reason for the difference is because the FFT requires windowing (cosine taper), otherwise there will be discontinuities and ringing or nonreal frequencies in the spectra. Bottom is the same 10 Hz, 10 μV peak-to-peak as shown in Figure 1.9 as produced by the same signal generator.

absolute values then it is important to describe the procedure and method of linear scaling. If a scaling factor is used to equate the JTFA and FFT absolute values, then it is important to describe the procedure and method of linear scaling. If no FFT windowing is used, then this too should be stated. Without windowing, discontinuities at the beginning and end of the epoch will produce ringing and false frequencies. Neuroguide uses a cosine taper to window the FFT. A simpler approach is to use the instantaneous means and standard deviations from the outset and not the FFT means and standard deviation, because if the exact same method is used to compute both the means and the Z scores then there is no question that in fact apples are compared to apples and oranges are compared to oranges. The between subject variance using instantaneous means and standard deviations to calculate instantaneous Z scores is valid although with significantly lower degrees of freedom. The use of the instantaneous means is not more computationally taxing and it avoids the need to use FFT means and standard deviations from age regression norms.

In summary, a violation of statistical sampling theory occurs when one uses different sampling populations to compute the statistics of a single sample. For example, a violation of statistical sampling theory occurs if one computes the mean and standard deviation of a barrel of oranges and then uses these statistics to compute the Z score of an individual apple. On the surface, this seems ok because both the apple and orange are round and have similar weights and therefore there is superficial overlap of features and properties. However, the fact is that apples are fundamentally different than oranges and any violation of sampling introduces error. This analogy holds when one uses FFT means and standard deviations to compute a Z score of a single JTFA measure. This introduces unnecessary error since it is easy to use a barrel of apples to compute Z scores of individual apples and there is no reason to use oranges to begin with.

APPENDIX

Complex Demodulation and JTFA

Complex demodulation is used in a JTFA to compute instantaneous power, coherence, amplitude asymmetry, and phase differences (Bloomfield, 2000; Granger & Hatanka, 1964; Otnes & Enochson, 1978; Thatcher et al., 2007) and then to compute a Z score based on these instantaneous values. Complex demodulation is an analytic linear shift-invariant transform that first multiplies a time series by the complex function of a sine and cosine at a specific center frequency (see Table 1.1) followed by a low-pass filter (sixth-order low-pass Butterworth) which removes all but very low frequencies (shifts frequency to 0) and transforms the time series into instantaneous amplitude and phase and an "instantaneous" spectrum (Bloomfield, 2000). We place quotations around the term "instantaneous" to emphasize that, as with the Hilbert transform, there is always a trade-off between time resolution and frequency resolution. The broader the bandwidth, the higher the time resolution, but lower the frequency resolution and vice versa. Mathematically, complex demodulation is defined as an analytic transform that involves the multiplication of a discrete time series $\{x_t, t = 1,\ldots, n\}$ by $\sin \omega_0 t$ and $\cos \omega_0 t$ giving

$$x'_t = x_t \sin \omega_0 t \tag{1.1}$$

and

$$x''_t = x_t \cos \omega_0 t \tag{1.2}$$

and then apply a low-pass filter F to produce the instantaneous time series, Z'_t and Z''_t where the sine and cosine time series are defined as

$$Z'_t = F(x_t \sin \omega_0 t) \tag{1.3}$$

$$Z''_t = F(x_t \cos \omega_0 t) \tag{1.4}$$

and

$$2[(Z'_t)^2 + (Z''_t)^2]^{1/2} \tag{1.5}$$

is an estimate of the instantaneous amplitude of the frequency ω_0 at time t and

$$\tan^{-1} \frac{Z'_t}{Z''_t} \tag{1.6}$$

is an estimate of the instantaneous phase at time t. At this step, the complex demodulation transform is the same as the Hilbert transform (Oppenheim & Schafer, 1975; Pikovsky, Rosenblum, & Kurths, 2003, p. 362).

The instantaneous cross-spectrum is computed when there are two time series $\{y_t, t = 1,\ldots, n\}$ and $\{y'_t, t = 1,\ldots, n\}$ and if $F[\cdot]$ is a filter passing only frequencies near zero, then, as above $R_t^2 = F[y_t \sin \omega_0 t]^2 + F[y_t \cos \omega_0 t]^2 = |F[y_t\, e^{i\omega_0 t}]^2|$ is the estimate of the amplitude of frequency ω_0 at time t and $\varphi_t = \tan^{-1}(F[y_t \sin \omega_0 t]/F[y_t \cos \omega_0 t])$ is an estimate of the phase of frequency ω_0 at time t and therefore,

$$F[y_t\, e^{i\omega_0 t}] = R_t\, e^{i\varphi_t} \tag{1.7}$$

and likewise,

$$F[y'_t\, e^{i\omega_0 t}] = R'_t\, e^{i\varphi_t} \tag{1.8}$$

The instantaneous cross-spectrum is

$$V_t = F[y_t\, e^{i\omega_0 t}]F[y_t'\, e^{-i\omega_0 t}] = R_t R_t'\, e^{i[\varphi_t - \varphi_t']} \quad (1.9)$$

and the instantaneous coherence is

$$\frac{|V_t|}{R_t^2 R_t'^2} \equiv 1 \quad (1.10)$$

The instantaneous phase difference is $\varphi_t - \varphi_t'$. That is, the instantaneous phase difference is computed by estimating the instantaneous phase for each time series separately and then taking the difference. Instantaneous phase difference is also the arctangent of the imaginary part of V_t divided by the real part (or the instantaneous quadspectrum divided by the instantaneous cospectrum) at each time point.

References

Bloomfield, P. (2000). *Fourier analysis of time series: An introduction*. New York, NY: John Wiley & Sons.

Box, G. E. P., & Cox, D. R. (1964). An analysis of transformations. *Journal of the Royal Statistical Society*, 211–243 (discussion 244–252).

Brazis, P. W., Masdeu, J. C., Biller, J., et al. *Localization in clinical neurology*. Philadelphia, PA: Williams and Wilkins.

Cooley, W. W., & Lohnes, P. R. (1971). *Multivariate data analysis*. New York, NY: John Wiley & Sons.

Duffy, F., Hughes, J. R., Miranda, F., Bernad, P., & Cook, P. (1994). Status of quantitative EEG (QEEG) in clinical practice. *Clinical Electroencephalography*, *25*(4), VI–XXII.

Gasser, T., Jennen-Steinmetz, C., Sroka, L., Verleger, R., & Mocks, J. (1988). Development of the EEG of school-age children and adolescents. II: Topography. *Electroencephalography Clinical Neurophysiology*, *69*(2), 100–109.

Granger, C. W. J., & Hatanka, M. (1964). *Spectral analysis of economic time series*. Princeton, NJ: Princeton University Press.

Heilman, K. M., & Valenstein, E. (1993). *Clinical neuropsychology* (3rd ed.). New York, NY: Oxford University Press.

John, E. R. (1990). *Machinery of the mind: Data, theory, and speculations about higher brain function*. Boston, MA: Birkhauser.

John, E. R., Prichep, L. S., & Easton, P. (1987). Normative data banks and neurometrics: Basic concepts, methods and results of norm construction. In A. Remond (Ed.), *Handbook of electroencephalography and clinical neurophysiology: Vol. III. Computer analysis of the EEG and other neurophysiological signals* (pp. 449–495). Amsterdam: Elsevier.

John, E. R., Prichep, L. S., Fridman, J., & Easton, P. (1988). Neurometrics: Computer assisted differential diagnosis of brain dysfunctions. *Science*, *293*, 162–169.

Matousek, M., & Petersen, I. (1973). Frequency analysis of the EEG background activity by means of age dependent EEG quotients. In P. Kellaway, & I. Petersen (Eds.), *Automation of clinical electroencephalography* (pp. 75–102). New York, NY: Raven Press.

Oppenheim, A. V., & Schafer, R. W. (1975). *Digital signal processing*. London: Prentice-Hall.

Otnes, R. K., & Enochson, L. (1972). *Digital time series analysis*. New York: John Wiley and Sons.

Otnes, R. K., & Enochson, L. (1978). *Applied time series analysis*. New York, NY: John Wiley & Sons.

Pikovsky, A., Rosenblum, M., & Kurths, J. (2003). *Synchronization: A universal concept in nonlinear sciences*. New York, NY: Cambridge University Press.

Robinett, R. W. (1997). *Quantum mechanics: Classical results, modern systems and visualized examples*. New York, NY: Oxford University Press.

Thatcher, R. W. (1998). EEG normative databases and EEG biofeedback. *Journal of Neurotherapy*, 2(4), 8–39.

Thatcher, R. W. (1999). EEG database guided neurotherapy. In J. R. Evans, & A. Abarbanel (Eds.), *Introduction to quantitative EEG and neurofeedback*. San Diego, CA: Academic Press.

Thatcher, R. W. (2000a). EEG operant conditioning (biofeedback) and traumatic brain injury. *Clinical EEG*, *31*(1), 38–44.

Thatcher, R. W. (2000b). An EEG least action model of biofeedback. *Eighth Annual Society for Neuronal Regulation*, Minneapolis, MN, September 23, 2000.

Thatcher, R. W. (2000c). 3-Dimensional EEG biofeedback using LORETA. *Eighth Annual Society for Neuronal Regulation*, Minneapolis, MN, September 23, 2000.

Thatcher, R. W. (2011a). Neuropsychiatry and quantitative electroencephalography in the 21st Century. *Neuropsychiatry*, *1*(5), 495–514. Available from http://dx.doi.org/doi:10.2217/npv.11.

Thatcher, R. W. (2011b). LORETA *Z* score biofeedback and traumatic brain injury. *NeuroConnections Newsletter*, (Part 3), 9–12.

Thatcher, R. W. (2012). Latest developments in live Z-score training: symptom check list, phase reset and LORETA Z score biofeedback. *Journal of Neurotherapy*, *17*(1), 69–87.

Thatcher, R. W., & Lubar, J. F. (2008). History of the scientific standards of QEEG normative databases. In T. Budzinsky, H. Budzinsky, J. Evans, & A. Abarbanel (Eds.), *Introduction to QEEG and neurofeedback: Advanced theory and applications*. San Diego, CA: Academic Press.

Thatcher, R. W., North, D., & Biver, C. (2005a). EEG inverse solutions and parametric vs. non-parametric statistics of Low Resolution Electromagnetic Tomography (LORETA). *Clinical EEG and Neuroscience*, *36*(1), 1–9.

Thatcher, R. W., North, D., & Biver, C. (2005b). Evaluation and validity of a LORETA normative EEG database. *Clinical EEG and Neuroscience*, *36*(2), 116–122.

Thatcher, R. W., North, D., & Biver, C. (2009). Self-organized criticality and the development of EEG phase reset. *Human Brain Mapping*, *30*(2), 553–574.

Thatcher, R. W., Walker, R. A., Biver, C., North, D., & Curtin, R. (2003). Quantitative EEG normative databases: Validation and clinical correlation. *Journal of Neurotherapy*, *7*(3/4), 87–122.

Thatcher, R. W., Walker, R. A., & Guidice, S. (1987). Human cerebral hemispheres develop at different rates and ages. *Science*, *236*, 1110–1113.

CHAPTER

2

Network Connectivity and LORETA Z Score Biofeedback

Robert W. Thatcher, Carl J. Biver and Duane M. North

Applied Neuroscience Research Institute, Seminole, FL, USA

The advent of modern neuroimaging methods such as positron emission tomography (PET), functional magnetic resonance imaging (fMRI) and electrical neuroimaging (electroencephalography (EEG)/magnetoencephalography (MEG)) in the late 1980s and early 1990s to 2014 has confirmed and extended the nearly two centuries of studies of space occupying lesions, tumors, strokes, and brain stimulation. In the last century with studies of strokes and penetrating head wounds (Broca, 1861; Jackson, 1876; Wernicke, 1881) and especially the last two decades with neural imaging technologies, there has been considerable progress in linking patient's symptoms to networks in the brain represented by structural/functional "modules" and "hubs" and subsystems of the brain for a wide variety of disorders as well as normal and optimal functioning of the human brain. Early and primitive hypotheses about function being located in particular centers have been replaced by neural network models where subsystems are dynamically phase locked for brief instances of time (e.g., 100–600 ms) across vast areas of the human brain. For example, simple localization of function in the brain has been replaced by collections of "functional systems" that are cross-frequency phase locked in subgroups of neurons in distributed network nodes. The synchronization of billions of neurons distributed across widespread nodes are recruited in about 40–80 ms as marked by a phase shift followed by a prolonged period of phase lock (e.g., 100–600 ms) followed by a subsequent phase shift recruiting a different neural resource at that instant of time in an ever cascading sequence of

Z Score Neurofeedback.
DOI: http://dx.doi.org/10.1016/B978-0-12-801291-8.00002-9

meta-stabile states (Rabinovich, Afraimovich, Christian, & Varona, 2012; Thatcher, 2012). Phase reset is a nonlinear "chaotic" event characterized by an abrupt, sudden, and unexpected onset followed by a prolonged period of phase lock or "stability" and is an important part of homeostasis in which the ratio of chaos/stability is correlated with the efficiency of information processing (Thatcher, North, & Biver, 2008a). This is one of the reasons that real-time Z scores were developed, i.e., to reinforce a balance of chaos and stability of instances of time as a part of the homeostatic normative reference or reinforcement toward $Z = 0$. Like using an M&M to reinforce quiet behavior of an unruly child in a class room that is disrupting the entire class, Z score biofeedback is designed to reinforce stability and efficiency of information processing in nodes and connections linked to the symptoms.

NEUROTOPOLOGY

In order to understand the network nature of the human brain today, we rely upon structural MRI that includes diffusion tensor imaging (DTI) which is a 3D measure of the flow of water in axons and tractography that counts and vectorizes 3D cortical axons. DTI has quantified the total number of cortical axons at around 80 billion with a few billion that are organized in a relatively small set of clusters which are nodes of a network (about 6–8) and the fiber connections between the nodes (Catani & de Schotten, 2012). Hagmann et al. (2008) demonstrated six major clusters called "modules" using a rigorous and anatomically based reference for quantifying structure–function relationships of the neocortex. Hagmann et al. (2008) used diffusion spectral imaging (DSI) and tractography to trace the cortico-cortical white matter connections of the human cerebral cortex between 66 cortical regions with clear anatomical landmarks, using the same gyri and sulci as described by Korbian Brodmann in 1909 (Brodmann, 1909) that are still in use today. Network spectral analyses of nodes and edges of the regions of interest (ROIs) were grouped into six anatomical "modules" with maximum centrality or high within density connectivity (Hagmann et al., 2008). A further subclassification into two groups of intra- versus extra-modular connection density labeled as "provincial hubs" and "connector hubs" were hypothesized to be likely switching nodes between modules. The participant coefficient was defined by the ratio of intra- to extra-modular connection density.

Catani and coworkers (Catani and de Schotten, 2012; Catani et al., 2012a,b, 2013) in a series of DTI studies produced an Atlas of the human cortical white matter. This work added detail to the conventional optical microscope neuroanatomy of cadavers to *in vivo* living brains with excellent clarity. The Catani and de Schotten (2012) Atlas mapped the white matter to Brodmann areas using the Montreal Neurological & Talaraich Atlas coordinate standard that co-registers the sources of the scalp EEG/MEG. In this context, Brodmann areas are functional subnodes connected by specific white matter fiber bundles, such as the cingulum (C), inferior fronto-occipital fasciculus (IFOF), uncinate fascculus (UF), superior longitudinal fasciculus (LF) (anterior and posterior segments—AS & PS) and multiple "U" shaped local fibers (approximately 1–6 cm). The long distance fiber bundles and "U" shaped fibers connect cortical gyri and constitute the cerebral white matter.

Pyramidal neurons are exclusively excitatory neurons with excitatory neurotransmitters and neuromodulators and excitatory axons that travel in both directions and therefore represent a massive and nested intracortical self-referential loop system. The concept of the neocortex as a self-referential loop system was emphasized by Braitenberg and Schuz (1998) and Nunez (1981). That is, small excitatory loops nested inside of longer distant excitatory loops with different conduction velocities and conduction delays between long and short distance loops are evident in both anatomy and the EEG (Nunez, 1981, 1995; Thatcher, Krause, & Hrybyk, 1986; Braitenberg and Schuz, 1998). Neural excitatory loops oscillate based on factors such as conduction velocity, distance between sender and receiver, synaptic rise times and synaptic integration times, as well as the pyramidal neuron membrane potential. If we assume that the average membrane potential and excitability of the pyramidal neurons is constant, then loop dynamics can be represented by $T = K(NA)$, where T = transit time in a loop, N = the number of neurons in the loop, A = the delay between the neurons, and K = iterations or recurrence in the loop. Recurrence in excitatory loops is critical for the production of long-term potentiation (LTP) and long-term depression (LTD) involved in the creation of new memory and learning.

Figure 2.1 is an example of the DTI derived axonal connections between different brain regions in the Catani and de Schotten Atlas of Human Connections.

Figure 2.2 is an example of low-resolution electromagnetic tomography (LORETA) EEG measures of the cortico-cortical cross-frequency couplings and resonances. The y-axis is distance from a reference ROI (e.g., posterior central gyrus) with respect to spatially ordered ROIs to the cuneus in the occipital lobes 62.75 mm distant. The x-axis is the frequency spectrum from 1 to 40 Hz and the color bar is the correlation between ROIs over an approximate 2 min period of time.

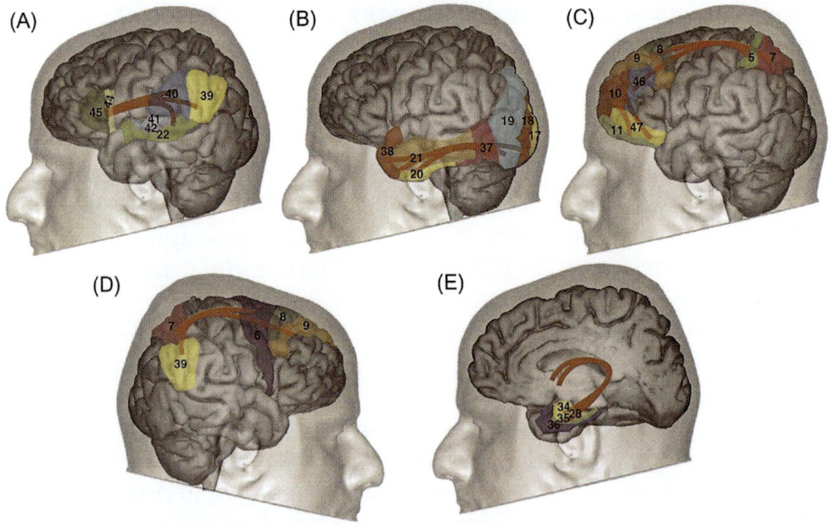

FIGURE 2.1 Examples of network connections via white matter tracks of various Brodmann areas. Each collection of nodes and connections represent functional networks in the brain. The use of DTI has provided the "wiring diagrams" of the brain with Talairach atlas coordinates of the beginning and ends of fasciculi and "U" shaped fibers that correspond to the ordered changes in LORETA source correlation and LORETA coherence and phase. *From Catani and de Schotten (2012).*

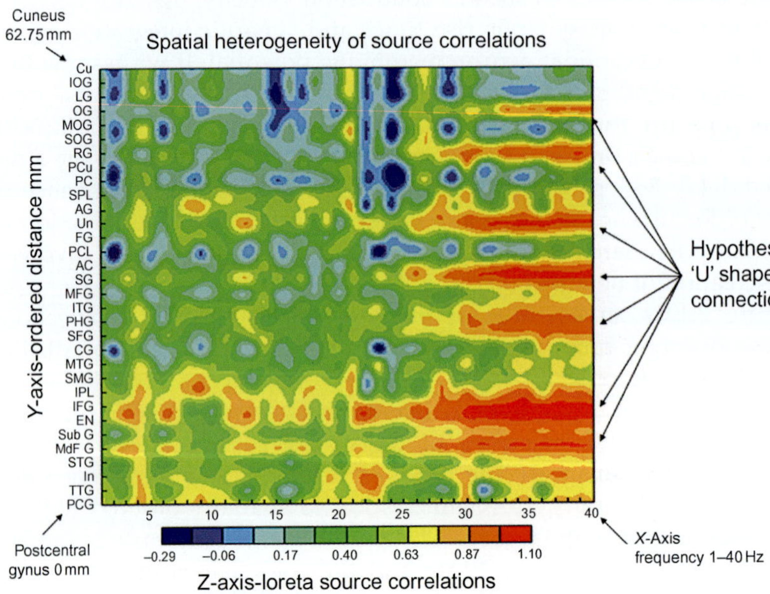

FIGURE 2.2 An example of one of the subjects demonstrating spatial heterogeneity of LORETA source correlations which cannot be explained by volume conduction. The ROIs

LORETA LINKAGE BETWEEN STRUCTURE AND FUNCTION

The same scientific literature review of the fMRI, PET, and EEG/MEG literature that links symptoms and neuropsychological diagnoses to functional specialization in the brain was used to provide a linkage to the 3D sources of the scalp EEG. We use "LORETA" that has a 7 mm cubic spatial resolution and adequately measures all of the Brodmann areas (see Figures 2.2 and 2.3) as evidenced by 795 peer reviewed journal articles that can be read at

http://www.appliedneuroscience.com/LORETA%20publications.pdf.

CROSS-MODAL VALIDATION OF LORETA

Cross-validation of LORETA includes over 2000 peer reviewed publications that include phantom head validations and mathematical simulations and physiological validations tests. Some of the physiological validation tests involved visual, auditory, and motor tasks (e.g., Mulert et al., 2001; Tuch, Wedeen, Dale, George, & Belliveau, 1999), epileptic discharges (e.g., Lantz et al., 1997), and cognitive tasks tapping specific brain regions (e.g., Pizzagalli et al., 2002).

Additional important cross-modal validation of LORETA has also come from studies directly combining LORETA with fMRI (Mulert et al., 2004;

◀ are ordered as a function of distance from the reference Brodmann area 1 or left post-central gyrus to the left cuneus (Brodmann area 17 that is 62.75 mm distant). The x-axis is frequency (1–40 Hz), the y-axis are ROIs, and the ROIs are ordered as a function of distance from the post-central gyrus. The z-axis is the magnitude of the LORETA source correlation as represented by the color bar of the contour map. The alternating horizontal red and blue lines represent a regular spacing of increases and decreases in coupling with a spacing consistent with the "U" shaped fiber system of the human cortex. The "U" shaped fibers are strongly coupled at 20–40 Hz. The alternating vertical red and blue represent a regular spacing of frequency in which a specific Brodmann area is coupled to many other Brodmann areas but only within a particular frequency band, e.g., theta and beta and alpha and gamma. The cortico-cortical fiber system is highly coupled in gamma band frequencies at 20–40 Hz and less in the lower frequency ranges. PCA = posterior pentral gyrus, TTG = transverse temporal gyrus, In = insula, STG = superior temporal gyrus, MdFG = middle frontal gyrus, Sub G = subgyral region, EN = extranuclear frontal gyrus, IFG = inferior frontal gyrus, IPL = inferior parietal lobule, SMG = supramaginal gyrus, MTG = middle temporal gyrus, CG = cingulate gyrus, SFG = superior frontal gyrus, PHG = parahippocampal gyrus, ITG = inferior temporal gyrus, MFG = medial frontal gyrus, SG = subcallosal gyrus, AC = anterior cingulate, PCL = paracentral lobule, FG = fusiform gyrus, UN = uncus, AG = angular gyrus, PC = posterior cingulate, PCu = precuneus, RG = rectal gyrus, SOG = superior occipital gyrus, MOG = middle occipital gyus, OG = orbital gyrus, LG = lingual gyrus, IOG = inferior occipital gyrus, Cu = cuneus. *From Thatcher, North, and Biver (2011).*

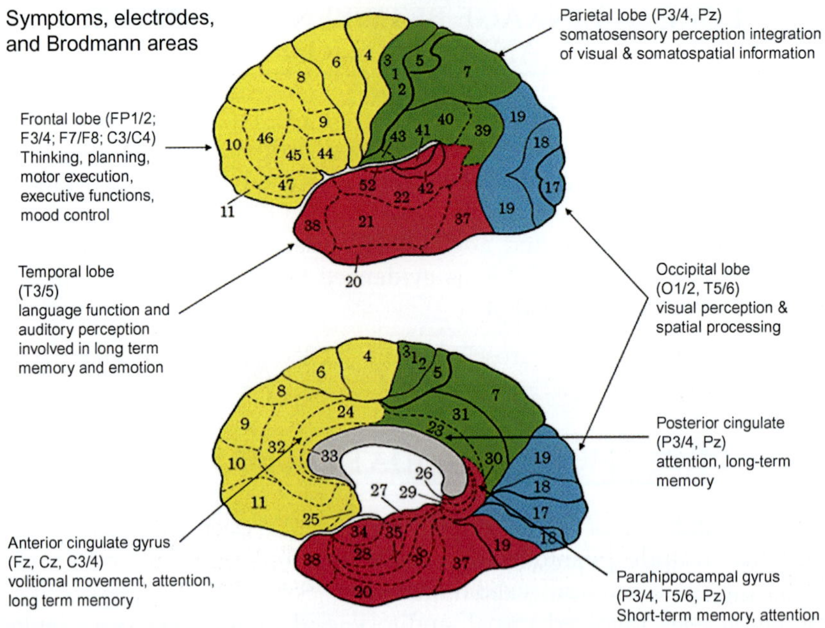

FIGURE 2.3 Illustration of Brodmann areas and related functions.

Vitacco, Brandeis, Pascual-Marqui, & Martin, 2002), structural MRI (Worrell et al., 2000), PET (Pizzagalli et al., 2004), and intracranial recordings (Seeck et al., 1998). Pizzagalli and colleagues have published a series of physiological validation studies demonstrating that theta current density in the rostral anterior cingulate cortex (ACC) was associated with treatment response in major depression (Pizzagalli et al., 2001). In two recent EEG/fMRI studies, LORETA localizations were on average 16 mm (Mulert et al., 2004) and 14.5 mm (Vitacco et al., 2002) from fMRI activation loci, a discrepancy that is in the range of the spatial resolution of LORETA (1–2 cm) that is commonly reported in the literature.

LORETA SYMPTOM CHECKLIST

To activate the LORETA symptom checklist, one must download, install, and launch the free Neuroguide from http://www.appliedneuroscience.com/ContactDownloadDemo.htm, then click File > Open > Lexicor > Lexicor NRS24 and then type in age 55, select the eyes closed condition, and click OK. Then click Edit > Select All, then click Report > Create Symptom Check List Match and then save the .scl file in a folder. Then click Collection > Setup & Monitor and then click

OK. Click Collection > Neurofeedback > LORETA Neurofeeback. Click Symptom Check List in the settings panel and open the .scl file that was previously saved. Scroll down to "Spatial Perception Problems" and double click on the Severity and type 10 because the EEG is from a patient with right parietal lobe damage and has symptoms of spatial neglect and left-sided paresis. The Symptom Check List (SCL) generates a list of likely Brodmann areas expected to be related to the patient's symptoms in the "Hypotheses" in the lower right list. The "Match" list shows the statistically significant Brodmann areas in the patient's record that match the hypothesized locations and the "Mismatch" shows the Brodmann areas that failed to match the hypothesized locations. It is possible that the mismatches represent "compensatory" processes and in this way one can focus on the most likely "weak" brain systems linked to the patient's symptoms as discussed by Alexander Luria (1973). Click OK to return to the settings panel and view the Brodmann areas and ROIs that were automatically generated by the symptom checklist match. For further details, click Help > NeuroGuide Help and then open the Chapter on Neurofeedback and Symptom Check list inside of the Neuroguide Manual. Figure 2.4 is an example

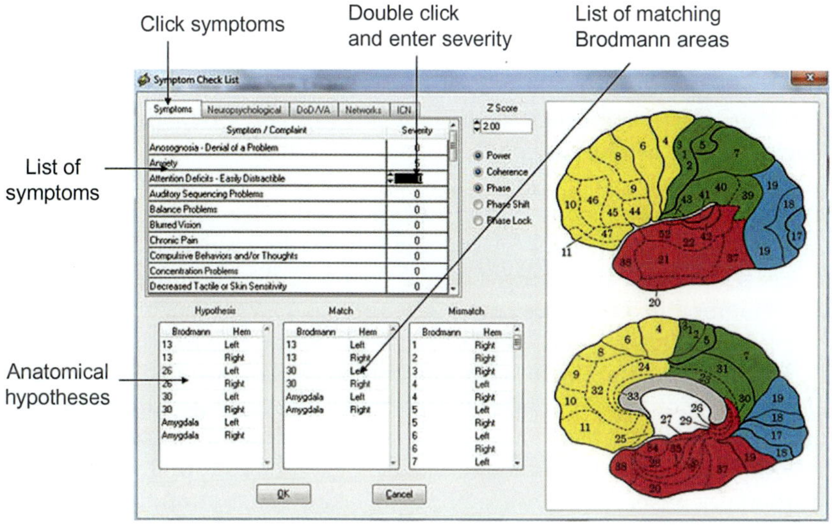

FIGURE 2.4 Illustration of the symptom checklist panel. Patient's symptoms and clinical history are first assessed and the clinician forms hypotheses as to which brain networks are most likely related to the patient's symptoms prior to recording EEG. The qEEG is then recorded and LORETA and the symptom checklist are used to confirm or disconfirm the hypotheses. Dysregulation as measured by Z scores from the Brodmann areas (nodes) and connections between Brodmann areas linked to the patient's symptoms are then selected as targets for EEG biofeedback.

of the SCL panel with the "Symptoms" selected and the Brodmann areas selected based on the match of symptoms and regions of the brain. The second screen is the SCL panel with "Neuropsychological Diagnoses" selected. A listing of these two different symptom checklists is available in Thatcher (2012).

INTRINSIC CONNECTIVITY NETWORKS

Recently, Laird et al. (2011) summarized the various "intrinsic connectivity networks" or ICNs into 18 specific groupings based upon 30,000 fMRI and PET studies, which, as previously mentioned, also dominate the EEG literature and show correlated infra-slow oscillations. This section copies directly from Laird et al. (2011) for each of the 18 ICNs (20 ICNs are present in the total survey; however, ICNs 19 and 20 are believed to be artifacts of the Blood-Oxygen-Level-Dependent (BOLD) procedure itself and therefore they are omitted). The ICNs have also been cross-validated using quantitative EEG (qEEG) methodology (Wisner, Atluri, Lim, & MacDonald, 2013). See the ICN locations in Figure 2.5.

ICN 1 (limbic and medial–temporal areas) included primary olfactory and limbic association cortices (BA 28/34/35/36/38), including parahippocampal gyri. This network was strongly associated with discrimination of emotional faces and pictures, particularly those that elicited fear, happiness, or humor. In addition, ICN 1 was strongly weighted toward interoceptive processing elicited during air-hunger and, more weakly, olfactory and gustatory responses (from Laird et al., 2011).

ICN 2 (subgenual ACC and orbital frontal cortex (OFC)) included BA 25 and BA 10/11/12 and was loaded toward olfaction, gustation, and emotion, with a strong preference for reward and thirst tasks (from Laird et al., 2011).

ICN 3 (bilateral BG and thalamus) was found to be linked to a wide range of mental processes, most strongly to reward tasks, nonpainful thermal stimulation, and interoceptive functions (e.g., bladder, sexuality, hunger, and thirst). In addition, this network was also found to be relevant to motor, pain, and somatosensory processing, with preference for a few cognitive tasks such as classical conditioning, go/no-go, film viewing, syntactic discrimination, and delay discounting. ICN 3 was additionally associated with emotional tasks, most strongly to anxiety and olfaction (from Laird et al., 2011).

ICN 4 (bilateral anterior insula/frontal opercula and the anterior aspect of the body of the cingulate gyrus) encompassed BA 13/16 and BA 24. These regions accounted for a complex set of language, executive function, affective, and interoceptive processes corresponding to the Stroop, go/no-go, Flanker, and Simon tasks, as well as auditory, pain, and gustatory processes. Other paradigms included deception, music,

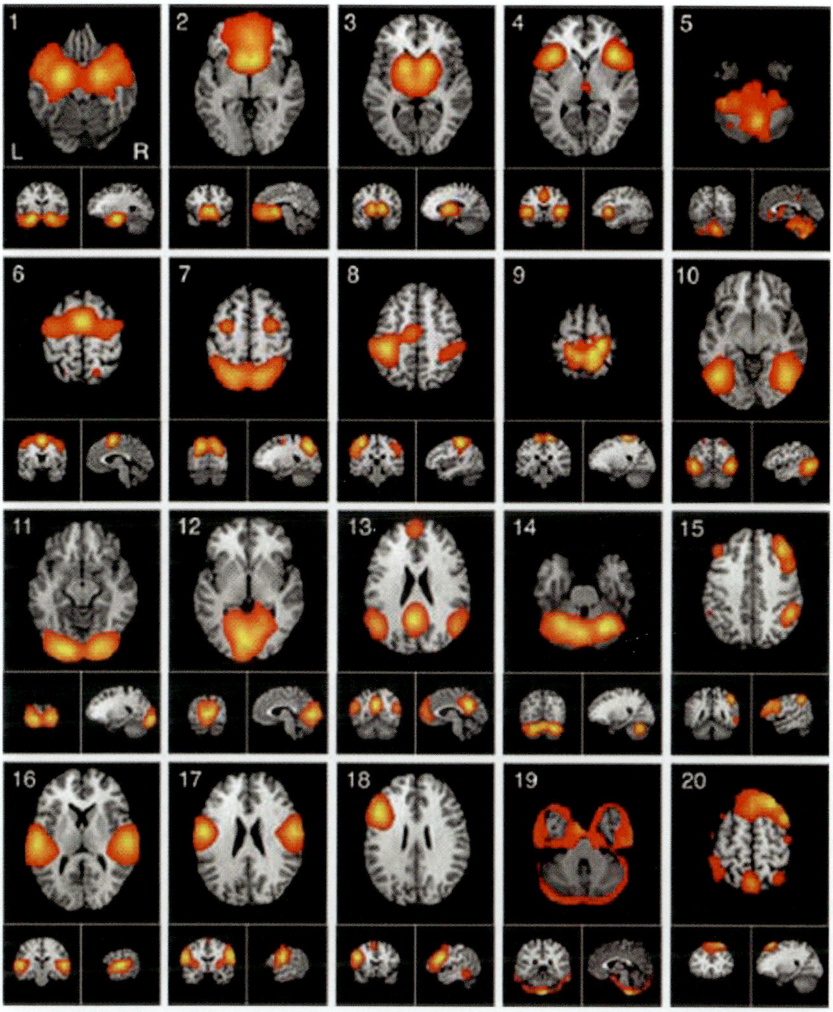

FIGURE 2.5 ICA was used to decompose 8637 experiment images extracted from the BrainMap database into 20 spatially cooccurring maps of ICNs. ICA maps were converted to z statistic images via a normalized mixture model fit, thresholded at $z > 4$, and viewed in standard (Talairach) brain space. Orthogonal slices of the most representative point in space are shown. *From Laird et al. (2011).*

and classical conditioning. This wide range of network functions was elicited across all possible stimulus modalities. Given the heterogeneous range of functions associated with ICN 4, we consider it to be a transitional network linking cognition and emotion/interoception (from Laird et al., 2011).

ICN 6 (superior and middle frontal gyri) included the premotor and supplementary motor cortices (supplemental motor area (SMA); BA 6) and frontal eye fields (FEFs) (BA 8/9) and was related to cognitive control of visuomotor timing and preparation of executed movements. Strongly weighted behavioral domains included action imagination and preparation and visual motion, and important paradigms were the Flanker task, saccades, antisaccades, and the learning and recall of complex sequences. Stimulus types tended toward visual targets, fixation points, and LEDs, to which subjects were frequently instructed to fixate, imagine, and track.

ICN 7 middle frontal gyri and prefrontal (BA 46) and posterior parietal cortices (BA 7) involving visuospatial processing and reasoning, with a strong weighting for tasks such as the Wisconsin Card Sorting Test, saccades, antisaccades, mental rotation, and counting or calculation. Notably, metadata functions for ICNs 7 and 4 agree with the systems differentiated in a dual-network model of top-down attentional control proposed by Dosenbach et al. (2007) wherein fronto-parietal and cinguloopercular networks are responsible for adaptive control and stable maintenance functions, respectively (from Laird et al., 2011).

ICN 8 (ventral precentral gyri, central sulci, post-central gyri, superior and inferior cerebellum) included primary sensorimotor cortices for upper extremities (M1; S1; BA 4/3/1/2). This network was associated with action and somesthesis corresponding to hand movements and included tasks such as finger tapping, grasping, pointing, electrical and vibrotactile stimulation, and TMS (from Laird et al., 2011).

ICN 9 (superior parietal lobule) included the medial posterior parietal association area (BA 5). This network was not observed as a separate component in our previous analysis but split from the previous ICN 8 component (hand region of the primary sensorimotor cortex) because of the increased number of papers in BrainMap accumulated between analyses. Support for the decomposition of ICNs 8 and 9 into two separate components is provided by a previous study indicating that medial superior parietal cortex (BA 5) is functionally distinct from primary sensorimotor cortices. Interestingly, the heat map for this network was strongly negative, indicating the range of cognitive and emotional functions that were anticorrelated, rather than correlated, with this region. A weak positive preference was found for motor execution and learning, particularly involving drawing and reaching, in agreement with previous research on the integration of body movements and hand–eye coordination (from Laird et al., 2011).

ICN 10 (middle and inferior temporal gyri) included the middle temporal visual association area (MT, middle superior temporal (MST), V5; BA 37/39) at the temporo-occipital junction. This network was elicited by viewing complex, often emotional, stimuli (e.g., faces, films), as well as action observation, overt picture naming, and visual tracking of moving objects, particularly random dot formations. Other tasks included mental rotation and the discrimination of locations in space (from Laird et al., 2011).

ICNs 11 and 12 (lateral and medial posterior occipital cortices) included the primary, secondary, and tertiary visual cortices (V1, V2, V3; BA 17/18/19). When viewed together, ICNs 12, 11, and 10 extended from medial to lateral aspects of the occipital and temporal cortices. ICN 12 was strongly linked to simple visual stimuli such as flashing checkerboards, and ICN 11 involved higher level visual processing associated with orthography and covert reading. ICN 11 also corresponded to Braille reading, demonstrating observed plasticity of these cortical regions in blind subjects. ICNs 11 and 12 displayed relatively weak loadings across many fields, such as behavioral domain, paradigm, and several of the condition fields. Rather than reflecting a functional non-specialization, further inspection of the heat map for the field "experimental contrast" revealed that many reported activations in these lateral and medial visual networks resulted from experiments in which the visual stimulation was not properly controlled. Because these visual activation patterns were not the primary effect sought and were classified under some other functional class (e.g., a delayed match to sample task contrasted with a resting baseline would be classified with a behavioral domain of "working memory" not "vision"), the functional descriptors relating to vision were, therefore, diluted across other metadata classes (from Laird et al., 2011).

ICN 13 (medial prefrontal and posterior cingulate/precuneus areas) was the component known as the default mode network and strongly corresponded to theory of mind and social cognition tasks. Weaker correspondence was observed for fixation, episodic recall, imagined scenes, and delay discounting tasks (from Laird et al., 2011).

ICN 14 (cerebellum), commonly associated with action and somesthesis, demonstrated a distributed range of sensorimotor, autonomic, and cognitive functions. Interestingly, both overt and covert naming showed a preference for cerebellar activity, despite the fact that no other language or speech tasks were associated with this region. Similarly ICN 14 showed preference for processing of humorous stimuli, yet no other emotional responses were observed (from Laird et al., 2011).

ICN 15 (right-lateralized fronto-parietal regions) included right BA 44/45 and 22/39/40. This network involved multiple cognitive processes, such as reasoning, attention, inhibition, and memory, and showed preference for n-back, delay discounting, and divided auditory attention tasks (from Laird et al., 2011).

ICN 16 (transverse temporal gyri) included the primary auditory cortices (A1; BA 41/42) and was related to audition (including tone and pitch discrimination), music, and speech. Other processes included phonological discrimination and oddball discrimination (from Laird et al., 2011).

ICN 17 (dorsal precentral gyri, central sulci, post-central gyri, superior and inferior cerebellum) included primary sensorimotor cortices for mouth (M1, S1; BA 4/3/1/2) and was associated with action and somesthesis corresponding to speech, such as overt reading or recitation, chewing or swallowing, and flexion/extension of the tongue (from Laird et al., 2011).

ICN 18 (left-lateralized fronto-parietal regions) included Broca's (BA 44/45) and Wernicke's (BA 22/39/40) areas and strongly mapped to a host of semantic, phonologic, and orthographic language tasks such as word generation and covert reading, as well as working and explicit memory tasks, such as paired associate recall, cued encoding and recognition, and the Sternberg task. Surprisingly, this network displayed a stronger preference toward working memory than did ICN 7. Stimulus types included words, pseudowords, letters, and Asian characters, with a dominance of button press responses (from Laird et al., 2011) (Figure 2.6).

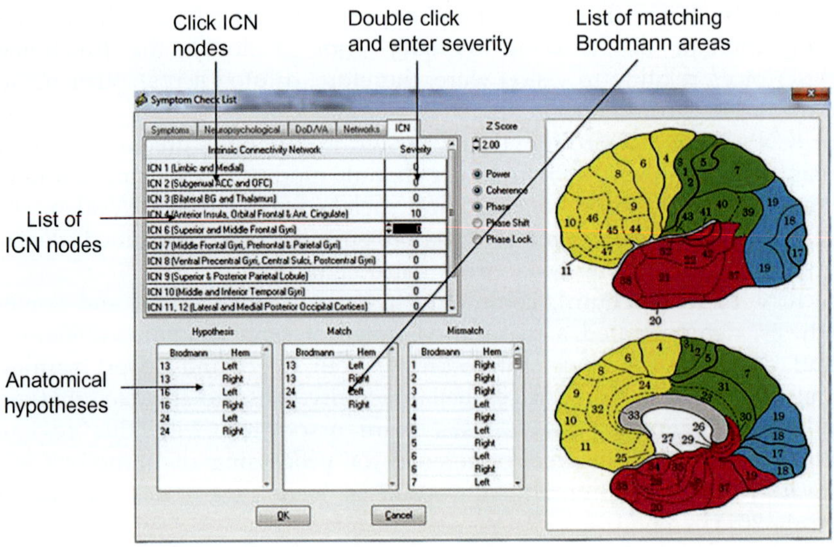

FIGURE 2.6 Illustration of the intrinsic connectivity (ICN) panel. Patient's symptoms and clinical history are first assessed and the clinician forms hypotheses as to which ICN brain networks are most likely related to the patient's symptoms prior to recording EEG. The qEEG is then recorded and LORETA and the ICN are used to confirm or disconfirm the hypotheses. Dysregulation as measured by Z scores from the Brodmann areas (nodes) and connections between Brodmann areas in ICNs linked to the patient's symptoms are then selected as targets for EEG biofeedback.

sLORETA AND LORETA Z SCORES AND THE CROSS-SPECTRUM

The computation of instantaneous Z scores for sLORETA and LORETA is different than for the surface EEG. This is because LORETA produces three orthogonal 3D current vectors from each voxel. That is, there are three time series in the x, y, and z directions. The resultant vector is the square root of the sum of squares. A problem with the resultant vector is that the square of x, y, and z rectifies the EEG current source time series or produces only positive values which double the frequency of the time series. In order to avoid frequency doubling, Neuroguide computes the mean time series or $(\sum x + y + z)/3 =$ mean current source in each voxel. Neuroguide also computed the x, y, and z means and standard deviations and compared the average of the means to the average of the x, y, and z vectors and found that they are essentially the same. Transforms were then applied to the average current source instantaneous time series in order to obtain Gaussian mean and standard deviation current sources from each voxel.

The mathematical details of using or not using complex numbers must be described and the methods of computation at each step. The case of the Neuroguide instantaneous norms of the cross-spectrum is calculated in the x, y, and z directions. The Z scores are computed from the mean of the x, y, and z real and imaginary components and the resultant vector is not used in the calculation of coherence and phase differences. The first and second derivatives of the phase difference time series is used to compute phase shift and phase lock duration with the same mathematics and methods as described by Thatcher et al. (2008a) and Thatcher, North, and Biver (2009). The resultant vector is useful for co-modulation or covariant magnitudes between Brodmann areas computed by a correlation coefficient.

NETWORK NODES AND CONNECTIONS

The 3D spatial Laplacian operator maximally smoothes the current source space in alignment with the physiological constraint of simultaneously active neurons that generate a spatially smeared distribution of current densities (see Pascual-Marqui et al., 1999). This means that adjacent voxels will be positively correlated and decrease smoothly with distance and as a consequence the center voxel of any given functional node will be representative of that node. For example, the correlation between the center voxel of a Brodmannn area and an adjacent voxel is about 0.99 and the correlation at the boundary or edge voxel is about 0.85 which is the case for all center voxels. Also, computing 6230 combinatorial is a matrix of 19 million by 19 million in the complex domain which is not feasible to compute in real time. As a consequence, an accepted method of computing sLORETA coherence and phase of the EEG sources is by using the center voxel of each functional ROI or Brodmann area or node of an interconnected network (Langer et al., 2011). The cross-spectrum is then calculated for all combinations of 88 Brodmann areas ($N = 3828$) for each frequency band which is handled easily with today's computers in real time.

STRUCTURAL, FUNCTIONAL, AND EFFECTIVE CONNECTIVITY

Karl Friston (1994) defined connectivity in three categories of (1) anatomical, (2) functional, and (3) effective connectivity. Anatomical connections are determined by cell staining methods, tract tracing methods, and DTI and diffusion spectrum imaging (Hagmann et al., 2008). Linkages between anatomical features and the qEEG are important, e.g., short versus long distance connections and EEG coherence or between EEG source magnitudes and the density of connections and phase lock and phase shift are linked to distance between hubs and modules (Nunez, 1981, 1994; Thatcher, Biver, & North, 2007; Thatcher et al., 1986, Thatcher, North, & Biver, 2008a,b). However, anatomy alone while providing indication of functional connectivity does not tell one how hubs and modules are dynamically connected in the millisecond domain. Functional connectivity is based on the analysis of the temporal correlations between separated neurophysiological events. Coherence, correlation, phase shift, phase lock, phase slope index (PSI), phase entropy transfer, and related measures provide estimates of time delays and coupling magnitude in the space–time frequency domain of hubs and modules (e.g., Joint-Time-Frequency-Analysis (JTFA)). Effective connectivity is aligned with "causal" connectivity and relies on directional information, e.g., the influence of one neural system on another (Friston, 1994; Nolte, Ziehe, & Nikulin, 2008). Estimates of causal connectivity includes measures of information flow such as with Granger causality (1969) and multivariate autoregressive modeling and conditional information measures (Greenblatt, Pflieger, & Ossadtchi, 2012; Kaminski, Ding, Truccolo, & Bressler, 2001) and the PSI (Ewald, Avarvand, & Nolte, 2013; Nolte et al., 2008). A problem with Granger causality is high noise sensitivity and reliance on multivariate model fitting.

PSI and phase transfer entropy (PTE) are a different class of causality metrics because they are based on the physics of phase differences or the imaginary part of the complex number. Mathematically, phase difference in a connective system is a function of distance and conduction velocity which means that when adjustments are made for relative phase, then all frequencies propagate at the same velocity according to volume conduction. Therefore, the phase difference due to volume conduction is equal to zero and hence only the imaginary part of the complex number is not equal to zero due to network delays. Network time delays are measured by the imaginary components of the cross-spectrum due to structural and functional connectivity with the direction of information flow determined by the spatial and temporal derivatives of the imaginary component describing the electricity of the EEG in a network. This is what is achieved by the PSI and PTE. The PSI is simple to compute and accurate and does not rely upon multivariate statistics. The PTE is more complicated to compute and is based on the Bayesian statistics of x influencing y like Granger causality but without the need to use autoregression as a first step. Both PSI and PTE can be used for cross-frequency causality, but again PSI is easier to compute and no systematic studies contrasting these two physics-based versus Granger-based effected connectivity studies have been conducted to date. The mathematical simulations of these various methods indicate high similarity but higher practical preference and simplicity to implement PSI and PTE which is driving the development of EEG effective connectivity going forward.

Z score neurofeedback of effective connectivity is one of a wide range of metrics soon to be available for neurofeedback. The scientific and mathematical foundations have been published and the application of these methods provides a reference to help determine the threshold and guide the direction of neurofeedback using effective connectivity at the level of Brodmann areas. The relative safety of a conservative approach toward reinforcement toward a standard of healthy individuals is foundational and unifying. The responsibility for good clinical outcome depends on the experience and competence of the practitioner and the ability to reinforce increased stability in networks of the brain related to the patient's symptoms.

References

Braitenberg, V., & Schüz, A. (1998). *Cortex: Statistics and geometry of neuronal connections* (2nd ed.). Heidelberg: Springer.

Broca, P. (1861). Perte de la parole, ramollissement chronique et destruction partielle du lobe antérieur gauche du cerveau. *Bulletins de la Société d'Anthropologie de Paris, 2*. 235e8 and 301e321

Brodmann, V. K. (1909). *Localization in the cerebral cortex: The principles of comparative localisation in the cerebral cortex based on cytoarchitectonics* (L. J. Garey, Trans.). London: Springer, 1994.

Catani, M., & de Schotten, M. T. (2012). *Atlas of human brain connections*. New York, NY: Oxford University Press.

Catani, M., Dell'Acquaa, F., Bizzi, A., Forkel, S. J., Williams, S. C., Simmons, A., et al. (2012a). Beyond cortical localization in clinico-anatomical correlation. *Cortex, 48*, 1262.

Catani, M., Dell'Acquaa, F., & de Schotten, M. T. (2013). A revised limbic system model for memory, emotion and behaviour. *Neuroscience and Biobehavioral Reviews, 37*, 1724–1737.

Catani, M., Dell'Acquaa, F., Vergani, F., Malik, F., Hodge, H., Roy, P., et al. (2012b). Short frontal lobes of the human brain. *Cortex, 48*, 273–291.

Dosenbach, N. U. F., Fair, D. A., Miezin, F. M., Cohen, A. L., Wenger, K. K., et al. (2007). Distinct brain networks for adaptive and stable task control in humans. *Proceedings of the National Academy of Sciences of the United States of America, 104*, 11073–11078.

Ewald, A., Avarvand, F. S., & Nolte, G. (2013). Identifying causal networks of neuronal sources from EEG/MEG data with the phase slope index: A simulation study. *Biomedical Technology, 58*(2), 165–178.

Friston, K. J. (1994). Functional and effective connectivity in neuroimaging. *Human Brain Mapping, 2*, 56–78.

Greenblatt, R. E., Pflieger, M. E., & Ossadtchi, A. (2012). Connectivity measures applied to human brain electrophysiological data. *Journal of Neuroscience Methods, 207*(1), 1–16.

Hagmann, P., Cammoun, L., Gigandet, X., Meuli, R., Honey, C. J., Wedeen, V. J., et al. (2008). Mapping the structural core of human cerebral cortex. *PLoS Biology, 6*, e159.

Jackson, H. (1876). Case of large cerebral tumour without optic neuritis and with left hemiplegia and imperception. In J. Taylor (Ed.), *Selected writings of John Hughlings Jackson* (p. 1876). London: Hodden and Stoughton.

Kaminski, M., Ding, M., Truccolo, W. A., & Bressler, S. L. (2001). Evaluating causal relations in neural systems: Granger causality, directed transfer function and statistical assessment of significance. *Biological Cybernetics, 85*, 145–157.

Laird, A. R., Fox, P. M., Eickhoff, S. B., Turner, J. A., Ray, K. L., McKay, D. R., et al. (2011). Behavioral interpretations of intrinsic connectivity networks. *Journal of Cognitive Neuroscience, 23*(12), 4022–4037.

Langer, N., Pedroni, A., Gianotti, A. R., Hanggi, J., Knoch, D., & Jancke, L. (2011). Functional brain network efficiency predicts intelligence. *Human Brainmapping, 33*(6), 1393e1406.

Lantz, G., Michel, C. M., Pascual-Marqui, R. D., Spinelli, L., Seeck, M., Seri, S., et al. (1997). Extracranial localization of intracranial interictal epileptiform activity using LORETA (low resolution electromagnetic tomography). *Electroencephalography & Clinical Neurophysiology, 102*, 414–422.

Mulert, C., Gallinat, J., Pascual-Marqui, R., Dorn, H., Frick, K., Schlattmann, P., et al. (2001). Reduced event-related current density in the anterior cingulate cortex in schizophrenia. *Neuroimage, 13*, 589–600.

Mulert, C., Jager, L., Schmitt, R., Bussfeld, P., Pogarell, O., Moller, H. J., et al. (2004). Integration of fMRI and simultaneous EEG: Towards a comprehensive understanding of localization and time-course of brain activity in target detection. *NeuroImage, 22*, 83–94.

Nolte, G., Ziehe, A., Nikulin, V., et al. (2008). Robustly estimating the flow direction of information in complex physical systems. *Physical Review Letters, 100*, 234101.

Nunez, P. L. (1981). *Electrical fields of the brain*. New York, NY: Oxford University Press.

Nunez, P. L. (1995). *Neocortical dynamics and human EEG rhythms*. New York, NY: Oxford University Press.

Pascual-Marqui, R. D., Lehmann, D., Koenig, T., Kochi, K., Merlo, M. C. G., Hell, D., et al. (1999). Low resolution brain electromagnetic tomography (LORETA) functional imaging in acute, neuroleptic-naive, first-episode, productive schizophrenia. *Psychiatry Research-Neuroimaging, 90*, 169–179.

Pizzagalli, D. A., Lehmann, D., Hendrick, A. M., Regard, M., Pascual-Marqui, R. D., & Davidson, R. J. (2002). Affective judgments of faces modulate early activity (approximately 160 ms) within the fusiform gyri. *NeuroImage, 16*, 663–677.

Pizzagalli, D. A., Oakes, T. R., Fox, A. S., Chung, M. K., Larson, C. L., Abercrombie, H. C., et al. (2004). Functional but not structural subgenual prefrontal cortex abnormalities in melancholia. *Molecular Psychiatry, 9*, 393–405.

Pizzagalli, D. A., Pascual-Marqui, R. D., Nitschke, J. B., Oakes, T. R., Larson, C. L., Abercrombie, H. C., et al. (2001). Anterior cingulate activity as a predictor of degree of treatment response in major depression: Evidence from brain electrical tomography analysis. *American Journal of Psychiatry, 158*, 405–415.

Rabinovich, M. I., Afraimovich, V. S., Christian, B., & Varona, P. (2012). Information flow dynamics in the brain. *Physics of Life Reviews, 9*, 51–73.

Seeck, M., Lazeyras, F., Michel, C. M., Blanke, O., Gericke, C. A., Ives, J., et al. (1998). Noninvasive epileptic focus localization using EEG-triggered functional MRI and electromagnetic tomography. *Electroencephalography and Clinical Neurophysiology, 106*, 508–512.

Thatcher, R. W. (2012). *Handbook of quantitative electroencephalography and EEG biofeedback*. St. Petersburg, FL: Anipublishing Co.

Thatcher, R. W., Biver, C. J., & North, D. (2007). Spatial-Temporal current source correlations and cortical connectivity. *Clinical EEG and Neuroscience, 38*(1), 35–48.

Thatcher, R. W., Krause, P., & Hrybyk, M. (1986). Corticocortical association fibers and EEG coherence: A two compartmental model. *Electroencephalography and Clinical Neurophysiology, 64*, 123–143.

Thatcher, R. W., North, D., & Biver, C. (2008a). Development of cortical connectivity as measured by EEG coherence and phase. *Human Brain Mapping, 29*(12), 1400–1415.

Thatcher, R. W., North, D., & Biver, C. (2008b). Intelligence and EEG phase reset: A two-compartmental model of phase shift and lock. *NeuroImage, 42*(4), 1639–1653.

Thatcher, R. W., North, D., & Biver, C. (2009). Self organized criticality and the development of EEG phase reset. *Human Brain Mapping, 30*(2), 553–574.

Thatcher, R. W., North, D. M., & Biver, C. J. (2012). Diffusion spectral imaging modules correlate with EEG LORETA neuroimaging modules. *Human Brain Mapping, 33*(5), 1062–1075.

Tuch, D. S., Wedeen, V. J., Dale, A. M., George, J. S., & Belliveau, J. W. (1999). Conductivity mapping of biological tissue using diffusion MRI. *Annals of the New York Academy of Sciences, 888*, 314–316.

Vitacco, D., Brandeis, D., Pascual-Marqui, R., & Martin, E. (2002). Correspondence of event-related potential tomography and functional magnetic resonance imaging during language processing. *Human Brain Mapping, 17*, 4–12.

Wernicke, K. (1881). *Text book of cerebral diseases*. Berlin: Karger.

Wisner, K. M., Atluri, G., Lim, K. O., & MacDonald, A. W. (2013). Neurometrics of intrinsic connectivity networks at rest using fMRI: Retest reliability and cross-validation using a meta-level method. *NeuroImage, 76*, 236–251.

Worrell, G. A., Lagerlund, T. D., Sharbrough, F. W., Brinkmann, B. H., Busacker, N. E., Cicora, K. M., et al. (2000). Localization of the epileptic focus by low-resolution electromagnetic tomography in patients with a lesion demonstrated by MRI. *Brain Topography, 12*, 273–282.

CHAPTER

3

Optimal Procedures in Z-Score Neurofeedback: Strategies for Maximizing Learning for Surface and LORETA Neurofeedback

Joel F. Lubar

Southeastern Neurofeedback Institute, Pompano Beach, FL, USA

In this chapter I will discuss the basic concepts of operant conditioning and present examples of how it has been for many years applied to neurofeedback. Historically, the concepts go back more than 100 years. Edward Thorndike proposed "law of effect" which stated that "any behavior that is followed by pleasant consequences is likely to be repeated and any behavior followed by unpleasant consequences is likely to be stopped," (Thorndike, 1898). Hilgard (1948), Hilgard and Marquis (1961) stated that "learning is an increase in the probability of a response as a result of reinforced practice." BF Skinner has been given the greatest credit for the development of operant theory and published many papers and books over a number of decades elaborating the concept of operant or instrumental learning (Ferster & Skinner, 1957; Skinner, 1936, 1938). Basically operant is a response that can either be reinforced either positively or negatively or punished. As Skinner and his colleagues had shown in their many publications the strength of increasing the probability of a reinforced response depends on what he termed "schedules of reinforcement" (Ferster & Skinner, 1957). Negative reinforcement is another term described by Skinner. In negative reinforcement, a response or behavior is strengthened by removing or avoiding a negative outcome or aversive stimulus.

In the context of neurofeedback or more broadly biofeedback, one reinforces a particular physiological response to increase its probability.

Z Score Neurofeedback.
DOI: http://dx.doi.org/10.1016/B978-0-12-801291-8.00003-0

In the case of biofeedback, this could be a decrease in muscle tension for specific muscle groups, an increase in hand or leg temperature, a change in electrodermal response (EDR), heart rate variability, or blood pressure, as a few examples. In neurofeedback, we either reinforce positively or negatively certain aspects of EEG, such as a particular frequency, or frequency band, the magnitude of this frequency band (amplitude averaged over time), or more complex parameters, such as coherence, phase, and recently phase shift and phase lock durations. The measurement can be based on the actual values of these parameters or on their Z-score deviation from a normative database which has been used very successfully in the Neuroguide program.

The determination of what parameters should be trained depends on many factors. A very detailed clinical history for helping to determine which clinical disorders needs to be considered. This information can be gleaned from patient's information gathered in conjunction with family members, psychometric or neuropsychological testing. Accurate clinical diagnosis is essential in order to provide the best outcome. Along with this accurate assessment of the patient's clinical status is the quantitative EEG (QEEG) analysis which may involve anywhere from 1 to 19 or more channels compared with a normative database. The normative database may contain eyes open and eyes closed information or if one is available a database can be evaluated under task conditions. A detailed discussion of databases and the development is presented in my edited publication (Lubar, 2003).

SCHEDULES OF REINFORCEMENT

Introductory experimental psychology courses discuss in detail Skinner's concept of schedules of reinforcement. Although there are a number of these that have been employed in both animal and human studies for nearly 100 years in biofeedback and neurofeedback, the one which is used almost exclusively is the continuous reinforcement schedule (CRF). In the context of neurofeedback, when a particular pattern of activity occurs usually, such as a spindle of sensorimotor rhythm (SMR), beta burst, or some other pattern, a feedback signal in the form of a simple or complex visual display, paired sometimes with sound and sometimes with a counter, is presented to the subject—patient. However, the feedback is withheld when the signal is contaminated by artifact including EMG, tongue movements, and head or body movements. This is akin to the animal model where the rat presses a lever, or pigeon pecks at a button and the pellet of food reward or birdseed is delivered. After a period of time, the animal subjects will become satiated and the rate of response decreases. In the human analog, the reinforcement is delivered rapidly and too often fatigue occurs and the rate of response decreases.

Another schedule of reinforcement which leads to faster learning and is more resilient to fatigue is the fixed ratio schedule. In this context, the subject must make a certain number of responses in order to receive a reward. In our early work with epileptic patients, I employed a form of fixed ratio conditioning which was described by Lubar and Culver (1978). This methodology employed a burst detector which was designed so that when a specified number of single cycles of a waveform occurred, reward was delivered. This was used in the context of SMR training and was set so that if six cycles of activity between 12 and 15 Hz occurred within half a second, both auditory and visual reward occurred. If the patient produced four cycles of 12 Hz activity which represented a time period of 0.3 s, then there was no reward. So effectively a fixed ratio schedule of six EEG events in half a second was the criterion for reward to occur. The same methodology could be used for any discrete event such as a burst of 10 Hz activity in the alpha band lasting for a specified time such as 1 or 2 s would be the criterion for reward of that frequency. The use of this approach based on a fixed ratio schedule led to powerful learning curves and long-term amelioration of seizures in the majority of patients trained.

Another schedule of reinforcement is known as the fixed interval schedule. In the animal model as long as the subject responds within the fixed interval, then a reward was obtained. For example, in a fixed interval schedule of 1 min as long as the response occurs at the end of that 1 min interval, there is a reward. Responses occurring early in the 1 min interval do not lead to reward and as a result the subject learns to produce most of the responses close to the 1 min end point. The human analog of the fixed interval schedule would be working on a production line in a factory with an instruction to produce at least one "widget" every minute and you will be paid $.10. Very soon the worker learns that they can relax for the first 55 s then produce the widget and receive the payment for that minute. The fixed interval schedule is good for developing timing behavior but is very inefficient and as far as I know not employed in neurofeedback.

Although there are many other schedules of reinforcement that can be used individually, combined or chained together, the most powerful schedule is the variable ratio schedule. If it wasn't for the variable ratio schedule, casinos would not be operating as lucratively as they are. In a variable ratio 50 and reward is delivered on the average when 50 responses have occurred but the range could be very great in terms of the time interval from almost instantaneous to many minutes or even hours. Every fisherman quickly learns that you cannot predict how many casts will lead to a strike. It could be one after another or many hours in between but when it occurs the effects are very rewarding and the behavior continues (probably maintained by the release of dopamine producing structures which are part of our reward circuit). An example of a variable reward ratio in neurofeedback would be a burst detector which on the average would produce a reward for a given number of responses. So in the example cited earlier for SMR, the reward might occur after three cycles of SMR the first time, six cycles next time, and nine cycles after that with many additional cycles averaging to six events. Since we know that variable interval schedules lead to very sustained response rates, they should be employed in neurofeedback training but as far as I know have not been.

LEARNING CURVES

There are many ways in which we can judge whether neurofeedback has been successful. The rather mechanistic but important approach is to see if learning curves are generated across training sessions both within a single session and over the totality of sessions trained. The training may be done under a single condition, such as eyes open or eyes closed, or during task conditions. An example of some learning curves employing a single pair of electrodes with one reward and two inhibit conditions is shown in Figure 3.1.

These graphs were generated automatically by the Autogenics A620 neurofeedback system. The feedback consisted of auditory and visual displays with fixed thresholds throughout the entire training course of sessions. Training occurred at the same time of day (late afternoon) after school two times a week. The last four sessions were spaced over a longer period of 6 months which was part of our follow-up procedure. Electrodes were placed at locations FCZ and CPZ where the latter location was the reference. A ground electrode was placed on the left earlobe. For these graphs, the individual, a 14-year-old male with attention-deficit/hyperactivity disorder (ADHD) was trained to increase 16–20 Hz and simultaneously to inhibit 4–8 Hz. A second inhibit channel blocked EMG activity between 80 and 120 Hz. The training was administered over five conditions, an initial baseline without feedback with the individual looking at a dot in the middle of the screen, a feedback condition by itself, a feedback condition combined with reading and only auditory feedback, another feedback only condition, and finally a feedback during listening to material read to the individual with a simple visual display. In order to obtain feedback, the child had to meet all criteria for 0.5 s. The first graph shows a steady increase in the microvolt levels of the reward frequency over sessions even during the phaseout, the next graph an

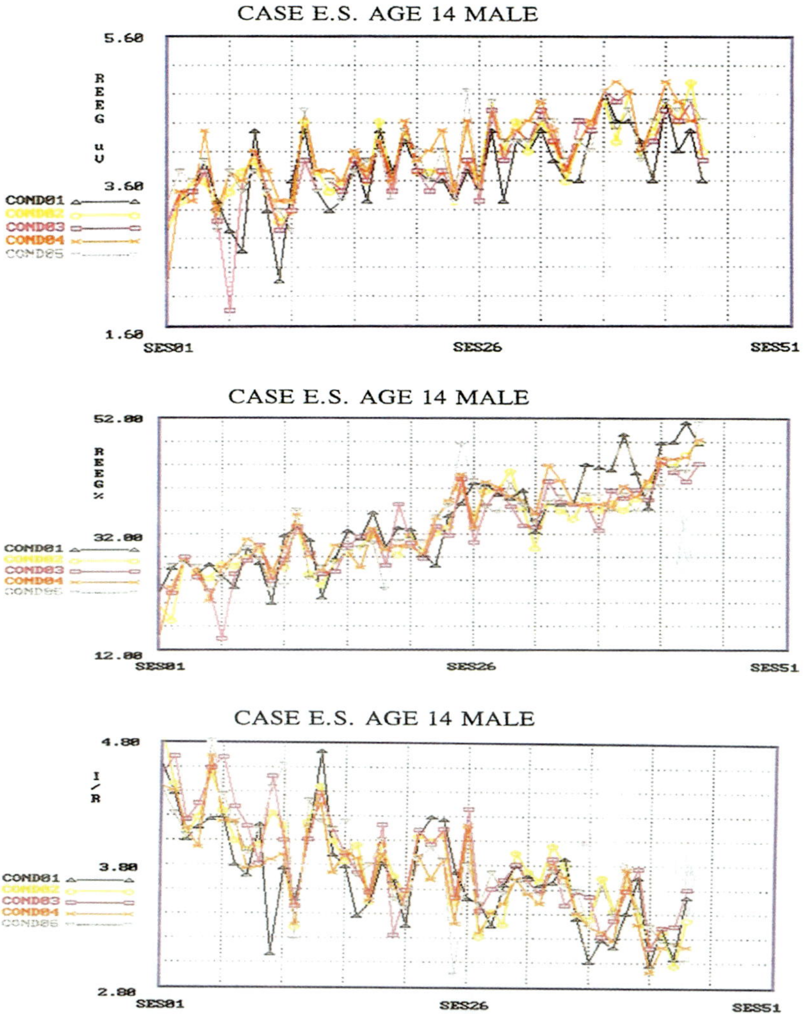

FIGURE 3.1 An example of learning curves employing a single pair of electrodes with one reward and two inhibit conditions.

increase in the percentage time that reward was obtained when there was no inhibit activity detected, the third graph a decrease in the ratio of the reward to the inhibit frequency over sessions.

These and additional graphs showing the percent of inhibit frequencies over sessions and microvolt levels of inhibit frequencies and threshold settings were obtained for all of our patients for the many years that we used this particular feedback system. Graphing of these parameters clearly demonstrate the power of operant conditioning. Judith Lubar worked with many of the patients and their families integrating individual and family therapy often guided by the graphing of the data. She has shown in her numerous workshops over the years how the use of graphs are important for signaling that it may be necessary to use other interventions to help patients especially when the graphing indicates that they are having difficulty with either feedback or feedback combined with academic tasks. Graphing intersession data is extremely important whether one is employing this in a clinical context or in a randomized controlled study in single or double-blind conditions. The numbers that generate the graphs can be used for statistical analyses as simple as rank order correlation across sessions or more complex statistics such as ANOVA comparing different conditions over sessions. Periodic full QEEGs obtained at various points throughout training and after long-term follow-up can be compared and evaluated using programs such as Neurostat in Neuroguide to determine the effect of training individual locations on the total QEEG distribution. Additional measures including phase, coherence, and more recently phase lock and phase shift can be evaluated and compared either with the Neuroguide database or between different training conditions.

Figure 3.2 shows an example of a learning curve generated over nine sessions in a middle-age female patient with anxiety and depression. The upper portion of the graph shows the percentage of reward

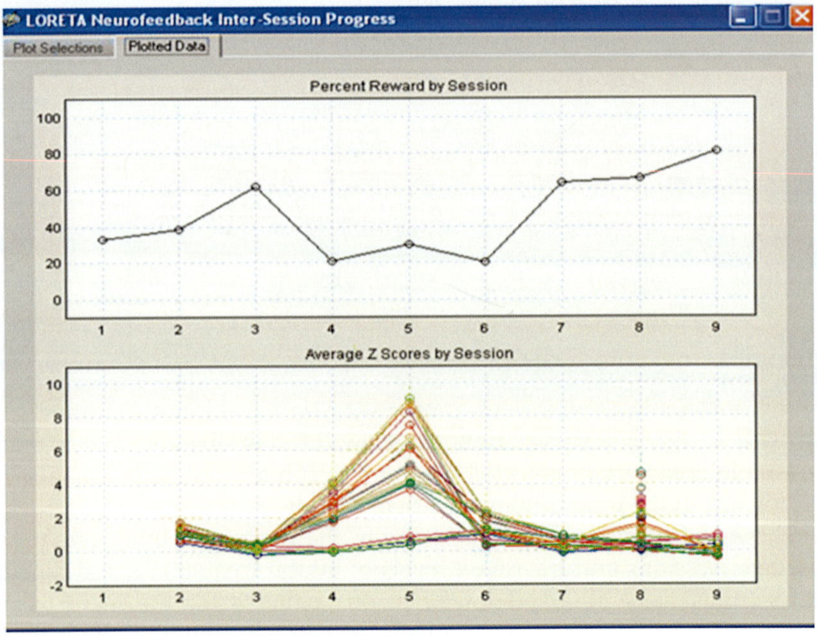

FIGURE 3.2 An example of a learning curve generated over nine sessions in a middle-age female patient with anxiety and depression.

averaged over all parameters trained for each session. The different parameters are graphed individually in the lower portion of the graph. There are also tables listing all the parameters that were used in composing the graphs.

These graphs were automatically generated in the Neuroguide NF2 LORETA neurofeedback program based on the symptom checklist.

CONTINGENCY OF FEEDBACK

I have already discussed briefly some of the schedules of reinforcement that had been employed for nearly 100 years to promote learning. The contingency between the event and operant to be reinforced needs to be considered in more detail. In the simplest case of continuous reinforcement (CRF schedule), the reward should be discreet and rapidly follow the physiological event which is to be either enhanced or inhibited. Some physiological events change very slowly, e.g., peripheral skin temperature which is related to blood flow. In this case, a proportional type of feedback such as a sound which changes as the temperature changes has been used for many years quite successfully. One could set a threshold such as 92°F for digital skin temperature which could result in a discreet second tone or visual feedback stimulus when the threshold line is crossed for a specific period of time. The tonic EDR also changes slowly and can be trained with similar feedback procedures. Interestingly, feedback based on the BOLD response (blood oxygen level dependent response) leads to very rapid learning often in a matter of a small number of sessions (De Charms et al., 2005). They reported decreased sensitivity to two painful noxious stimuli with training in the anterior cingulate. Even though the bold response is slow, the accuracy for localization in subcortical structures is even better than it is for LORETA, S LORETA, or even E LORETA, the latter claiming zero localization error.

In the case of EEG, changes occur very rapidly. A burst of SMR rarely lasts for more than 0.75 s, gamma bursts are usually shorter, whereas beta spindles may occur for 1−2 s and alpha bursts may last for many seconds. One of the features of Neuroguide's training paradigm is that the required duration of the trained event can now be set from 0.25 to 3.0 s. If one is training an event such as a beta burst, which is known to last for 1.0 s, then the clinician can start where the required time duration window can be slowly increased in stages up to 1.0 s before a discreet stimulus is provided. Specifically, the clinician can begin with 0.25 s and progress over time to 0.5 and 0.75 and finally up to 1.0 s. If the goal is to either increase or decrease Z-score of long alpha bursts, then longer durations up to 3 s can be trained.

TYPES OF FEEDBACK

The Neuroguide program allows for many types of feedback stimuli depending on the input amplifier. Neuroguide itself has a green dot which changes in size and when maintained at maximal size for the selected time from 0.25 to 3 s, it can be paired with a tone or several selected musical instruments. There are also a variety of multimedia displays that are essentially little movie clips that can be used for feedback. Different input amplifiers also have displays of their own, so for example the Deymed Truscan system has approximately 20 "game displays," the Brain Master Discovery has a series of displays that can be linked to Neuroguide and other amplifiers also have their displays as well. One popular type of feedback is the use of the DVD which in terms of contingency can be problematic. Most DVD displays allow the stimulus to change either in size, brightness, or color saturation. The sound associated with the DVD can also very as a function of changes in these parameters. In order to be really contingent when the EEG changes rapidly, the use of sound or changing size will occur so rapidly that it will create significant problems for the ability of the patient to learn. A rapidly changing size or brightness can be like photic stimulation and might lead to seizures in patients who are either photo or sound sensitive or a less severe example would be migraine headaches that are often set off by rapidly changing brightness or sounds. If the brightness or size change slowly, the feedback will be noncontingent with rapidly changing events in the EEG. The use of color saturation is interesting because the DVD continues to play, but its properties change from a color movie to a black-and-white movie. For children watching a cartoon, they will desire it to be colorful; therefore, this display might be the best one to use but again unless it changes very rapidly it could become noncontingent. As far as I know there are no randomized controlled studies comparing DVD with simple sound and light displays which are discreet and tied to the event which is to be trained in the EEG.

THRESHOLDING

An important consideration concerns when to use fixed or changing threshold settings. Figure 3.1 illustrates clear learning curves where the threshold was the same throughout training overall sessions. However, threshold settings have also to be calibrated with the number of discrete rewards per unit time. So for example, if one is getting 30 rewards per minute measured by either a point counter or visual and auditory feedback, on the average reward is being presented every 2 s. This can lead to saturation or a "ceiling" effect where it be very difficult to increase the number of rewards per unit time. In contrast, if the patient is only getting four rewards per minute, this would mean approximately one reward every 15 s on the average and might lead to frustration or a feeling of inability to learn. I have found over many years of experience with different types of EEG-based feedback that for adults initially between approximately 10 and 15 rewards per minute and for children 15 to 20 rewards per minute seem to be reasonable initial values. Many clinicians will then adjust the threshold making it more difficult if the number of rewards becomes excessive per unit time. One possibility that was recently suggested by Dr. Thatcher is to have a set number of rewards, e.g., 15 per minute and automatically change the threshold settings to achieve this. One has to be very careful when using any kind of autothresholding program because if it is done incorrectly it can lead to laziness, in that the threshold is continuously made easier until eventually events other than that desired in the EEG are being reinforced including artifact. If one changes the threshold automatically to maintain a fixed number of rewards, then the threshold settings can be graphed and as long as they show that the threshold settings are associated with more challenge then this might be acceptable. Sometimes clinicians will change thresholds within a session especially if the session is divided up into discrete rounds and the patient is having difficulty in a particular round getting a reasonable number of rewards. Again one has to be very careful not to allow the patient to allow artifact to be reinforced as a result of making the program too easy.

NUMBER OF PARAMETERS TRAINED

This is an area where a lot of information is not well established. For example if one uses the Neuroguide symptom checklist and several related symptoms are indicated such as executive function, and those involving attention, several hundred parameters might be chosen for training if one includes power, phase, coherence, and more recently phase lock and phase shift. The clinician can deselect any of these categories or in the recent versions of the program can select only a subset of these for training. Occasionally, when one performs an initial QEEG before training, one may find that in the case of surface EEG, there are many abnormalities in absolute power with phase and coherence being relatively normal. In the case of LORETA, one can import the tab delimited text (TDT) tables for power, coherence, and phase and maybe eventually phase lock and phase shift. Again if current density is very abnormal but the connectivity measures are quite normal, then based on the symptom checklist perhaps only absolute power for surface or LORETA power will be chosen for training. The opposite can also occur where current density or surface power is quite normal, but the connectivity measures are very abnormal.

Many of us have observed that when using the Z tunes program, those parameters which are below threshold even when there are several hundreds of them usually remain so over sessions. The main emphasis then will be to bring the "outliers" down toward the threshold with the rest of the group. One could also determine who the outliers are and set up a separate protocol just for them. If there are relatively few outliers, then the "all or none" program might be useful. Phase lock requires a longer time to compute than phase shift and the other measures. As a result, one often finds that the threshold has to be set very high in order for phase lock and sometimes phase shift to be reinforced in conjunction with the other measures. At this point, we need to gather a lot more information on how to set up a triage for training all of these parameters either individually, or in small groups, or all combined.

USE OF ROUNDS FOR TRAINING

In our initial work, which is illustrated in Figure 3.1, we usually used five, 5 min rounds. Many patients after several rounds of training begin to get lower scores which they claim is due to fatigue or sometimes boredom. I have found a very easy way to assess this. One should record the entire session during training by activating the red record button at the beginning of the session. Later after the session is completed, it can be reassessed in the playback mode. As an example, if the session was 30 min long consisting of six, 5 min rounds, play the session back with 30, 1 min rounds and only 5 s between rounds. At the end of each round, a bar graph representing the number of rewards for that round will appear. In this example, a bar graph showing increase in the number of rewards for the first 15 rounds and then a decrease for the remaining 15 rounds could indicate that fatigue or boredom was developing halfway through the session. As a result, the clinician could then start out with shorter rounds, perhaps 10, 3 min rounds with 30 or more seconds of rest between rounds. The whole concept is to be able to increase the round length and eventually the session length where all the training parameters can be sustained for longer periods. I recommend that each session be recorded if at all possible.

TRANSFER OF TRAINING

How does one learn a complex task in such a way that the results can be transferred into real-world situations. There have been arguments going back to the 1960s as to whether one has to develop a cognitive, emotional, or some other strategy in order for a physiological variable to be trained in a biofeedback or neurofeedback setting. Kober, Witte, Ninaus, Neuper, and Wood (2013) trained individuals to either increase SMR or gamma over 10 sessions and to report what strategies they used in order to obtain feedback. Some people were able to elaborate strategies they used to obtain physiological control, but others could not. Some using "vivid reports" involving cognitive strategies found that it may be counterproductive in terms of increasing SMR power. During training itself, there is a point counter which resets at the end of each round. I have found that if we simply asked the individual being trained to try to beat their previous round score, this often generated excellent learning curves. This is particularly the case when you are trying to increase attention or executive function or using the attention network tab. If one is trying to train for sustained attention over long periods of time, increasing the duration of the rounds and the duration of the session would also be an important goal. In contrast, working with the patient with obsessive-compulsive disorder (OCD) or anxiety, such a goal directed strategy might be counterproductive. In one of our studies (Lubar, 2005) we had a professional person using the Connors symptom checklist and telephone interview rate individuals that had been in training on their experience. These individuals varied from less than 1 year up to 10 years post-training. Many of them found that the neurofeedback had been of significance in terms of their amelioration of symptoms and their success in pursuing academic or career paths. I have always believed the treatment is not successful it doesn't last. How many procedures, medical, psychological, even surgical lead to very promising initial results only to be followed by relapse to the initial state. This has certainly been true of the addiction field, dealing with traumatic brain injury and posttraumatic stress disorder (PTSD) as just a few examples.

I have already discussed several ways of monitoring patient progress including looking at the intersession graphs or comparing the initial QEEG or LORETA findings with those after training. Recently I have suggested to people who consult with me that they take a 3–5 min initial baseline where the patient is simply asked to look at a fixation point on a wall in front of them but not to look at the EEG scrolling across the screen which produces excessive eye movement. Then when training is initiated to record the entire training session and then finally at the end of training to record another 3–5 minute post-baseline. Each of these three conditions can be analyzed separately and compared.

The best-case scenario is where there is considerable normalization of the surface and/or LORETA measures which are maintained during the post-baseline recording. The post-baseline recording can then be compared with the pre-baseline recording of the next session to see if the changes were maintained during the nontraining interval. Another scenario is where there is normalization of many of the parameters during training but regression back to pre-baseline QEEG and LORETA during the post-baseline measurement. This is an example of "state dependent learning" where the positive changes only occur during training, but the patient regresses to the pre-baseline level. If this happens consistently over sessions, there is very little evidence that the patient will show a long-term amelioration of symptomatology. It is important that the clinician shares these findings with the patient and to develop strategies to help the patient maintain without feedback and the improvements that were obtained during the training session itself. Figure 3.3 shows changes obtained in surface coherence with 5 min of LORETA neurofeedback training in a 48-year-old female employing the anxiety network. All decreased coherences seen in the initial baseline disappeared during feedback and only one coherence in high beta reappeared between F8 and PZ during the 5 min post-training baseline.

TRAINING PHASE SHIFT AND PHASE LOCK DURATIONS

Thatcher, North, and Biver (2008) built a database for individuals with low, normal range, and high IQs. In this study, they demonstrated that phase shift duration and phase lock duration are strongly related to IQ and also depend on distances between different nodes based on Brodmann areas. Phase shift duration is correlated with allocating or bringing together resources from different brain regions or hubs in order for an individual to comprehend and develop schema for complex problem solving. As the phase shift duration increases between specific regions that are associated with different tasks, more resources are allocated or assembled. The complexity of this operation is highly correlated with increased IQ. Although it is no longer fashionable to think of a "G" factor to explain intelligence especially since intelligence has many different components, it is interesting that there is a QEEG measure that is correlated with this concept. Once resources have been pulled together or allocated, they need to be utilized in order to successfully complete a complex operation. This is mirrored by the phase lock duration which tends to be shorter and highly intelligent individuals. As an analogy, think of taking a difficult multiple-choice examination. In order to decide which of the detractors is the correct answer, one has

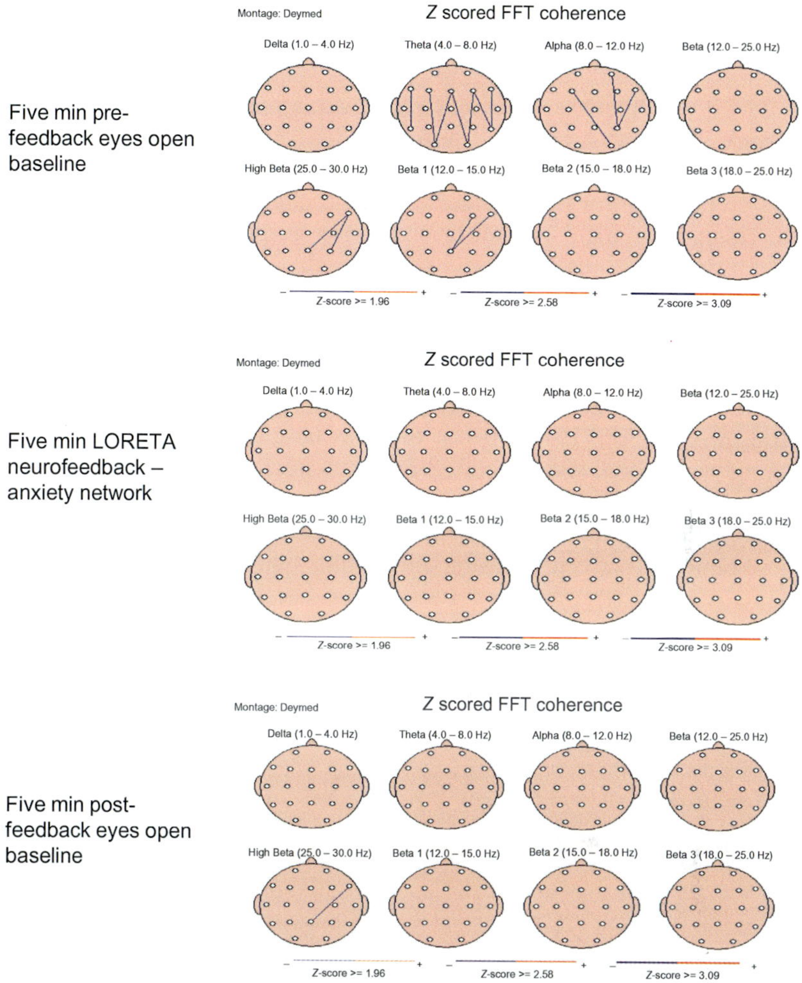

FIGURE 3.3 Changes obtained in surface coherence with five minutes of LORETA neurofeedback training in a 48-year-old female employing the anxiety network.

to pull together a lot of memory and other types of information before marking the choice on an answer sheet. Once a decision is made, one has to progress rapidly to the next question and pull together necessary resources again in order to make the correct choice. If these two processes are not completed efficiently, the individual may not complete the examination in the allotted time. The interplay of phase shift duration and phase lock duration for the different areas of the brain that are involved in allocating resources is of paramount importance.

Even though phase shift and phase lock are very complex measures, Figure 3.4 shows that within one session it is possible this to change the shift duration from too short to virtually normal. In this example, a female with problems in memory recall experienced, in a 12 min neurofeedback session, substantial improvement in phase shift duration. Although the illustration shows the changes using the Neuroguide connectivity suite for delta, there were also changes in theta and beta as well. This person also showed improvement in phase lock duration.

OVERVIEW

Changing your brain doesn't change your life unless there are a whole series of supportive interventions to maintain the effects of the physiological intervention. Examples of this can be gleaned by looking at the learning curves that are generated by intersession graphs. The ideal case is where a patient comes in having read a number of articles about neurofeedback and really believes that it can help them. In addition, this patient generates strong learning curves and when they are shown to the patient by the therapist reinforces his or her belief that this is really working and it is going to continue to work. But what about the patient who is extremely skeptical, has read articles that are critical of neurofeedback, and nevertheless shows excellent learning curves. In this case,

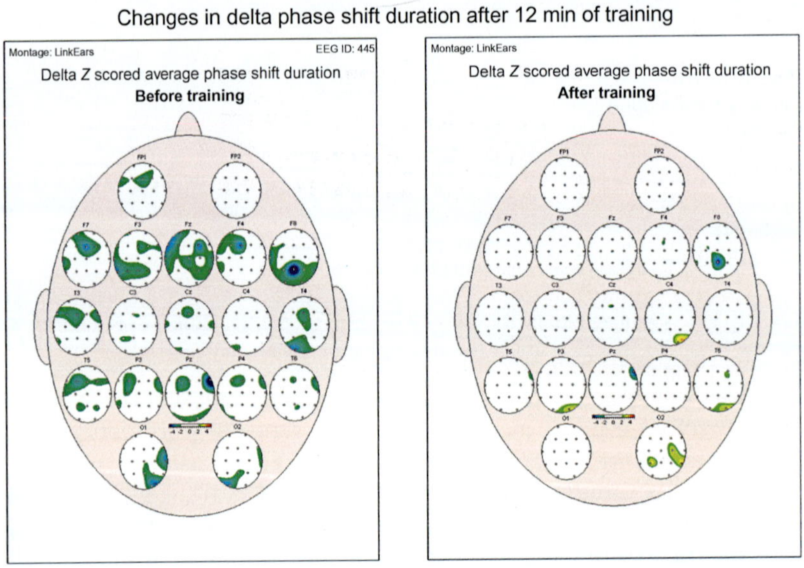

FIGURE 3.4 Changes in delta phase shift duration after 12 min of training. This figure shows that within one session it is possible this to change the phase shift duration from too short to virtually normal.

a skilled clinician can help the patient reframe their belief system that if the physiology has changed perhaps the change in viewpoint may begin to overcome any negative feelings regarding the effectiveness of neurofeedback. The opposite scenario is a patient who has read many articles about the field and really believes that neurofeedback will be of great help to them but they just cannot learn to change the parameters trained. Their learning curves demonstrate a "flatline" situation. If the patient is feeling better, it may be necessary to point out that we are only graphing those parameters that were trained, but those parameters are linked to many others that are not graphed representing other kinds of brain networks or perhaps other peripheral physiological systems that may have changed and that is why he or she is feeling better. The most unfortunate scenario represents the patient who neither believes in neurofeedback nor cannot generate any evidence of learning. This patient runs the risk of dropping out of treatment and feeling it was totally useless. There may be circumstances in the individual's life, job, or family or medical situation that demonstrates to him the need for either psychotherapeutic or medical intervention including pharmacology if necessary.

In our field, we need more discussion and sharing of information regarding how we can help patients transfer what they have learned in the clinic or laboratory to their life circumstances. This gets into the controversial area of professional practice standards and minimal requirements for one to be able to engage in biofeedback. AAPB, ISNR, and BCIA have published standards of practice and B CIA (Biofeedback Certification International Alliance) has a comprehensive certification program for both technicians and practitioners. Since biofeedback and neurofeedback, when dealing with psychological and psychiatric disorders, have to be integrated with individual and family therapy in most cases, the whole question of who is qualified to provide such services has been an area of considerable and often vociferous debate. The APA (American Psychological Association) recognizes biofeedback including neurofeedback as a legitimate insupportable intervention. Recently mental health has achieved some parity in terms of recognition with treatment of medical disorders and more insurance companies are beginning to recognize and cover the services. The point of all this is that quality transfer of training will not occur if neurofeedback is performed mechanically and without complete and detailed evaluation of the patient's circumstances, diagnosis, and evaluation of any underlying medical and psychiatric disorders. Pharmacological considerations are extremely important as medications can affect the outcome of treatment and will sometimes have to be reduced as neurofeedback is performed because the patients react as if they are overmedicated. This is particularly true regarding ADHD with neurofeedback and sometimes anticonvulsants can be reduced if the neurofeedback is successful in helping patients with epilepsy.

STUDIES SUPPORTING Z-SCORE-BASED NEUROFEEDBACK

At present, there are no published studies comparing Z-score-based neurofeedback with conventional neurofeedback. However, there are many published studies involving individual cases or small numbers of cases that indicate that Z-score-based neurofeedback produces more rapid learning than conventional feedback and appears to be very effective for many different disorders. Examples of these are publications by Collura, Guan, Tarrent, Bailey, and Starr (2010) and Collura, Thatcher, Smith, Lambos, and Stark (2009). More recently Hammer, Colbert, Brown, and Ilioi (2011) have shown that Z-score training may be helpful for insomnia. In our early work with epilepsy Lubar et al. (1981) employed a double-blind cross-over approach showing that neurofeedback can be quite effective in reducing epileptic seizures. In our subsequent study, Whitsett, Lubar, Holder, Pamplin, and Shabsin (1982) showed that these changes in epileptiform activity could be maintained during sleep depending on which parameters were reinforced or inhibited. Koberda (2011) and Koberda, Hiller, Jones, Moses, and Koberda (2012) have worked with a number of epileptics using Z-score-based neurofeedback with very promising results.

Unfortunately for many scientists and particularly for those employing pharmacological treatments, the "gold standard" is a randomized controlled double-blind study. Usually these studies employ a condition known as "sham" which in the case of pharmacology involves a placebo and in the case of bio- or neurofeedback involves a group given noncontingent reinforcement compared with the actively reinforce group. One of the flaws of sham reinforcement is that it is not truly noncontingent and occasionally, based on a variable ratio schedule, the same pattern may be reinforced in the noncontingent group that is appropriately reinforced in the contingent group. When this occurs, the sham control group may not differ in terms of its "learning" from the experimental group because the appropriate pattern was inadvertently reinforced from time to time. It is very important (although this has not yet been done) to mark the EEG every time a reward is delivered for both the experimental and the control group. Although the procedure is tedious, one could determine the percentage time that the appropriate pattern was inadvertently reinforced in the sham control.

If one is working with either the attention network or attention, concentration, and executive function difficulties, clearly a sham group will be focusing on the feedback display even if it is relatively noncontingent and would be expected to show improvements although they may not last long after the treatment is completed. The group given totally contingent reinforcement as we have seen should show a long-term carryover of gains obtained during training. Since many of our neurofeedback interventions have been in effect for years combined with either medical or psychiatric approaches employing pharmacology or neuropharmacology, there is a much simpler experimental design that should be considered. This would involve three completely matched randomized groups with all of the appropriate pre-measures and post-measures and follow-up. One group would receive only pharmacological treatment where the dosages of the various medications are as constant as possible throughout the training. The second group would receive only neurofeedback without medication, the third group would receive constant medication dosages combined with neurofeedback. In this very straightforward design, one would know whether the neurofeedback is as effective or less effective than medication and to what extent the combination of the two is better than either by itself. Unfortunately studies like this have not yet been done for neurofeedback employing the Z-score approach.

In general, controlled randomized double-blind studies usually follow many years of clinical experience with a technique. This is because such studies have to be large, often involve multiple centers, and require extensive grant support which currently is very difficult to obtain. At present the best we can do is to work with our patients very carefully, document their learning, and follow their progress after training has been completed. Patients who have been successful are usually the best advocates to help gain government and insurance support for a new procedure. Eventually the controlled studies will probably be done although there are detractors who believe that a new procedure should not be administered until those studies are completed. In reality this is not the way even the scientific world works. In the surgery, new procedures and devices (often implanted) are carried out experimentally and after many years clinical trials are finally completed which may or may not support the initial clinical interventions. We should continue to move forward in the development of our new field of Z-score-based neurofeedback and continue to be innovative but very careful and to always work in the context of the old Hippocratic dictum of "do no harm."

References

Collura, T., Guan, J., Tarrent, J., Bailey, J., & Starr, R. (2010). EEG biofeedback case studies using live Z-score training and a normative database. *Journal of Neurotherapy, 14*(1), 22–46.

Collura, T., Thatcher, R., Smith, M. L., Lambos, W., & Stark, C. (2009). *EEG biofeedback training using live* Z-*scores and a normative database*. Philadelphia, PA: Elsevier.

De Charms, C., Maeda, F., Glover, G. H., Ludlow, D., Pauly, J. M., Soneji, D., et al. (2005). *Proceedings of the National Academy of Sciences of the United States of America, 51*, 18626–18631.

Ferster, C. B., & Skinner, B. F. (1957). Schedules of reinforcement. Englewood Cliffs, NJ.

Hammer, B. U., Colbert, A. P., Brown, K. A., & Ilioi, E. C. (2011). A neurofeedback for insomnia: A pilot study of Z-score SMR and individualized protocols. *Applied Psychophysiology and Biofeedback, 10*, 1007–1048.

Hilgard, E. R. (1948). *Theories of learning*. New York, NY: Appleton-Century-Crofts.

Hilgard, E. R., & Marquis, D. O. (1961). *Conditioning and learning* (2nd ed.). Prentice-Hall.

Kober, S. E., Witte, M., Ninaus, M., Neuper, C., & Wood, G. (2013). Learning to modulate one's own brain activity: The effect of spontaneous mental strategies. *Frontiers in Neuroscience, 18*, 1–12.

Koberda, J. L. (2011). A clinical advantages of quantitative electroencephalogram (QEEG) application in general neurology practice. *Neuroscience Letters, 500*(Suppl.), e32.

Koberda, J. L., Hiller, D. S., Jones, B., Moses, A., & Koberda (2012). A Application of neurofeedback in general neurology practice. *Journal of Neurotherapy, 16*(3), 231–234.

Lubar, J. F. (2003). Neurofeedback for the management of attention-deficit/hyperactivity disorders. In M. Schwartz, & F. Andrasik (Eds.), *Biofeedback: A practitioner's guide* (pp. 409–437). New York, NY: Guilford.

Lubar, J. F., & Culver, R. M. (1978). Automated EEG signal-detection methodologies for biofeedback conditioning. *Behavior Research Methods and Instrumentation, 10*, 607–616.

Lubar, J. F., Shabsin, H. S., Natelson, S. E., Holder, G. S., Whitsett, S. F., Pamplin, W. E., et al. (1981). EEG operant conditioning in intractable epileptics. *Archives of Neurology, 38*, 700–704.

Skinner, B. F. (1936). Conditioning and extinction and their relation to drive. *Journal of General Psychology, 14*, 296–317.

Skinner, B. F. (1938). *The behavior of organisms: An experimental analysis*. New York, NY: Appleton-Century-Crofts.

Thatcher, R. W., North, D. M., & Biver, C. J. (2008). Intelligence and phase reset: A two compartmental model of phase shift and lock. *NeuroImage, 42*(4), 1639–1653.

Thorndike, E. L. (1898). Animal intelligence: An experimental study of the associative processes in animals. *Psychological Monographs: General and Applied, 2*. (4), i-109.

Whitsett, S. F., Lubar, J. F., Holder, G. S., Pamplin, W. E., & Shabsin, H. S. (1982). Changes in the epileptic's sleep EEG following EEG biofeedback training. *Biofeedback and Self-Regulation, 7*, 193–209.

CHAPTER

4

Surface and LORETA Neurofeedback in the Treatment of Post-Traumatic Stress Disorder and Mild Traumatic Brain Injury

Dale S. Foster, Ph.D. and Robert W. Thatcher, Ph.D.

Memphis Integral Neurofeedback Institute (MINI), Cordova, TN and Applied Neuroscience Research Institute, Seminole, FL, USA

SURFACE AND LORETA NEUROFEEDBACK OF POST-TRAUMATIC STRESS DISORDER

Peniston and Kulkosky (1991) treated 15 combat veterans suffering from chronic post-traumatic stress disorder (PTSD) with 30 sessions of occipital alpha–theta neurofeedback, in addition to standard treatment, and demonstrated remediation of symptoms and improvements on minnesota multiphasic personality inventory (MMPI) clinical scales in comparison to a 14-member control group who received only standard treatment. A 30-month follow-up revealed that all 14 of the control group had experienced relapse of their symptoms, while only 3 of the 15 members of the treatment group had experienced relapse.

In a second uncontrolled study, Peniston, Marrinan, Deming, and Kulkosky (1993) trained 20 veterans with chronic PTSD symptoms as well as comorbid alcohol abuse with 30 sessions of alpha–theta neurofeedback resulting in elimination of symptoms. Monthly follow-up interviews conducted with subjects and family members for 26 months after treatment revealed that 16 of the veterans remained symptom free, while the other four reported few (one to three) episodes of PTSD symptoms.

Pop-Jordanova and Zorcec (2004) treated 10 children with PTSD using a multimodal approach (supportive, play, and behavior–cognitive

Z Score Neurofeedback.
DOI: http://dx.doi.org/10.1016/B978-0-12-801291-8.00004-2

therapies), which featured electrodermal (EDR) biofeedback and neurofeedback training to increase 12–16 Hz. Using a battery of psychometric instruments, they identified high levels of anxiety and stress, somatization, and behavioral problems (aggressiveness, impulsivity, nonobedience, and nightmares) in the subjects. After 20 sessions of weekly EDR biofeedback and neurofeedback lasting 50 min each, subjects' symptoms of PTSD had been eliminated.

Smith (2008) trained 10 combat veterans diagnosed with PTSD utilizing a two-phased functional neural anatomy–based neurofeedback approach, wherein subjects initially received 10 daily 30-min sessions training increased left hemispheric 15–18 Hz and right hemispheric 12–15 Hz while suppressing theta. Phase two consisted of 20 daily sessions of 30 min of alpha–theta training followed by 10 min of the phase one training. Smith found significant decreases in PTSD symptoms of depression on the Hamilton Depression Rating Scale and improvements in attention as measured by the Test of Variables of Attention.

Walker (2009) used quantitative electroencephalogram (qEEG)-guided neurofeedback with 19 PTSD sufferers training them to simultaneously decrease high-frequency beta and increase alpha. Multiple training sites were chosen for each subject based on elevated high beta power identified through Thatcher normative database comparisons. Each subject received five to seven sessions of training at two to six sites, one site at a time. At the end of training as well as at 1-month follow-up, all 19 subjects reported decreased anxiety as a result of the training, from moderate to severe anxiety (5/10–7/10) to mild or no anxiety (0/10–2/10).

Nelson and Esty (2012) treated seven combat veterans with persistent symptoms of PTSD and traumatic brain injury (TBI) with Flexy Neurotherapy System and demonstrated reductions in PTSD symptom scale scores with effect sizes ranging from 0.62 to 0.93. Although this method uses pulsed electromagnetic stimulation linked to the subjects' EEG instead of operant conditioning, it is included here due to its apparent efficacy and to illustrate the need for continued basic research into the mechanisms underlying effective neurofeedback and neuromodulation.

Kluetsch et al. (2013), building upon their previous research with healthy normal subjects (Ros et al., 2013) in which they demonstrated functional magnetic resonance imaging (fMRI) salience network changes caused by neurofeedback, successfully trained 21 chronic PTSD sufferers to decrease alpha amplitude in a single 30-min session. Subjects reported improvements in relaxation, calmness, and clear-mindedness and demonstrated a post-training rebound of increased resting alpha. Additionally, fMRI measures quantified improved connectivity within both the salience network and the default mode network, both known to be dysregulated in sufferers of PTSD. Although they did not include a sham neurofeedback control group for "ethical reasons," this study clearly shows short-term modifications in the underlying neuropathology associated with PTSD as well as improvements in the subjective experience of PTSD symptoms. They also quantified a relationship between relative reduction of alpha during training and the amount of rebound alpha after training: the greater the alpha decrease during neurofeedback, the greater was the alpha amplitude rebound after training. This effect occurred globally, at all 19 channels, not just at the site of the single channel training, PZ. This study thus demonstrates both global and specific network effects of single channel neurofeedback on the specific neuropathology and symptomatology of PTSD.

Foster and Veazey-Morris (2013) utilized low-resolution EEG tomographic analysis (LORETA) Z-score neurofeedback (LZN) in conjunction with a symptom checklist, functional neural network match (SCL–FNM) method (Thatcher, 2012, 2013) to train eight combat veterans diagnosed with both PTSD and post-concussion syndrome. This method allows training of multiple EEG power and connectivity metrics within and among multiple neural networks simultaneously through real-time 3D neuroimaging and normative database comparisons, thus potentially providing the most individual-specific or personalized method of neurofeedback to date. They reported normalization of the PTSD-affected neural networks trained and reduction in PTSD symptoms.

These data indicate that neurofeedback is probably efficacious in the treatment of PTSD. However, as seen in this review, multiple methods of neurofeedback training have produced evidence of efficacy in the reduction of PTSD symptoms as well as improvements in the underlying neuropathology. It is apparent that the neurofeedback methods available have evolved dramatically since Peniston's initial 1991 work allowing increasingly personalized approaches to the treatment of PTSD symptoms, from single site one-size-fits-all methods to multiple site, normative database-guided, 3D tomographic functional neural anatomy–based methods. The rapidly growing cross-validated neuroimaging literature supporting the accuracy and utility of functional neural network models in the identification of mechanisms underlying the symptoms of PTSD suggests that the most rational approach to the treatment of this disorder will make use of this body of knowledge through approaches such as normative database-guided EEG tomographic Z-score neurofeedback with SCL–FNM methods. However, the questions concerning the relative efficacy of current and evolving approaches need to be asked and answered empirically through well-designed controlled comparative studies.

SURFACE AND LORETA NEUROFEEDBACK OF MILD TRAUMATIC BRAIN INJURY

A January 2014 Internet search for studies utilizing neurofeedback in the treatment of TBI yielded 27 peer reviewed studies, involving 605 subjects, all of which demonstrated positive outcomes. Outcome measures included self-report of improved symptoms (mood, fatigue, focus, ability to return to work), neuropsychological test scores (objective tests of attention, executive function, visual and auditory memory), and qEEG metrics (increased beta, SMR and/or alpha power; decreased theta, high beta, and/or EMG power; and normalization of coherence and/or phase). Five of the studies employed control groups, of which three utilized random assignment ($N=88$) (Ayers, 1993, $N=12$; Keller, 2001, $N=21$; $N=12$; Schoenberger et al., 2001, $N=12$; and Tinius and Tinius, 2000, $N=31$), six studies employed historical control ($N=91$) (Foster and Veazey-Morris, 2013, $N=8$; Hoffman et al., 1996, $N=14$; Laibow et al., 2001, $N=27$; Walker et al., 2002, $N=26$; Zelek, 2002, $N=10$; and Zorcec et al., 2011, $N=6$), and 14 studies involved uncontrolled individual case studies and case series ($N=405$) (Ayers, 1987, $N=250$; Bratic et al., 2007, $N=2$; Byers, 1995, $N=1$; Greuling et al., 1998, $N=1$; Hammond, 2006, $N=2$; Malkowicz and Martinez, 2009, $N=1$; Nash, 2005, $N=1$; Reddy et al., 2009, $N=1$; Thornton, 2000, $N=2$; Thornton, 2002, $N=4$; Thornton and Carmody, 2013, $N=15$; Wing, 2001, $N=1$; Surmeli, 2007, $N=24$; $N=100$).

The three studies, which utilized randomized assignment to control groups, included Ayers (1993), Keller (2001), and Schoenberger et al. (2001). Ayers (1993) conducted a study in which 12 outpatients in ongoing psychotherapy with right hemisphere closed head trauma and symptoms of emotional dyscontrol were randomly assigned to either neurofeedback inhibiting 4–7 Hz and rewarding 15–18 Hz in the right hemisphere ($N=6$) or a psychotherapy only control group ($N=6$). Only the neurofeedback group showed decreased symptomatology and progress in psychotherapy. A weakness of Ayers was the lack of information regarding her data analysis techniques.

Keller (2001) treated 21 inpatients with moderate TBI an average of 3.8 months post-injury randomly assigning them to either 10 sessions of neurofeedback training ($N=12$) or 10 computerized attention training sessions ($N=9$). Focusing primarily on attention measures and beta frequency (13–20 Hz) EEG power, he found that both groups demonstrated improvements in attention measures, but only the neurofeedback group showed improvement on a sustained attention task and in time spent producing beta.

Schoenberger et al. (2001) randomly assigned 12 subjects who had suffered mild to moderately severe closed head injuries at least 1 year previously to either a wait-list control group or 25 sessions of neurofeedback utilizing the Flexyx Neurotherapy System. The treatment group self-reported improvements in mood and fatigue and demonstrated improvements in working memory. Improvements in social and occupational function were also reported by a majority of the treatment group including reductions in need for medication and increased ability to return to work.

Tinius and Tinius (2000) did not use random assignment but compared 16 outpatients diagnosed with mild TBI with 15 healthy controls and demonstrated improvements on measures of attention, response control, executive function, and self-reported symptom severity after 20 sessions of neurofeedback training combined with computerized cognitive retraining exercises. The neurofeedback training involved single site power training along the sensorimotor strip. A weakness of this study is that the effects of neurofeedback were not differentiated from the possible effects of the cognitive retraining exercises.

Laibow et al. (2001) treated 27 brain injured subjects with neurofeedback training at CZ rewarding alpha and midrange beta while inhibiting theta and high beta. Subjects were classified according to symptom type, number, and severity. Improvements varied according to these symptom variables as did the number of sessions ranging from 23 to 132. They reported 59–87% rehabilitation, based on the improvement ratings of subject, physician, and caregiver.

In a departure from the usual method of training EEG power to remediate symptoms, Walker et al. (2002) employed qEEG-guided coherence training in the treatment of 26 outpatients with persistent post-traumatic symptoms 3–70 months after mild TBI. Training one coherence measure at a time, they reported that in an average of 19 sessions 88% of the patients reported greater than 50% improvement in self-reported symptoms. In addition, all patients employed prior to their injury were able to return to work. They added that these results were an improvement over their unpublished data analysis showing that beta training at CZ required an average of 38 sessions to achieve equivalent gains.

Thornton and Carmody (2013) trained 15 TBI patients to modify both power and connectivity at multiple sites based on functional neural network models and demonstrated improvements in both auditory and visual memory as well as qEEG power and connectivity measures. One of their findings revealed a 0.64 correlation between the amount of improvement in auditory memory and the number of sessions administered.

Foster and Veazey-Morris (2013) utilized LZN employing an SCL–FNM method in a case series of eight veterans with both TBI and PTSD who were an average of 8.8 years post-injury. They simultaneously trained multiple power and connectivity (coherence and phase) measures in multiple Brodmann areas with real-time normative database comparisons. Selection criteria for the measures trained relied on a symptom checklist developed from the cross-validated functional neuroimaging literature (Thatcher, 2013). Subjects demonstrated improvements in both self-report of symptoms and normalization of qEEG measures. This neurofeedback method offers the most specificity and personalization of training to date. Additionally, this method offers the added safety of decreased likelihood of overtraining due to training toward a normative database in real time (live Z-score training) rather than training a specific measure with off-line normative database comparisons or no normative comparison.

Based on the data available, neurofeedback training is probably effective in the treatment of TBI. However, the heterogeneity of traumatic brain injuries obviates the need for individualized treatment, and the accumulating data indicate that the effectiveness of neurofeedback in the treatment of TBI varies according to appropriateness of the training for the symptoms being treated. With the cross-validation of qEEG with other functional neuroimaging techniques, specific symptoms are being correlated with specific neural network abnormalities with increasing accuracy. This ability to identify specific neural network abnormalities behind the identified symptoms and renormalize them through operant conditioning with live normative database comparisons (Z-score training), training multiple measures simultaneously, appears to be the next step in the evolution of neurofeedback training for TBI. It also appears evident that the utilization of EEG tomography through LORETA and the resulting increased specificity of training that this allows is a move toward the needed personalization of training for such a varied problem as TBI. Further research is needed to demonstrate the efficacy and specificity of this approach.

THE STUDY

This case series presents data from 11 subjects diagnosed with PTSD and mild TBI referred to Dr. Dale Foster at Memphis Integral Neurofeedback Institute (MINI) by Dr. Katherine Veazey-Morris, a Veteran's Administration polytrauma psychologist, for LZN. The first case presented includes data from his first session as an example of the normal procedure and is considered typical in terms of how a responsive trainee is affected neurophysiologically by the process. The remaining 10 cases are presented in random order and trained in the same manner.

Subjects

The participants in this 11 case series were involved in multimodal treatment provided by the Veteran's Administration. Seeking additional help in overcoming their PTSD and TBI symptoms, they were made aware of the neurofeedback option by Dr. Veazey-Morris and volunteered to participate in LZN at MINI. They made their own appointments and provided their own transportation. The average time since the initial trauma was 8 years, and nine of the subjects had suffered multiple mild traumatic brain injuries.

Materials and Procedures

Sessions occurred once per week, for 45 min, scheduled by the participant, paid for by the Veteran's Administration, and conducted by Dr. Foster at MINI. The hardware and software used in the training were the same for each session: a Deymed TruScan 32 EEG encoder and NeuroGuide 2.7 EEG acquisition, analysis, and neurofeedback software. The NeuroGuide software module used was NF2 for the LZN.

During the initial meeting, a brief clinical interview was conducted, a brief introduction to neurofeedback was provided, and eyes open and eyes closed baseline 19-channel EEG data were acquired. Participants were also introduced to the Goal Monitoring Log and asked to begin to make a list of positive outcomes that would prove to them that this process is working and bring their ideas to the next session. They were encouraged to remain skeptical about rating their own improvements in order to assist in the process of adjusting the training parameters for maximal benefit.

Between the first and second meeting, EEG data were artifacted using a standardized process: (1) The record was "eyeballed" in order to confirm a valid record was obtained. (2) The NeuroGuide automatic editing routine was run with identical settings for each record ("High" artifact sensitivity, 2.00 Z-score EEG selection, and time constraints set to the first 2 min of artifact-free data). (3) The results of the automatic editing were "eyeballed" again to confirm their face validity. After the data were artifacted, they were analyzed with NeuroGuide software using normative database comparisons, and a LORETA Symptom Checklist was constructed within NeuroGuide based on those normative database comparisons. The NeuroGuide LORETA Symptom Checklist construction compares the current source density (CSD) of the subjects' data with the normative data and calculates the Z-scores in each of the Brodmann areas in each of the EEG frequency bands for later hypothesis testing utilizing the SCL–FNM process. This process involves the identification of the clinical symptoms of the subject, hypothesizing the neural network disturbances probably underlying the symptoms, and testing those hypotheses by matching the clinical symptoms with the abnormally functioning Brodmann areas that are likely to explain the symptoms, based on the available neuroimaging research. This process is currently the most rational procedure for identifying neurofeedback training targets.

The second meeting involved a brief review of the surface and LORETA neuroimages, construction of a Goal Monitoring Log, brief discussion of supportive "Positive Behaviors" listed on their Goal Monitoring Log known to promote neuroplasticity and neurogenesis, a brief introduction to Heart Rate Variability biofeedback, and the first LZN session.

At the beginning of the first LZN session, Dr. Foster and the trainee cooperatively selected the target symptoms from the Department of Defense/Veteran's Administration Symptom Checklist and identified the neural networks that would be targeted with the training. This process was repeated as needed in subsequent sessions based on the progress of symptom resolution. Subsequent LZN sessions began with a review of the Goal Monitoring Log and Positive Behavior list with the trainee providing a self-rating of each goal and behavior. The trainee then engaged in Heart Rate Variability biofeedback (emWave by HeartMath™) utilizing an infrared ear sensor while an ElectroCap™ was applied.

Each LZN session consisted of a number of rounds of feedback with brief pauses between rounds. The participant and clinician sat side by side, with the participant in a comfortable recliner in an upright position with feet either on the floor or on a footrest. Two computer monitors were used, one directly in front of the trainee and the other in front of the clinician and out of the trainee's view. The clinician monitored the ongoing raw EEG, impedance, percent reward, immediate Z-scores, and other data, while the participant observed the audio and video biofeedback. The participant was allowed to choose the graphic and sound from a selection based on his/her preferences. The trainee was shown his/her live raw EEG signal stream and educated about reducing artifact as needed.

Before each round, the participant's Z-score threshold was adjusted by the clinician to keep the percent reward between 30% and 60%. Participants were coached as needed to help them eliminate ineffective strategies and experience the natural success of effective biofeedback. Verbal instructions, encouragement, and education were provided as needed. Homework assignments were also provided based on the needs of the trainee. All trainees were encouraged to practice rehearsing the "state" they entered, when they were experiencing the most success with the biofeedback.

Regions for data analysis were selected based on the following procedure: the baseline EEG data were analyzed with NeuroGuide's LORETA Z-score normative database comparison, and the voxel with the most significant Z-score, which was also included in the symptom checklist as a region of training (ROT), was chosen for statistical analysis to determine neurophysiological outcome.

Rounding

Each LZN session consisted of a series of rounds of LZN based on the most recent symptom checklist. After each round of LZN, the session was paused, and the trainee was asked whether he thought the Z-score comparison graph will show that the round was better, the same, or worse than the previous round. Trainees were encouraged to not think about it too much but to just go with their first impression or gut feeling. As soon as they guessed, the comparison graph was shown to them in a quick, matter of fact, nonjudgmental way. The Z-score threshold was then adjusted by the clinician for the next round to maintain a percent reward between 30 and 60%, and the next round was begun. Rounds ranged from 2 to 5 min, and as many rounds as possible were made within the 45-min session. Trainees were allowed to terminate the session at will and were encouraged to generate interest in the process even in the face of fatigue.

Results of a Single Session

These are the results of the first LZN session of subject 11. They are considered typical of a good responder and representative of the neurophysiological effects of a single session of LZN. The LORETA neuroimages below compare the pre- and post-training eyes closed resting EEGs of the first session of subject 11. This typical first session consisted of eight 2-min rounds interspersed with brief pauses.

Analysis

The target voxel in the neuroimages shown in Figure 4.1 was chosen for this analysis, because it was the most deviant in terms of Z-score, and it was included in this subject's symptom checklist match. It is included in the hypothesized list of neural networks, because there is strong support for the role of the cingulate cortex in PTSD symptoms,

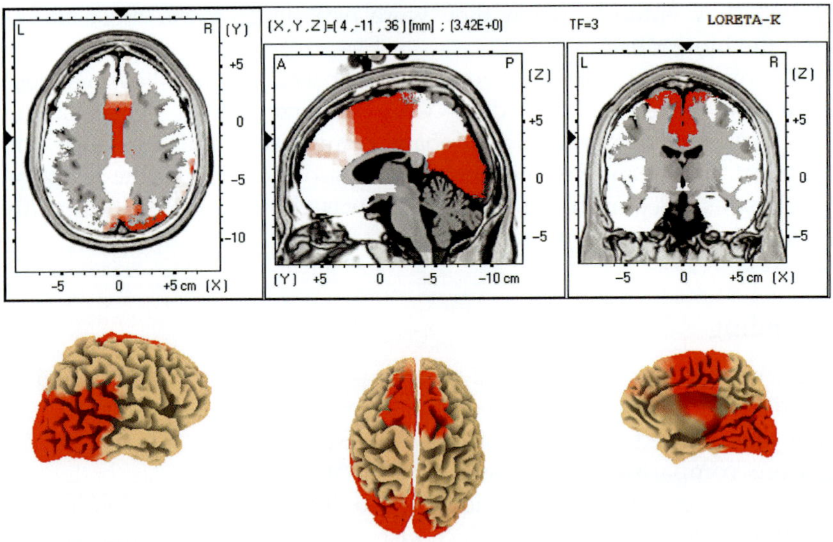

FIGURE 4.1 This is the pre-training LORETA Z-score neuroimage of the maximum Z-score in Brodmann area 24, in the cingulate gyrus. The target frequency is 3 Hz, the maximum Z = 3.42, and conditions were eyes closed, relaxed.

and it is included in this specific subject's symptom checklist, because it was found to deviate from norms in its function. Although this target voxel was chosen for analysis, it is understood that it functions in concert with multiple neural networks as a part of a specific network node. This most significant Z-score method used throughout this study is adopted as a reasonable approach to reducing the large amount of data available. Visual examination of the LORETA neuroimages in Figures 4.1 and 4.2 suggests that this single session of LZN produced a large effect on this subject's EEG. A paired *t*-test comparing the pre- and post-Z-scores of this voxel at this frequency produces $p < 0.0001$ (degrees of freedom = 37, one-tailed *t*-test). Using Cohen's d with the means and standard deviations of current density for this voxel at the same targeted frequency, the effect size of this single session for this individual on this voxel of his cingulate cortex is 1.042, a large effect size. Cohen categorized effect sizes as "small, $d = 0.2$," "medium, $d = 0.5$," and "large, $d = 0.8$."

Rounding Results

The LZN session that occurred between the two eyes closed relaxed EEGs analyzed above consisted of eight 2-min rounds interspersed with

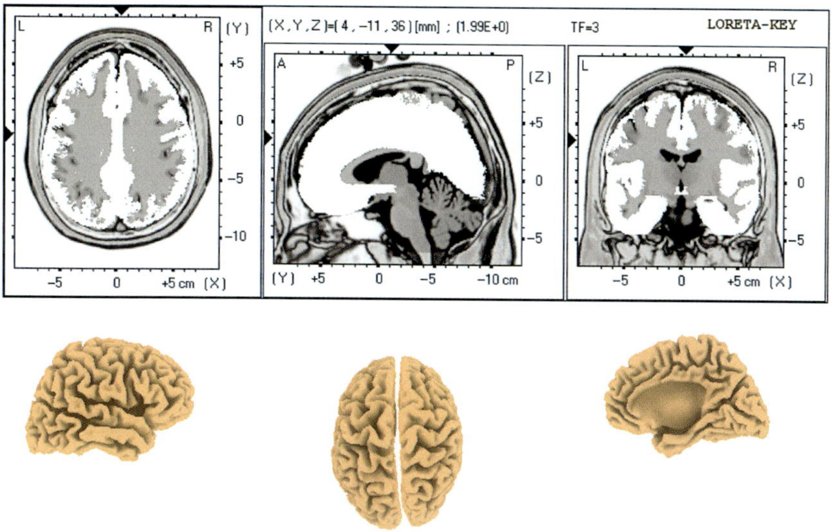

FIGURE 4.2 This is the post-training LORETA Z-score neuroimage under identical conditions and settings as the image in Figure 4.1, after a single session of LZN involving eight 2-min rounds.

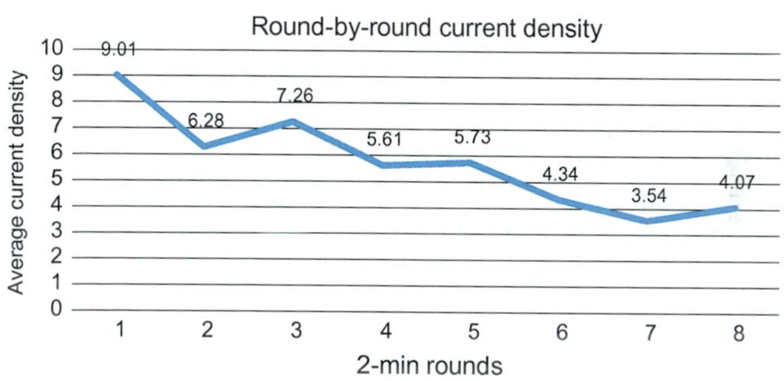

FIGURE 4.3 Progressive normalization of current density in BA 24, in the cingulate cortex.

brief pauses. Using the same location and frequency as the above analysis, the artifacted data from each of these 2-min rounds were analyzed. The average raw LORETA current density is plotted on the graph shown in Figure 4.3. The subject evidently progressively modified the neural activity in his cingulate cortex as the rounds progressed, normalizing the current density through the LZN process.

TABLE 4.1 Comparisons of Round 1 with Each Successive Round Illustrate Increasingly Significant Modification of Current Density and Increasingly Large Effects of the LZN Training

Paired *t*-test	*t* value	*p* value	Cohen's *d*
Round 1 vs. Round 2	2.38	0.0118	0.543
Round 1 vs. Round 3	1.49	0.073	0.403
Round 1 vs. Round 4	4.85	0.000017	1.186
Round 1 vs. Round 5	3.77	0.000345	0.961
Round 1 vs. Round 6	4.82	0.000016	1.224
Round 1 vs. Round 7	4.95	0.000012	1.606
Round 1 vs. Round 8	4.95	0.000014	1.303

Statistical analysis including paired *t*-tests and effect size estimations with Cohen's *d* indicate that each subsequent round was significantly better than Round 1 with effect sizes becoming increasingly large as the rounds progressed. Table 4.1 illustrates this progression.

Discussion

It is evident that subject 11 demonstrated learning within this single LZN training session. Along with the neurophysiological changes, one would expect that, if the SCL–FNM method works, there would be an accompanying improvement in symptoms. This, then, becomes the next hypothesis to test—that normalizing the deviant neuroelectric activity will be accompanied by a reduction in the subject's symptoms.

TEN CASE STUDIES

Method

The following cases are the first 10 subjects who voluntarily requested LZN from Dr. Foster after being referred by Dr. Veazey-Morris. Presented in random order, each subject was trained with the above procedures, and analysis was based on the most significant Z-score method described above.

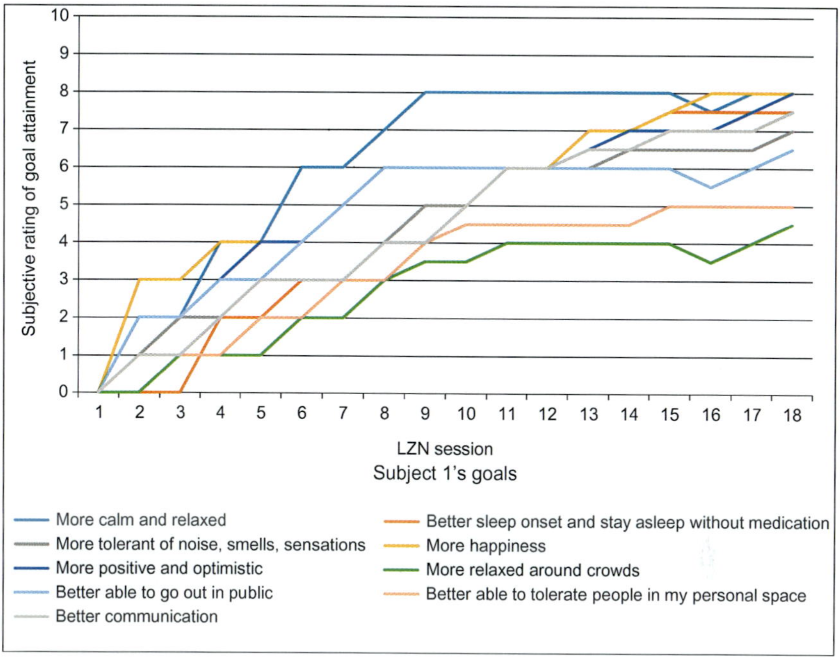

CHART 4.1 Subject 1: Subjective report of goal attainment by LZN session.

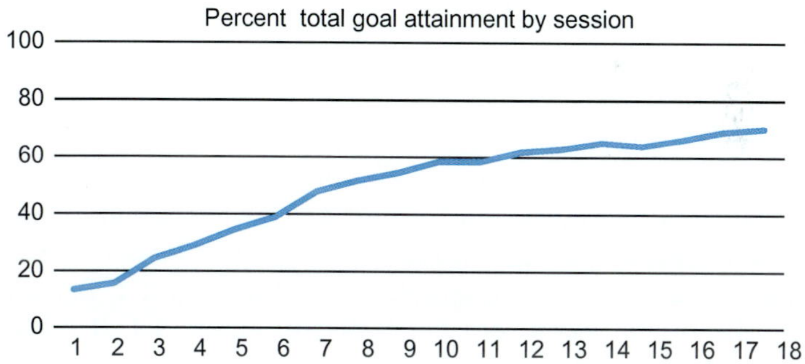

CHART 4.2 Subject 1: Total progress across sessions.

Subject 1

Using the procedures described above, Subject 1 constructed a Goal Monitoring Log, which included the items on the list in the chart below. As can be seen in Charts 4.1 and 4.2, consistent and significant progress was made in terms of goal attainment.

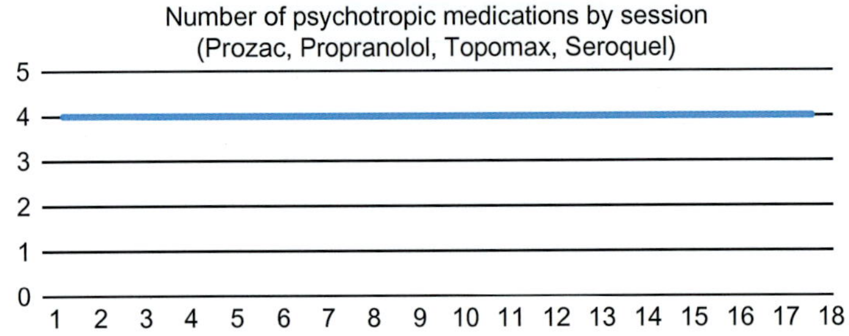

CHART 4.3 Subject 1: Psychotropic medication across sessions.

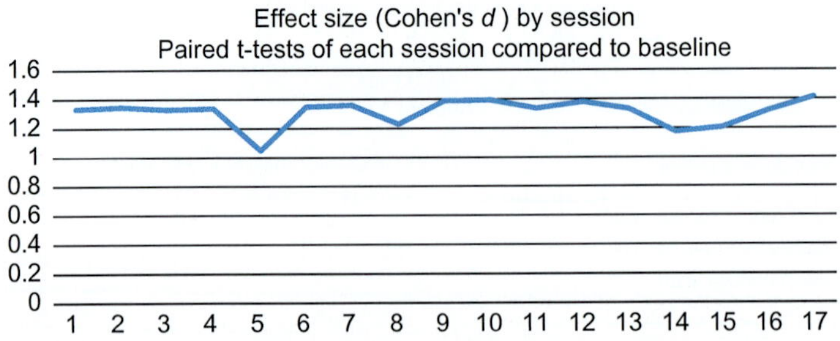

CHART 4.4 Subject 1: Effect size of each session compared to baseline.

Psychotropic medication was monitored across sessions in all subjects. Chart 4.3 indicates Subject 1 did not change his medications during LZN training.

Results

Paired *t*-tests were conducted comparing sessions 2–17 with the eyes open baseline data from session 1. Chart 4.4 illustrates that each of these LZN sessions resulted in significant differences and large effect sizes.

Changes in the CSD in the targeted ROT for Subject 1, BA 46, in the right middle frontal gyrus, are illustrated in Figure 4.4. It is clear that normalization occurred.

Paired *t*-test comparing the pre- and post-CSD of this ROT resulted in $p < 0.001$, and a large effect size as indicated by Cohen's $d = 1.414$.

Subject 2

Subject 2's goal attainment by session, percent total goal attainment, and psychotropic medications by session are illustrated in Charts 4.5–4.7.

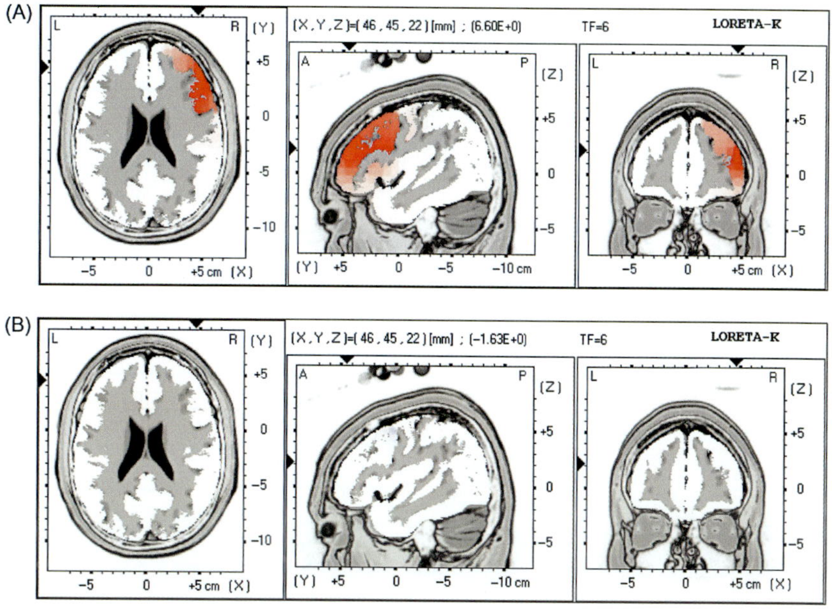

FIGURE 4.4 Subject 1: LORETA *Z* neuroimages demonstrating normalization in BA 46; (A) Pre: BA 46, right middle frontal gyrus: $(X, Y, Z) = (46, 45, 22)$; (B) Post: BA 46, right middle frontal gyrus: $(X, Y, Z) = (46, 45, 22)$.

Results

Changes in the CSD in the targeted ROT for Subject 2, BA 10, in the left middle frontal gyrus, are illustrated in Figure 4.5.

Paired *t*-test comparing the pre- and post-CSD of this ROT resulted in $p < 0.001$, and a large effect size as indicated by Cohen's $d = 4.625$.

Subject 3

Subject 3's goal attainment by session, percent total goal attainment, and psychotropic medications by session are illustrated in Charts 4.8–4.10.

Results

Changes in the CSD in the targeted ROT for Subject 3, BA 11, in the right middle frontal gyrus, are illustrated in Figure 4.6.

Paired *t*-test comparing the pre- and post-CSD of this ROT resulted in $p < 0.001$, and a large effect size as indicated by Cohen's $d = 1.272$.

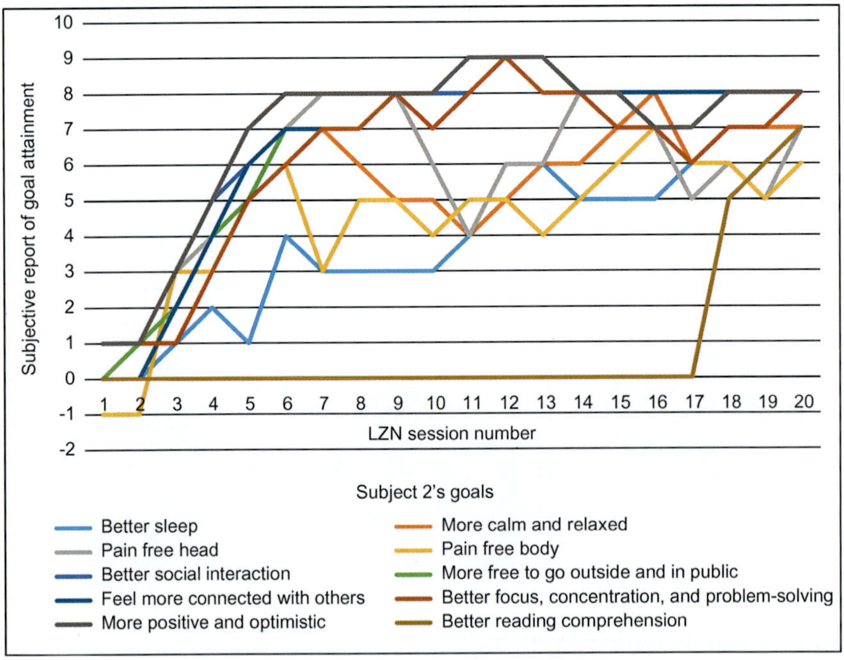

CHART 4.5 Subject 2: Subjective report of goal attainment by LZN session.

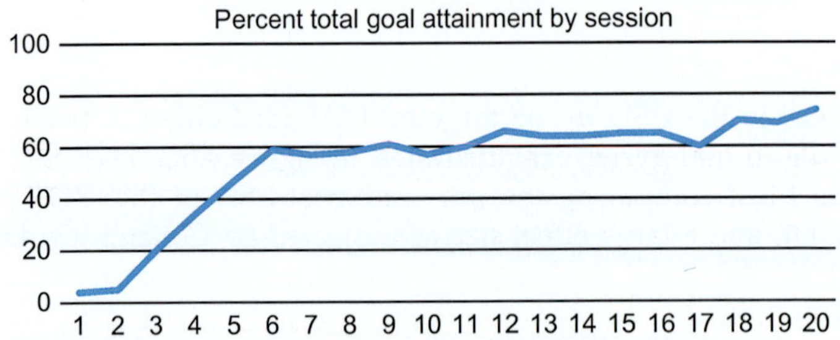

CHART 4.6 Subject 2: Percent total goal attainment by session.

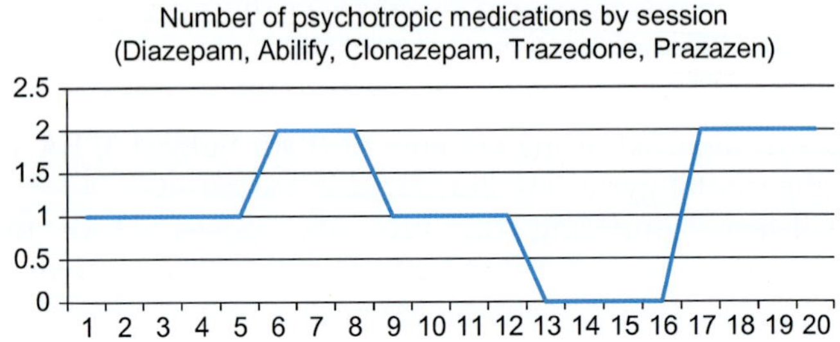

CHART 4.7 Subject 2: Psychotropic medications by session.

(A)
(B)

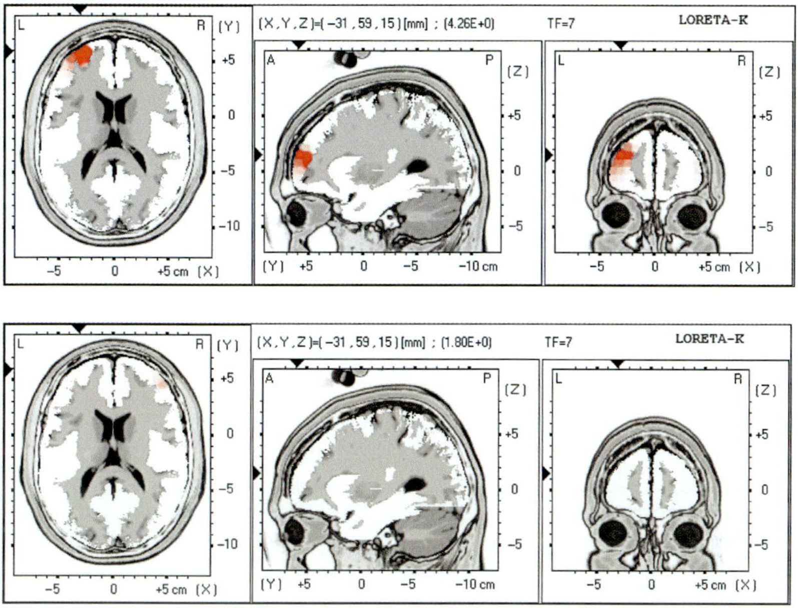

FIGURE 4.5 Subject 2: LORETA Z neuroimages demonstrating normalization in BA 10; (A) Pre: LORETA Z neuroimage: BA 10, $(X, Y, Z) = (-31, 59, 15)$, left middle frontal gyrus; (B) Post: LORETA Z neuroimage: BA 10, $(X, Y, Z) = (-31, 59, 15)$, left middle frontal gyrus.

Subject 4

Subject 4's goal attainment by session, percent total goal attainment, and psychotropic medications by session are illustrated in Charts 4.11–4.13. Note the correlation between memory improvement on his goal chart and the elimination of Zolpidem, a sleep medication found to cause cognitive impairment.

Results

Changes in the CSD in the targeted ROT for Subject 4, BA 9, in the right inferior frontal gyrus, are illustrated in Figure 4.7.

Paired *t*-test comparing the pre- and post-CSD of this ROT resulted in $p < 0.001$, and a large effect size as indicated by Cohen's $d = 1.42$.

Subject 5

Subject 5's goal attainment by session, percent total goal attainment, and psychotropic medications by session are illustrated in Charts 4.14–4.16.

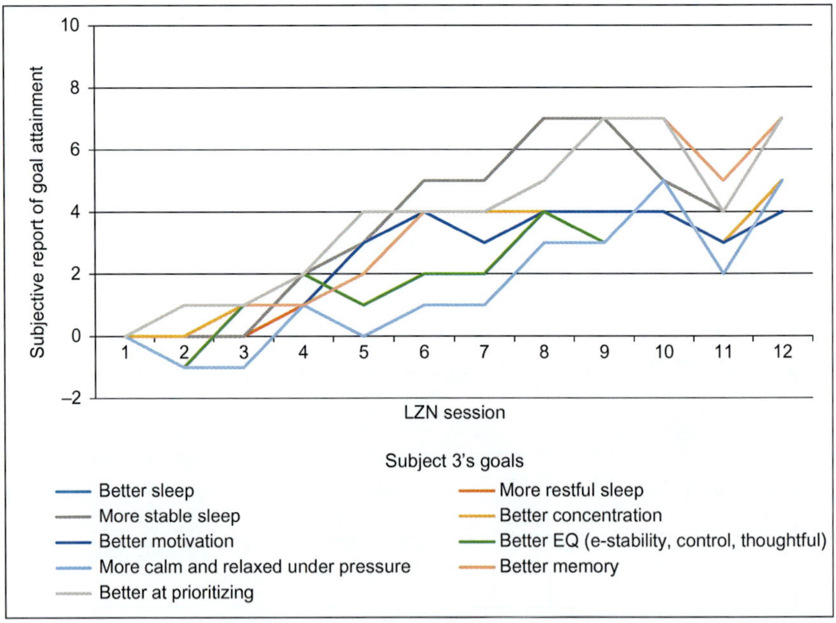

CHART 4.8 Subject 3: Subjective report of goal attainment by LZN session.

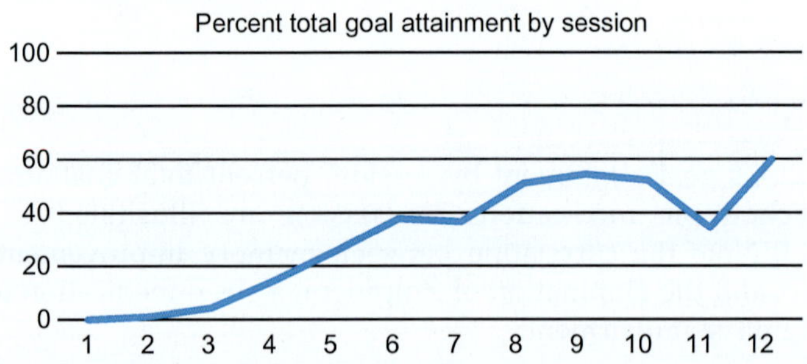

CHART 4.9 Subject 3.

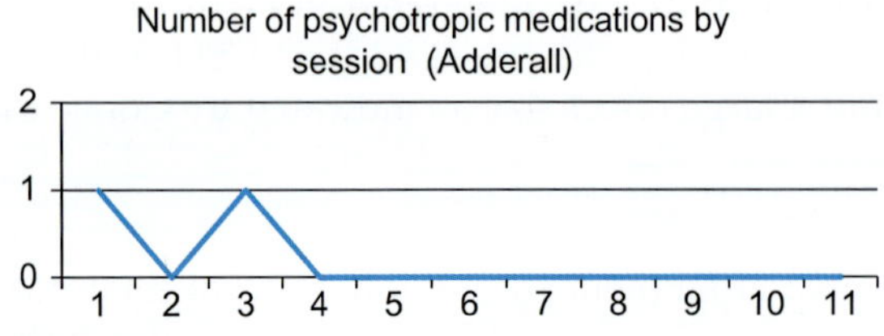

CHART 4.10 Subject 3.

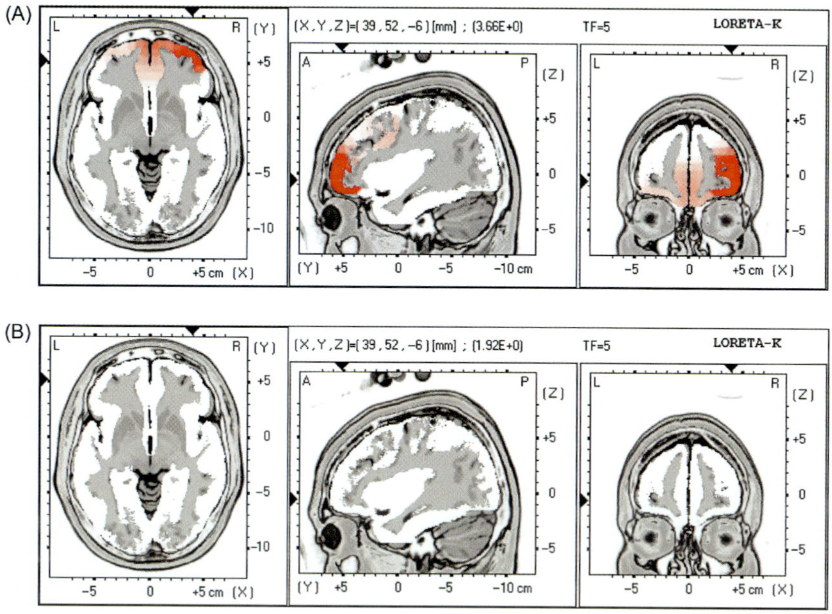

FIGURE 4.6 Subject 3: LORETA Z neuroimages demonstrating normalization in BA 11; (A) Pre: LORETA Z neuroimage: BA 11, $(X, Y, Z) = (39, 52, -6)$, right middle frontal gyrus; (B) Post: LORETA Z neuroimage: BA 11, $(X, Y, Z) = (39, 52, -6)$, right middle frontal gyrus.

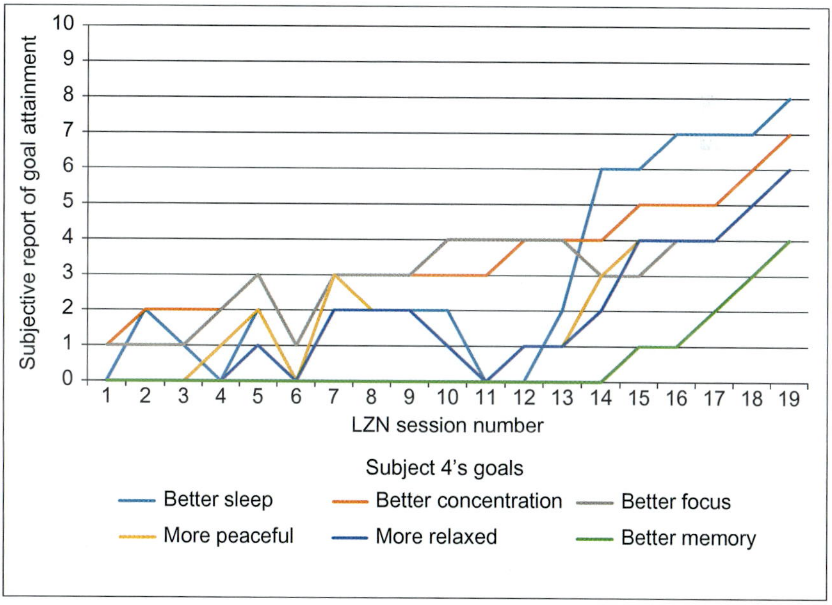

CHART 4.11 Subject 4: Subjective report of goal attainment by LZN session.

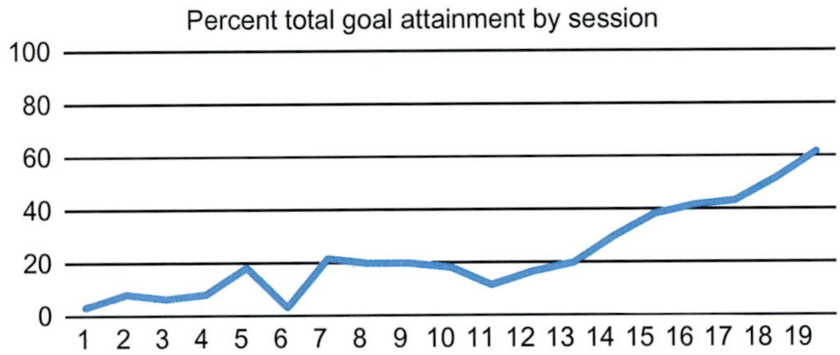

CHART 4.12 Subject 4.

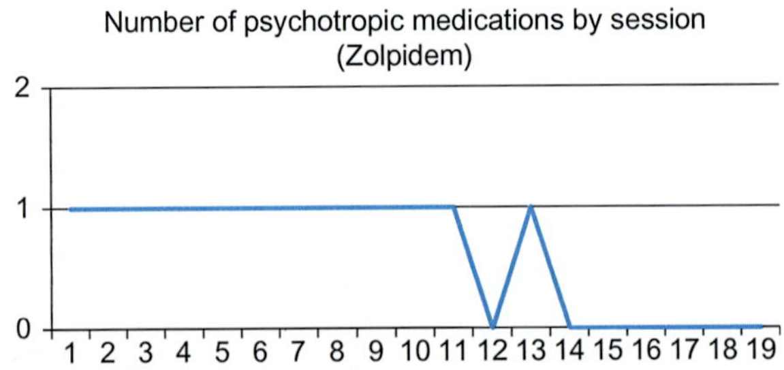

CHART 4.13 Subject 4.

Results

Changes in the CSD in the targeted ROT for Subject 5, BA 9, in the right inferior frontal gyrus, are illustrated in Figure 4.8.

Paired *t*-test comparing the pre- and post-CSD of this ROT resulted in $p < 0.001$, and a medium effect size as indicated by Cohen's $d = 0.474$.

Subject 6

Subject 6's goal attainment by session and percent total goal attainment are illustrated in Charts 4.17 and 4.18. Note that Subject 6 was not taking psychotropic medication.

Results

Changes in the CSD in the targeted ROT for Subject 6, BA 6, in the left middle frontal gyrus, are illustrated in Figure 4.9.

Paired *t*-test comparing the pre- and post-CSD of this ROT resulted in $p < 0.001$, and a large effect size as indicated by Cohen's $d = 2.291$.

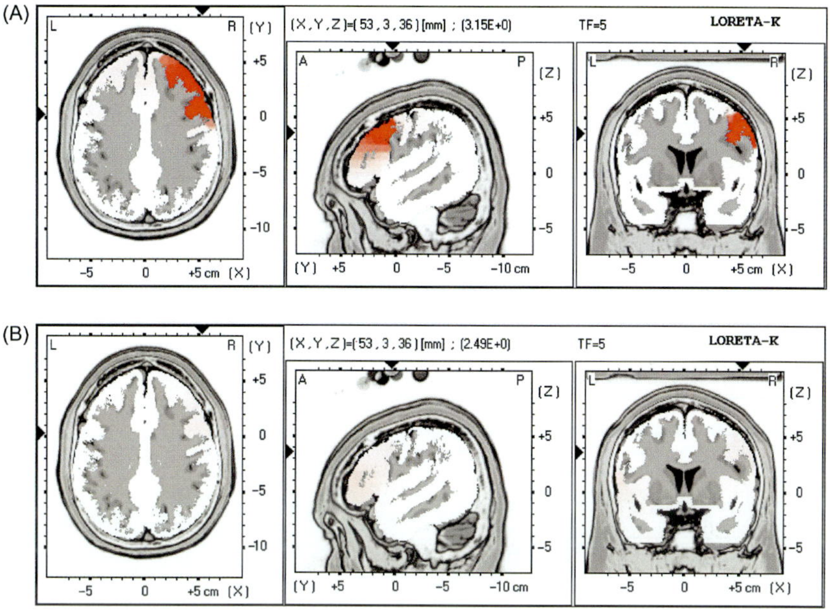

FIGURE 4.7 Subject 4: LORETA Z neuroimages demonstrating normalization in BA 9; (A) Pre: LORETA Z neuroimage: BA 9, (X, Y, Z) = (53, 3, 36), right inferior frontal gyrus; (B) Post: LORETA Z neuroimage: BA 9, (X, Y, Z) = (53, 3, 36), right inferior frontal gyrus.

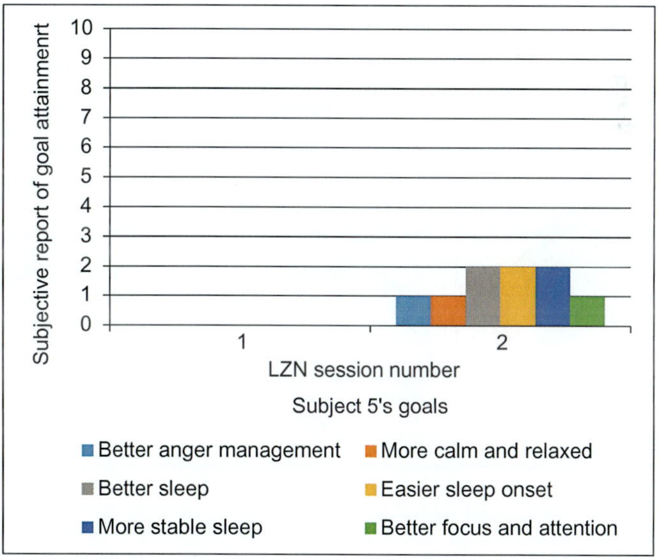

CHART 4.14 Subject 5: Subjective report of goal attainment by LZN session.

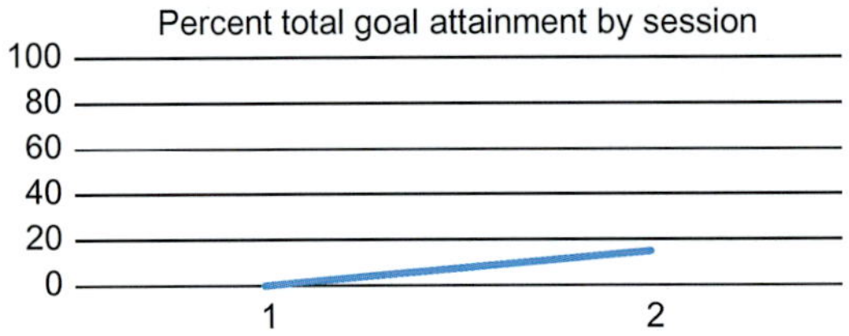

CHART 4.15 Subject 5.

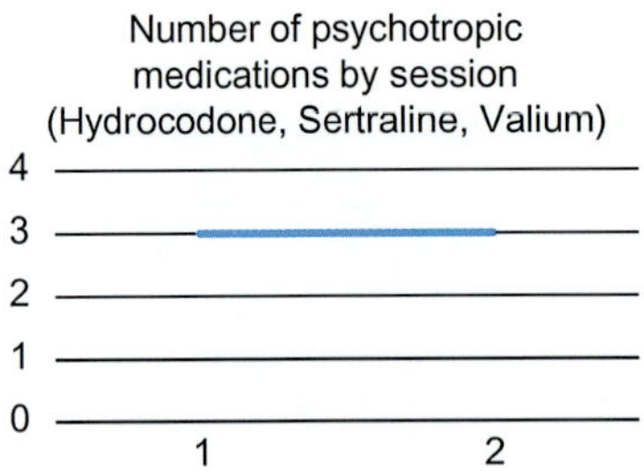

CHART 4.16 Subject 5.

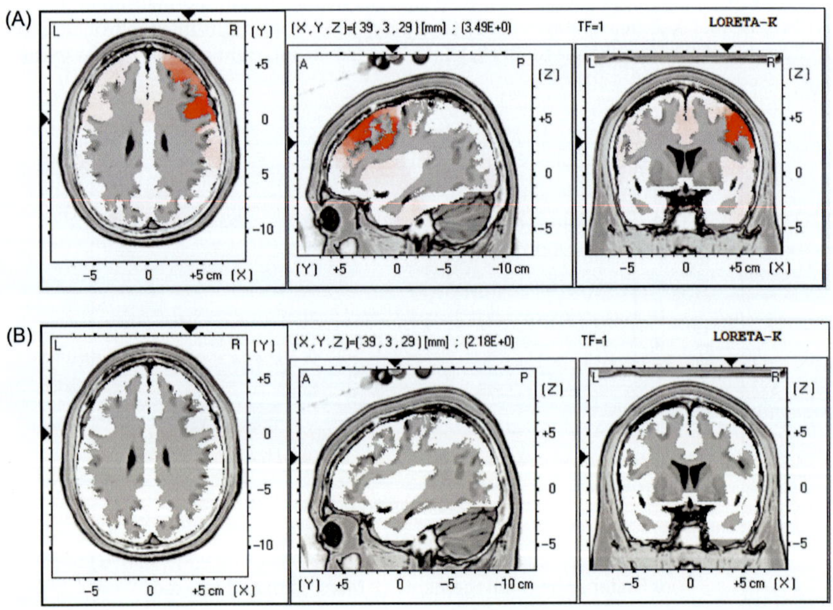

FIGURE 4.8 Subject 5: LORETA Z neuroimages demonstrating normalization in BA 9; (A) Pre: LORETA Z neuroimage: BA 9, (X, Y, Z) = (39, 3, 29), right inferior frontal gyrus; (B) Post: LORETA Z neuroimage: BA 9, (X, Y, Z) = (39, 3, 29), right inferior frontal gyrus.

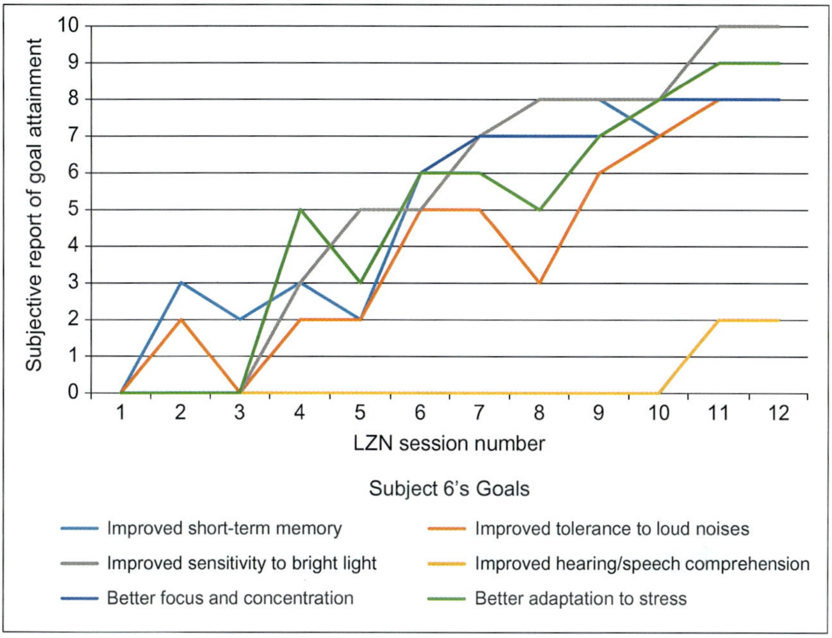

CHART 4.17 Subject 6: Subjective report of goal attainment by LZN session.

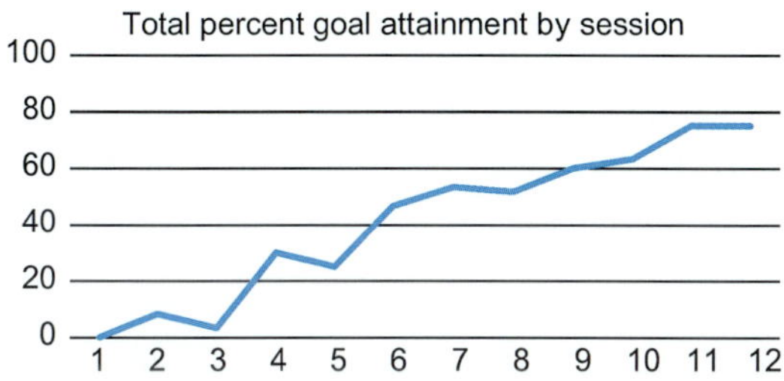

CHART 4.18 Subject 6.

Subject 7

Subject 7's goal attainment by session and percent total goal attainment by session are illustrated in Charts 4.19 and 4.20. Subject 7 was not taking psychotropic medication.

Results

Changes in the CSD in the targeted ROT for Subject 7, BA 9, in the right middle frontal gyrus, are illustrated in Figure 4.10.

Paired t-test comparing the pre- and post-CSD of this ROT resulted in $p < 0.001$, and a large effect size as indicated by Cohen's $d = 0.79$.

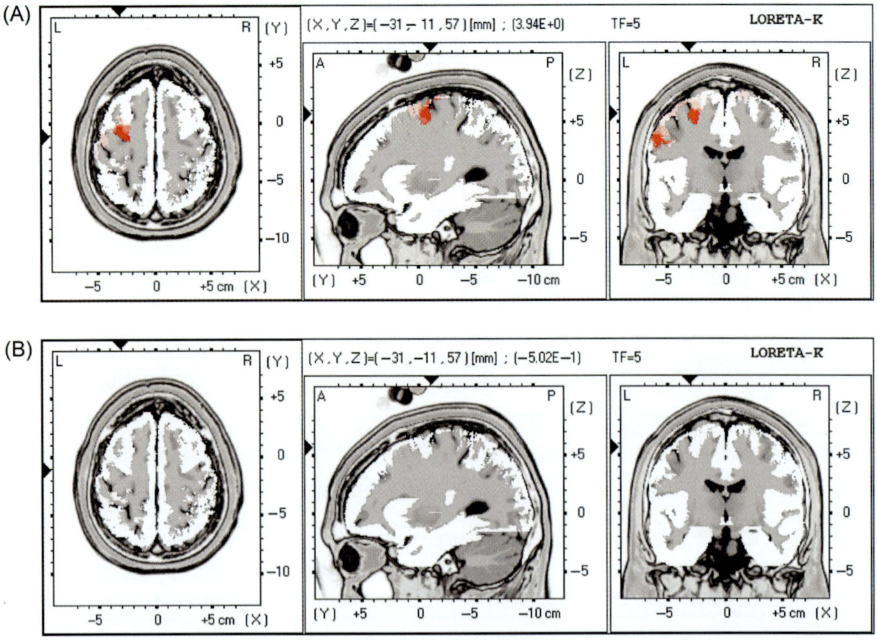

FIGURE 4.9 Subject 6: LORETA Z neuroimages demonstrating normalization in BA 6; (A) Pre: LORETA Z neuroimage: BA 6, $(X, Y, Z) = (-31, -11, 57)$, left middle frontal gyrus; (B) Post: LORETA Z neuroimage: BA 6, $(X, Y, Z) = (-31, -11, 57)$, left middle frontal gyrus.

Subject 8

Subject 8's goal attainment by session, percent total goal attainment, and psychotropic medications by session are illustrated in Charts 4.21–4.23.

Results

Changes in the CSD in the targeted ROT for Subject 8, BA 18, in the lingual gyrus, are illustrated in Figure 4.11.

Paired t-test comparing the pre- and post-CSD of this ROT resulted in $p < 0.001$, and a large effect size as indicated by Cohen's $d = 1.35$.

Subject 9

Subject 9's goal attainment by session, percent total goal attainment, and psychotropic medications by session are illustrated in Charts 4.24–4.26.

Results

Changes in the CSD in the targeted ROT for Subject 9, BA 11, in the left superior frontal gyrus, are illustrated in Figure 4.12.

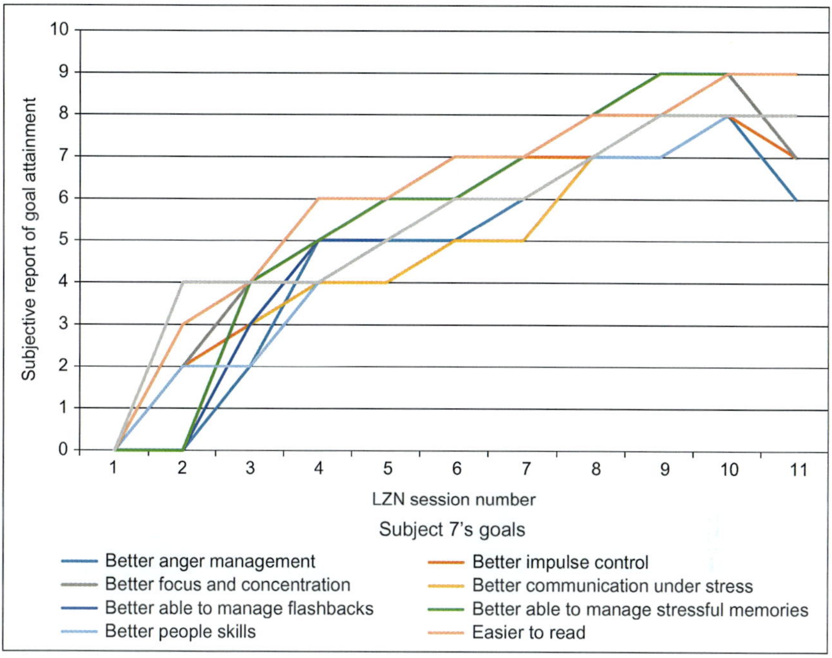

CHART 4.19 Subject 7: Subjective report of goal attainment by LZN session.

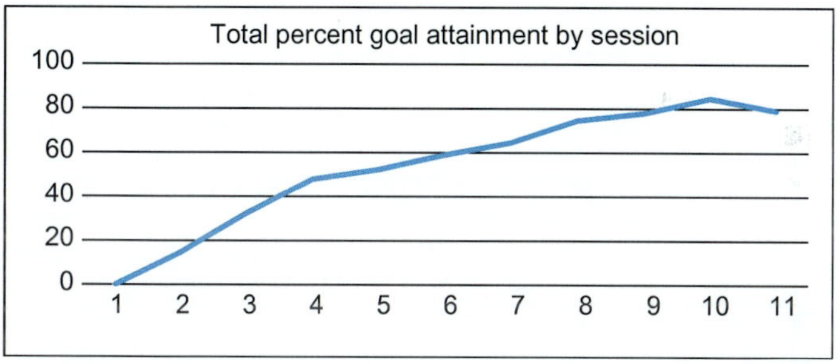

CHART 4.20 Subject 7.

Paired t-test comparing the pre- and post-CSD of this ROT resulted in $p < 0.01$, and a medium effect size as indicated by Cohen's $d = 0.458$.

Subject 10

Subject 10's goal attainment by session, percent total goal attainment, and psychotropic medications by session are illustrated in Charts 4.27–4.29.

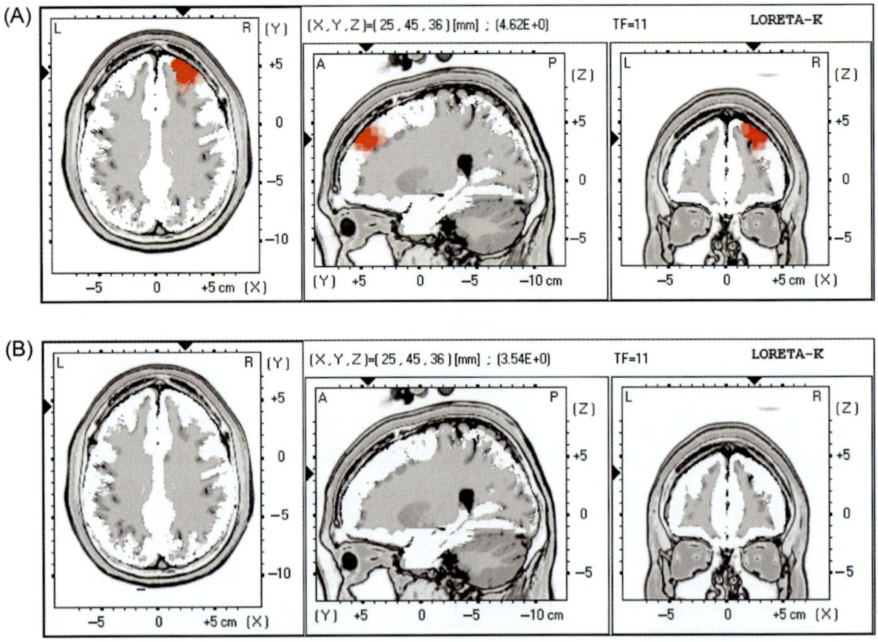

FIGURE 4.10 Subject 7: LORETA Z neuroimages demonstrating normalization in BA 9; (A) Pre: LORETA Z neuroimage: BA 9, (X, Y, Z) = (26, 45, 36), right middle frontal gyrus; (B) Post: LORETA Z neuroimage: BA 9, (X, Y, Z) = (26, 45, 36), right middle frontal gyrus.

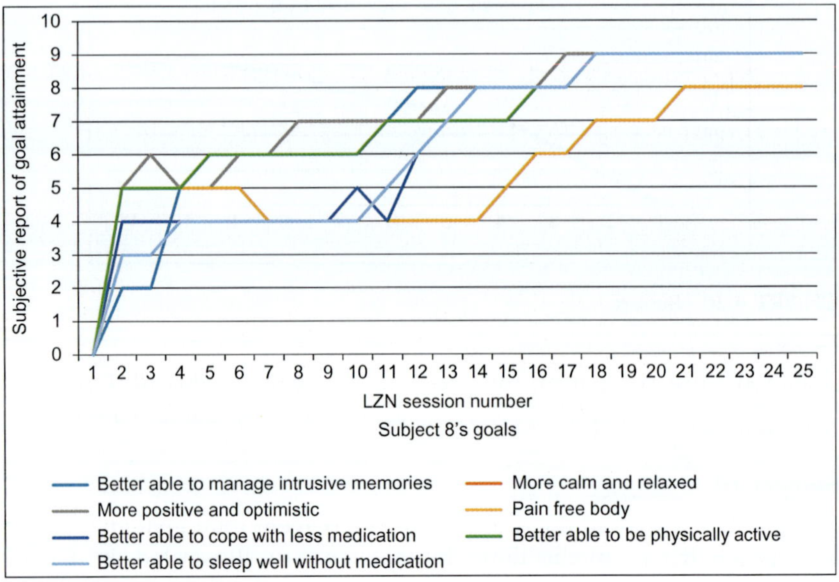

CHART 4.21 Subject 8: Subjective report of goal attainment by LZN session.

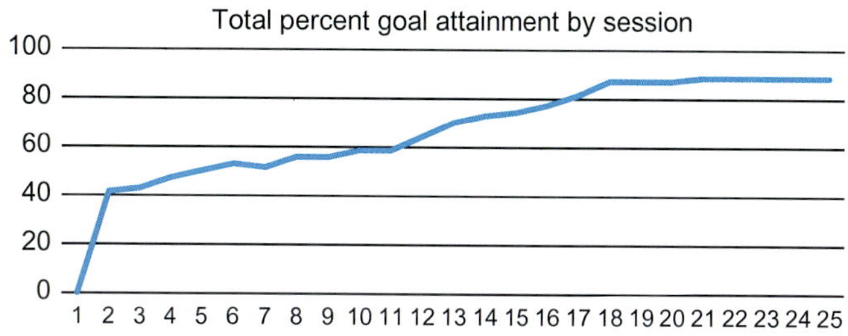

CHART 4.22 Subject 8.

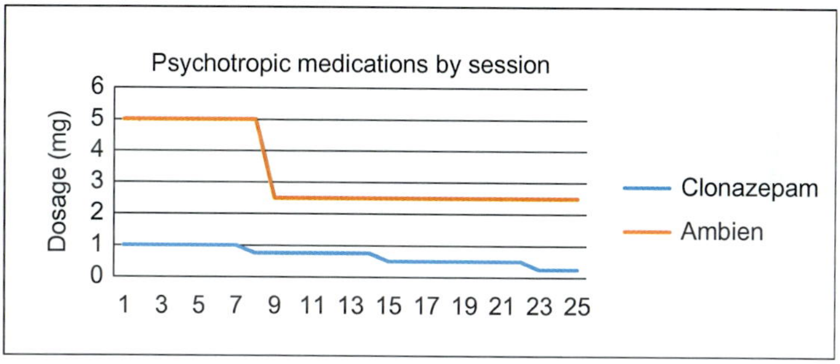

CHART 4.23 Subject 8.

Results

Changes in the CSD in the targeted ROT for Subject 10, BA 6, in the left superior frontal gyrus, are illustrated in Figure 4.13.

A paired *t*-test comparing the pre- and post-CSD of this ROT resulted in $p < 0.001$, and a large effect size as indicated by Cohen's $d = 1.85$.

Observations and Discussion

The data are clear that LZN using this SCL–FNM method is effective in alleviating symptoms and specific in its effect on the regions of training selected by the most significant Z-score method used here. It is also evident, as illustrated by Chart 4.30, that this training tends to elicit large effects.

Visual perusal of the psychotropic medication charts by subject suggests an interaction between medications and goal attainment as well as a trend toward decreasing medication as training progressed. Chart 4.31 graphically illustrates the interaction between number of psychotropic medications and total percent goal attainment.

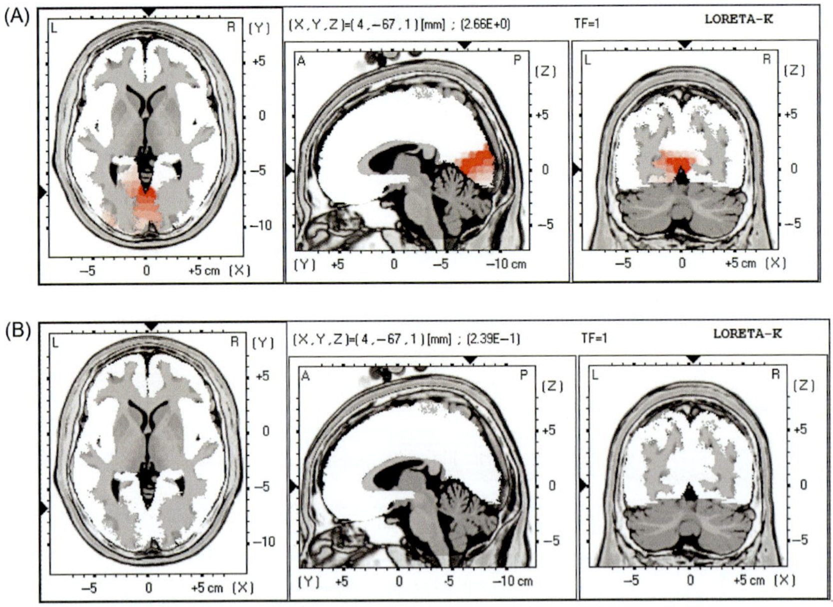

FIGURE 4.11 Subject 8: LORETA Z neuroimages demonstrating normalization in BA 18; (A) Pre: LORETA Z neuroimage: BA 18, $(X, Y, Z) = (4, -67, 1)$, lingual gyrus; (B) Post: LORETA Z neuroimage: BA 18, $(X, Y, Z) = (4, -67, 1)$, lingual gyrus.

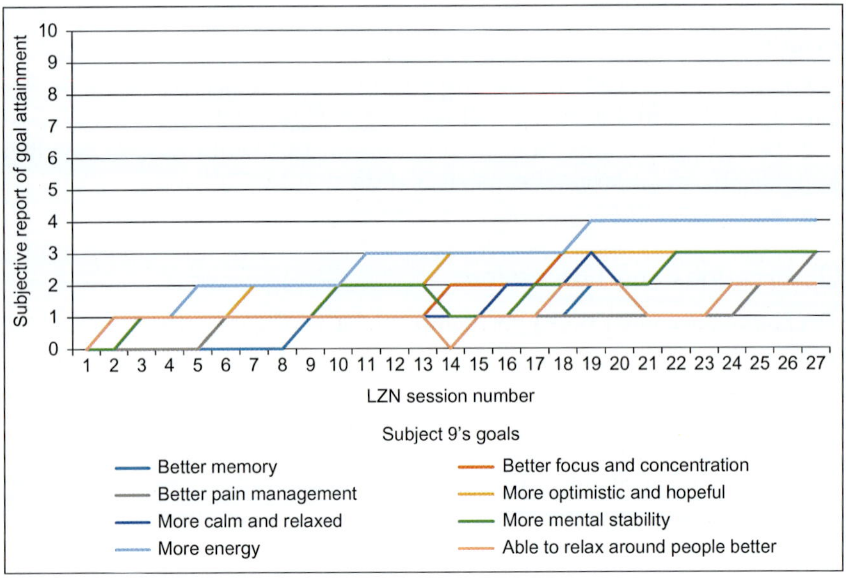

CHART 4.24 Subject 9: Subjective report of goal attainment by LZN session.

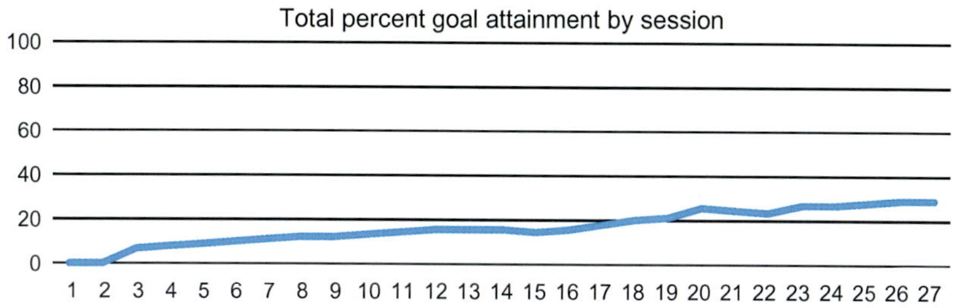

CHART 4.25 Subject 9.

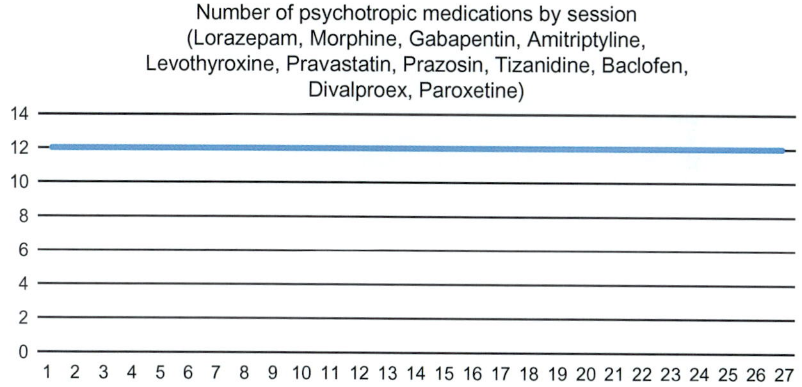

CHART 4.26 Subject 9.

An analysis of the correlation between psychotropic medications at the end of training and percent total goal attainment yields a Pearson $r = -55$, a large negative correlation that is significant at $p < 0.05$. Although severity of trauma probably correlates with number of psychotropic medications, many psychotropic medications tend to inhibit learning in general and operant conditioning during LZN. While all of the subjects in this study were interested in decreasing their reliance on or avoiding the need for psychotropic medications, 3 of the 10 were successful in eliminating medication, one decreased his reliance, and two were successful remaining medication free. It is also interesting to note that the two subjects who were medication free throughout their training demonstrated two of the three highest percent goal achievement per session scores. These observations illuminate the need for close collaboration between the trainee, the LZN trainer, and prescribing physicians to promote maximal benefit from the training.

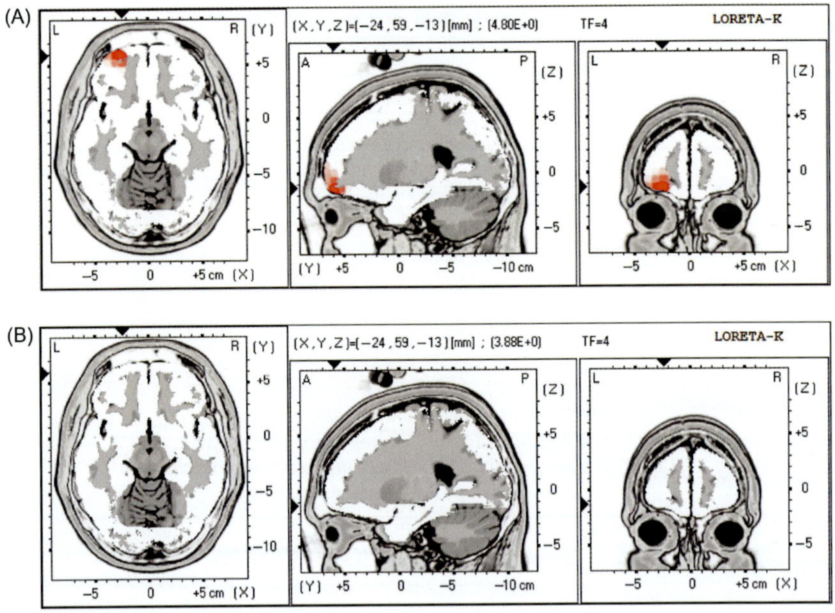

FIGURE 4.12 Subject 9: LORETA Z neuroimages demonstrating normalization in BA 11; (A) Pre: LORETA Z neuroimage: BA 11, (X, Y, Z) = (− 24, 59, −13), left superior frontal gyrus; (B) Post: LORETA Z neuroimage: BA 11, (X, Y, Z) = (− 24, 59, −13), left superior frontal gyrus.

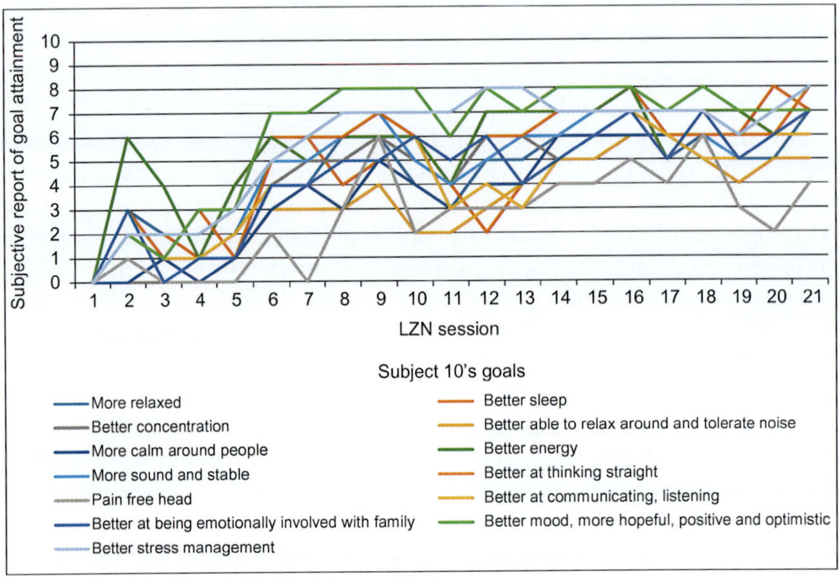

CHART 4.27 Subject 10: Subjective report of goal attainment by LZN session.

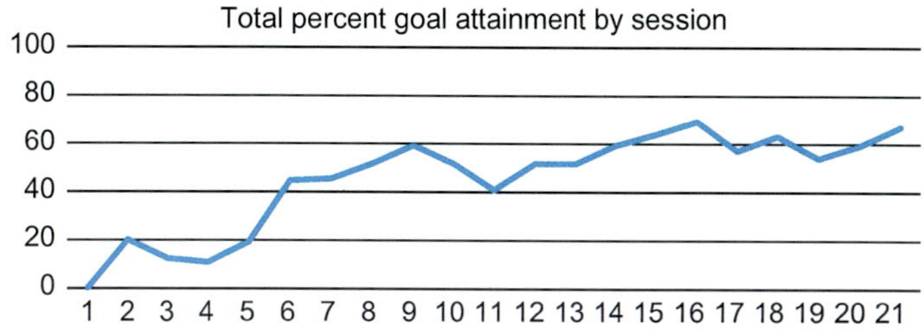

CHART 4.28 Subject 10.

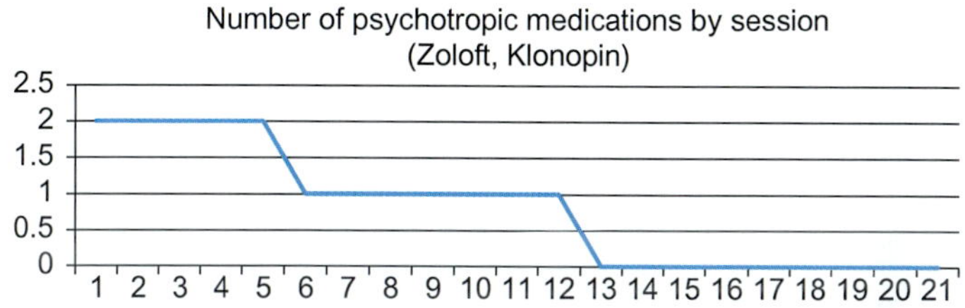

CHART 4.29 Subject 10.

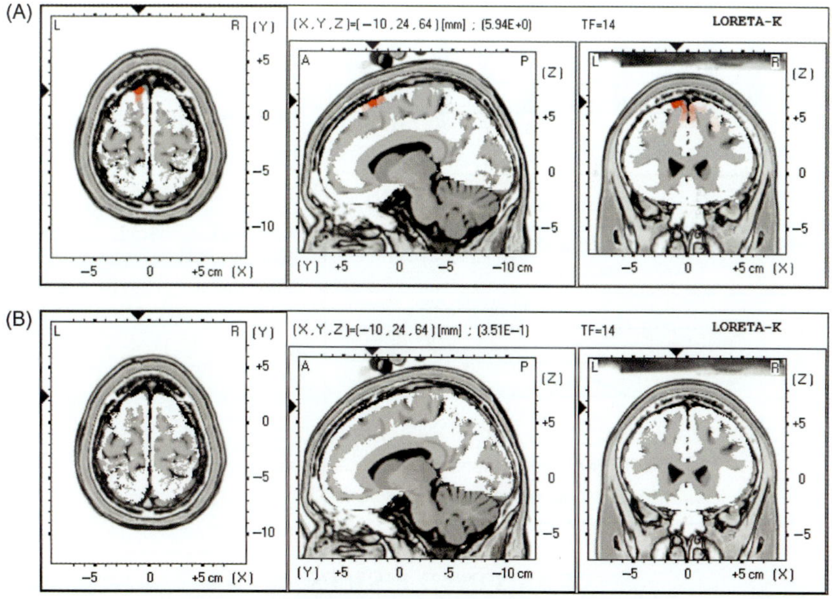

FIGURE 4.13 Subject 10: LORETA Z neuroimages demonstrating normalization in BA 6; (A) Pre: LORETA Z neuroimage: BA 6, $(X, Y, Z) = (-10, 24, 64)$, left superior frontal gyrus; (B) Post: LORETA Z neuroimage: BA 6, $(X, Y, Z) = (-10, 24, 64)$, left superior frontal gyrus.

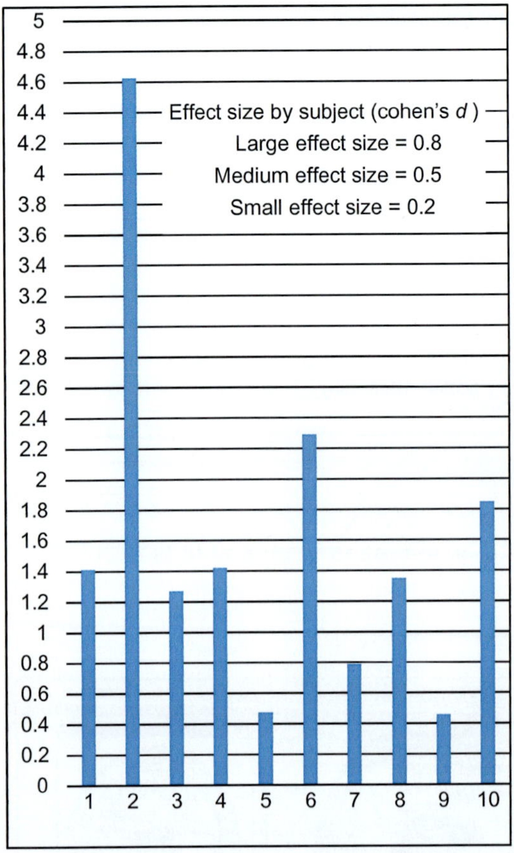

CHART 4.30 Effect size by subject.

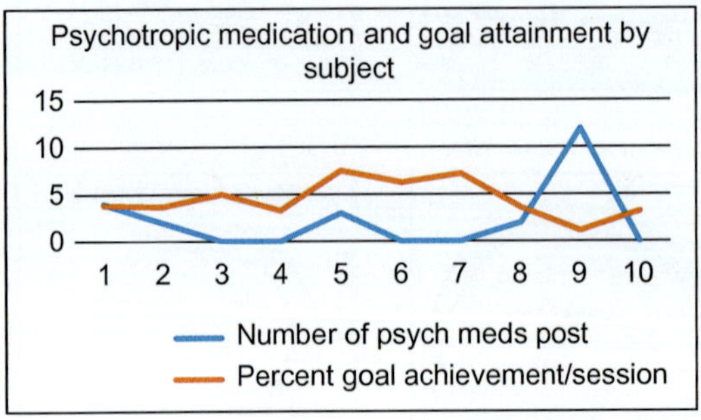

CHART 4.31 Interaction between medication and goal attainment.

CONCLUSION

LZN utilizing an SCL–FNM method is evidently effective and specific in the treatment of PTSD and mild TBI. Further research into and further development of these methods should be a high priority among health-care researchers and providers. Although double-blind, placebo-controlled studies are not necessary, and would probably be unethical at this point, to further elucidate the effectiveness of these methods, studies involving comparisons with other treatment methods and combinations of already proven methods are called for.

References

Ayers, M. (1993). A controlled study of EEG neurofeedback training and clinical psychotherapy for right hemispheric closed head injury. *Biofeedback and Self Regulation, 18*(3), 148–149.

Ayers, M. E. (1987). *Electroencephalic neurofeedback and closed head injury of 250 individuals.* Head injury frontiers. *National Head Injury Foundation*, 380–392.

Bratic, A., Orsillo, S., Esslen, M., & Jancke, L. (2007). Neurofeedback treatment of attention disorders after traumatic brain injuries. *Brain Topography, 20*, 41–53.

Byers, A. P. (1995). Neurofeedback therapy for a mild head injury. *Journal of Neurotherapy, 1*(1), 22–37.

Foster, D. S., & Veazey-Morris, K. (2013). LORETA Z score neurofeedback in the treatment of veterans with PTSD and TBI. *Proceedings of the 2013 ISNR conference, Journal of Neurotherapy*, 17: 276. Paper presented at: 21st Annual Conference of the International Society for Neurofeedback and Research. Dallas, TX..

Greuling, J. W., Lloyd, H. A., & Bowser, B. L. (1998). Neurofeedback treatment outcome of a severe closed head injury. *Archives of Clinical Neuropsychology, 13*, 139.

Hammond, D. C. (2006). Neurofeedback to improve physical balance, incontinence, and swallowing. *Journal of Neurotherapy, 9*(1), 27–48.

Hoffman, D. A., Stockdale, S., & Van Egeren, L. (1996). EEG neurofeedback in the treatment of mild traumatic brain injury. *Clinical Electroencephalography, 24*, 6.

Keller, I. (2001). Neurofeedback therapy of attention deficits in patients with traumatic brain injury. *Journal of Neurotherapy, 5*(1–2), 19–32.

Kluetsch, R. C., Ros, T., Theberge, J., Frewen, P. A., Calhoun, V. D., Schmahl, C., et al. (2014). Plastic modulation of PTSD resting-state networks and subjective wellbeing by EEG neurofeedback. *Acta Psychiatrica Scandinavica, 130*(2), 123–136.

Laibow, R. E., Stubblebine, A. N., Sandground, H., & Bounias, M. (2001). EEG neurobiofeedback treatment of patients with brain injury: Part 2: Changes in EEG parameters versus rehabilitation. *Journal of Neurotherapy, 5*(4), 45–71.

Malkowicz, D., & Martinez, D. (2009). Role of quantitative electroencephalography, neurotherapy, and neuroplasticity in recovery from neurological and psychiatric disorders. *Journal of Neurotherapy, 13*, 176–188.

Nash, J. K. (2005). Neurotherapy with adults. *Journal of Adult Development, 12*, 105–112.

Nelson, D. V., & Esty, M. L. (2012). Neurotherapy of traumatic brain injury/posttraumatic stress symptoms in OEF/OIF veterans. *Journal of Neuropsychiatry and Clinical Neuroscience, 24*, 237–240.

Peniston, E. G., & Kulkosky, P. J. (1991). Alpha-theta brainwave neurofeedback therapy for Vietnam veterans with combat-related post-traumatic stress disorder. *Medical Psychotherapy, 4*, 47–60.

Peniston, E. G., Marrinan, D. A., Deming, W. A., & Kulkosky, P. J. (1993). EEG alpha–theta synchronization in Vietnam theater veterans with combat-related post-traumatic stress disorder and alcohol abuse. *Advances in Medical Psychotherapy, 6*, 37–50.

Pop-Jordanova, N., & Zorcec, T. (2004). Child trauma, attachment, and biofeedback mitigation. *Macedonian Academy of Sciences and Arts, Section of Biological and Medical Sciences, 25*(1–2), 103–114.

Reddy, R. P., Jamuna, N., Devi, B. I., & Thennarasu, K. (2009). Neurofeedback training to enhance learning and memory in patient with traumatic brain injury: A single case study. *International Journal of Psychosocial Rehabilitation, 14*, 21–28.

Ros, T., Théberge, J., Frewen, P. A., Kluetsch, R., Densmore, M., Calhoun, V. D., et al. (2013). Mind over chatter: Plastic up-regulation of the fMRI salience network directly after EEG neurofeedback. *Neuroimage, 65*, 324–335.

Schoenberger, N. E., Shif, S. C., Esty, M. L., Ochs, L., & Matheis, R. J. (2001). Flexyx Neurotherapy System in the treatment of traumatic brain injury: An initial evaluation. *Journal of Head Trauma Rehabilitation, 16*(3), 260–274.

Smith, W. D. (2008). *The effect of neurofeedback training on PTSD symptoms of depression and attention problems among military veterans* (Doctoral dissertation, Capella University).

Surmeli, T. (2007). Efficacy of QEEG and neurofeedback in the assessment and treatment of post concussive syndrome: 24 cases. *Paper presented at 15th Annual Conference of the International Society for Neurofeedback and Research*; September 6–9, San Diego, CA.

Thatcher, R. W. (2012). *Handbook of quantitative electroencephalography and EEG biofeedback*. St. Petersburg, FL: Anipublishing, Inc..

Thatcher, R. W. (2013). Latest developments in Live Z-score training: Symptom check list, phase reset, and LORETA Z-score biofeedback. *Journal of Neurotherapy: Investigations in Neuromodulation, Neurofeedback and Applied Neuroscience, 17*(1), 69–87.

Thornton, K. (2000). Improvement/rehabilitation of memory functioning with neurotherapy/QEEG biofeedback. *Journal of Head Trauma Rehabilitation, 15*(6), 1285–1296.

Thornton, K. (2002). Rehabilitation of memory functioning with EEG biofeedback. *Neurorehabilitation, 17*(1), 69–81.

Thornton, K., & Carmody, D. (2013). The relation between memory improvement and QEEG changes in three clinical groups as a result of EEG biofeedback treatment. *Journal of Neurotherapy, 17*, 116–131.

Tinius, T. P., & Tinius, K. A. (2000). Changes after EEG biofeedback and cognitive retraining in adults with mild traumatic brain injury and attention deficit hyperactivity disorder. *Journal of Neurotherapy, 4*(2), 27–44.

Walker, J. E. (2009). Anxiety associated with post traumatic stress disorder—the role of quantitative electro-encephalograph in diagnosis and in guiding neurofeedback training to remediate the anxiety. *Biofeedback, 37*(2), 67–70.

Walker, J. E., Norman, C. A., & Weber, R. K. (2002). Impact of qEEG-guided coherence training for patients with a mild closed head injury. *Journal of Neurotherapy, 6*(2), 31–43.

Wing, K. (2001). Effect of neurofeedback on motor recovery of a patient with brain injury: A case study and its implications for stroke rehabilitation. *Topics in Stroke Rehabilitation, 8*, 45–53.

Zelek, V. (2002). QEEG brainwave amplitude and coherence values as predictors of cognitive improvement to neurofeedback after moderate-to-severe acquired brain injury. *Journal of Head Trauma and Rehabilitation, 23*, 339–355.

Zorcec, T., Demerdzieva, A., & Pop-Jordanova, N. (2011). QEEG, brain rate, executive functions and neurofeedback training in patients with traumatic brain injury. *Acta Informatica Medica, 9*, 23–28.

CHAPTER

5

Z-score LORETA Neurofeedback as a Potential Therapy in Depression/Anxiety and Cognitive Dysfunction

J. Lucas Koberda, MD, PhD[1]

Tallahassee NeuroBalance Center, Tallahassee, FL, USA

Major depressive disorder (MDD) is a common mental illness affecting approximately 2.5% of the general population. MDD is one of the leading causes of disability; it is projected to be the cause of the second highest burden of disease (measured in disability-adjusted life years) by 2020 (WHO). MDD has negative social consequences in terms of reduced employment and psychosocial impairment (Andersen, Thielen, Bech, Nygaard, & Diderichsen, 2011). The pathophysiology of depression involves both external social stressors and internal genetic vulnerability.

Depressed individuals frequently report multi-somatic complaints with poor memory and low cognitive functions. Cognitive impairment is a core endophenotype of MDD; difficulty with concentration is one of the defining criteria of the disorder (Pittenger, 2013). In addition to these deficits in concentration and attention, patients with major depression can exhibit difficulties with explicit memory, especially recollection memory (Pittenger, 2013). Disruption of explicit memory capacity is seen in a number of stress-associated disorders, such as MDD and post-traumatic stress disorder (PTSD). Chronic stress produces a number of abnormalities in brain circuitries that are required for explicit memory function, such as the hippocampus and dorsolateral prefrontal cortex, which provides a probable mechanism for these effects (Pittenger, 2013).

[1]www.TallahasseeNeuroBalanceCenter.com

Z Score Neurofeedback.
DOI: http://dx.doi.org/10.1016/B978-0-12-801291-8.00005-4

Anxiety disorders are among the most common of all mental disorders (Kessler, Chiu, Demler, Merikangas, & Walters, 2005). The diagnostic and statistical manual of mental disorders (DSM-IV-TR) includes generalized anxiety disorder (GAD, a chronic form of anxiety characterized by excessive, uncontrollable worry), panic disorder (PD, with recurrent, unexpected paroxysms of anxiety, somatic, and autonomic symptoms and fear), phobic disorders (e.g., specific phobias, agoraphobia, social phobia (SP)), PTSD (characterized by unwanted, intrusive remembrances—as daytime thoughts and nighttime dreams and nightmares—and avoidance of activities and other cues associated with prior life-threatening trauma) and obsessive–compulsive disorder (OCD, with recurrent obsessions and compulsions in this category).

In addition to psychotherapy and pharmacotherapy, other noninvasive modalities including neurofeedback (NFB), repetitive transcranial magnetic stimulation (rTMS) and transcranial direct current stimulation (tDCS) have been found effective in the treatment of these conditions (Alonzo, Chan, Martin, Mitchell, & Loo, 2013; Stevens, 2014). TMS has also been cleared by the FDA for the treatment of medically resistant depression (Stevens, 2014). In addition to noninvasive modalities for the treatment of depression and anxiety, other invasive techniques were introduced, including vagus nerve stimulation (VNS) and deep brain stimulation (DBS). DBS, especially with subcallosal cingulate (Brodmann's area 25), has been reported to be beneficial in depression cases resistant to conventional medical therapy (Riva-Posse, Holtzheimer, Garlow, & Mayberg, 2013 and Schlaepfer & Bewernick, 2013). Unfortunately, any invasive procedure carries a risk of potential complications and side effects including bleeding, infection, and misplacement of an active electrode (Williams & Okun, 2013). NFB (in contrast to the above invasive methods) is believed not to be associated with any major side effects and is relatively inexpensive when compared with DBS. Unfortunately, NFB has not yet gained wide acceptance in the clinical arena as a potential therapeutic modality. Standard one or two electrode NFB has been reported in a pilot study as beneficial in relieving depression symptoms in several investigations, including a randomized controlled study (Choi et al., 2011). The NFB training had profound effects on emotion and cognition. The authors replicated earlier findings that enhancing the left frontal activity led to alleviation of depressive symptoms (Choi et al., 2011). Moreover, cognitive tests revealed that the asymmetry training improved performance on executive function tests, whereas the placebo treatment did not show improvement (Choi et al., 2011).

In Z-score NFB, a real-time comparison to an age-matched population of healthy subjects is used for data acquisition, simplifying protocol generation, and allowing clinicians to target modules and hubs that indicate dysregulation and instability in networks related to symptoms

(Thatcher, 2013). Z-score NFB increases specificity in operant conditioning, providing a guide that links extreme Z-score outliers to symptoms and then reinforcing Z-score shifts toward states of greater homeostasis and stability. The goal is increased efficiency of information processing in brain networks related to the patient's symptoms (Thatcher, 2013).

A recently introduced method called low-resolution electromagnetic tomography (LORETA) Z-score NFB is capable of targeting specific dysregulated anatomical structures, many of which are in deep cortical locations (Koberda, Koberda, Bienkiewicz, Moses, & Koberda, 2013; Thatcher, 2013). For example, the insula and anterior cingulate (AC) have been identified as potential NFB target sites for improving pain control in patients who display electrical dysregulation of these areas (Koberda et al., 2013).

Our neurology center conducted Z-score LORETA NFB therapy for 31 patients with depression and/or associated anxiety. In addition to depression and anxiety, these patients frequently reported other coexisting problems including cognitive dysfunction, OCD, and chronic pain. Most patients were found to have quantitative electroencephalogram (QEEG) abnormalities including alpha power increase, asymmetry, or LORETA electrical dysregulation in frontal areas (Figure 5.1A and B).

Detailed analysis of our patients diagnosed with depression and/or anxiety showed that out of 31 included in the study, 24 (77%) were found to have both subjective and objective (improvement of QEEG abnormalities) improvement of the symptoms within 10 sessions of LORETA Z-score NFB. In this chapter, I would like to present some of our patients who successfully completed Z-score LORETA NFB with marked improvement in both depression and cognitive function. Cognitive function, which is often impaired in patients with depression, usually improves after NFB therapy.

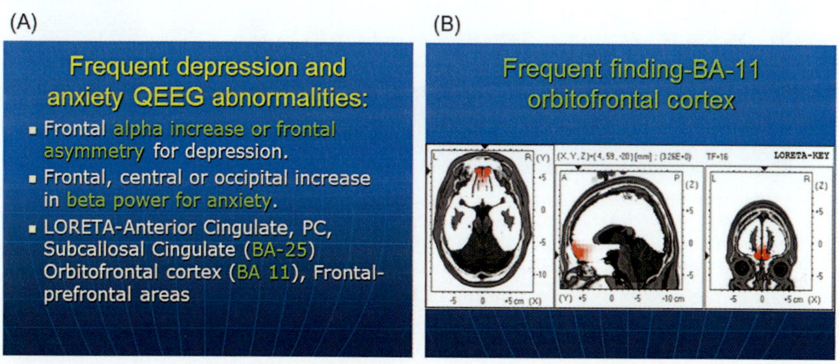

FIGURE 5.1 (A) Summary of frequently identified QEEG/LORETA abnormalities in patients suffering from depression and anxiety. (B) Orbitofrontal electrical (area in red) dysregulation (BA-11) seen in one of the patients with depression and anxiety.

CASE 1

Figure 5.2A and B shows LORETA images, as well as brain maps, before and after completion of 15 sessions of Z-score LORETA NFB for a 15-year-old female who suffered from extreme anxiety before and during horse riding competitions. Her symptoms included anxiety with palpitations, frequently associated with nausea and vomiting. Marked dysregulation of the AC subcallosal region—Brodmann's area (BA) 25—was identified during the pre-NFB LORETA (Figure 5.2A), manifesting as increased beta activity. Following 15 NFB sessions, this electrical dysregulation was corrected, as seen on the lower portion of Figure 5.2A.

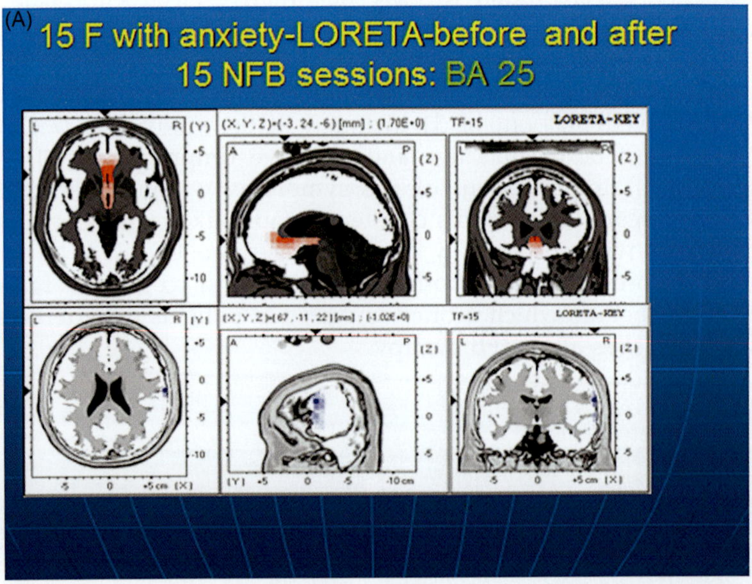

FIGURE 5.2 (A) Shows LORETA images of the 15-year female suffering from anxiety. Upper part of the picture shows area of electrical dysregulation (area in red) in the subcallosal cingulate (BA-25) before NFB therapy. Lower part of the picture shows resolution of previously identified dysregulation after 15 sessions of NFB.

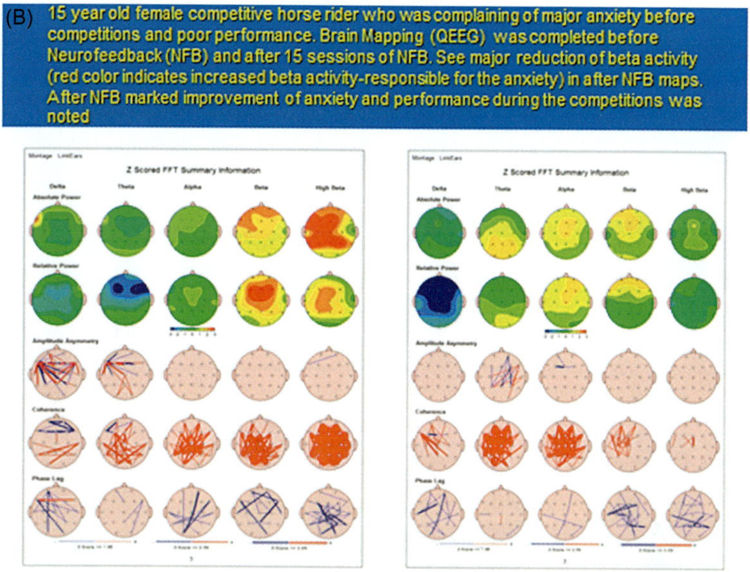

FIGURE 5.2 (B) QEEG maps of 15-year female suffering from anxiety. Left image shows brain maps before NFB, right image shows brain maps after 15 NFB sessions.

CASE 2

A 40-year-old female, who was previously treated by a psychiatrist for major depression and did not respond to pharmacological treatment, was referred to me for NFB therapy. Prior to NFB, she was treated with electro-convulsive therapy (ECT), which was not successful in relieving her depression. Instead, the individual sustained major memory impairment and visual–spatial difficulties. Since she was not responding to conventional therapy, her psychiatrist referred her to my practice for NFB therapy. The patient's cognitive and depressive dysfunction caused inability to continue her employment as a pharmaceutical representative. Initial LORETA showed several areas of electrical dysregulation including (Figure 5.3A) BA-5 (secondary sensorimotor cortex), BA-9 (prefrontal cortex) and temporal cortex (not shown).

Her computerized cognitive testing before NFB showed deficiency in memory, information processing speed, and visual–spatial domains.

continued

CASE 2 *(cont'd)*

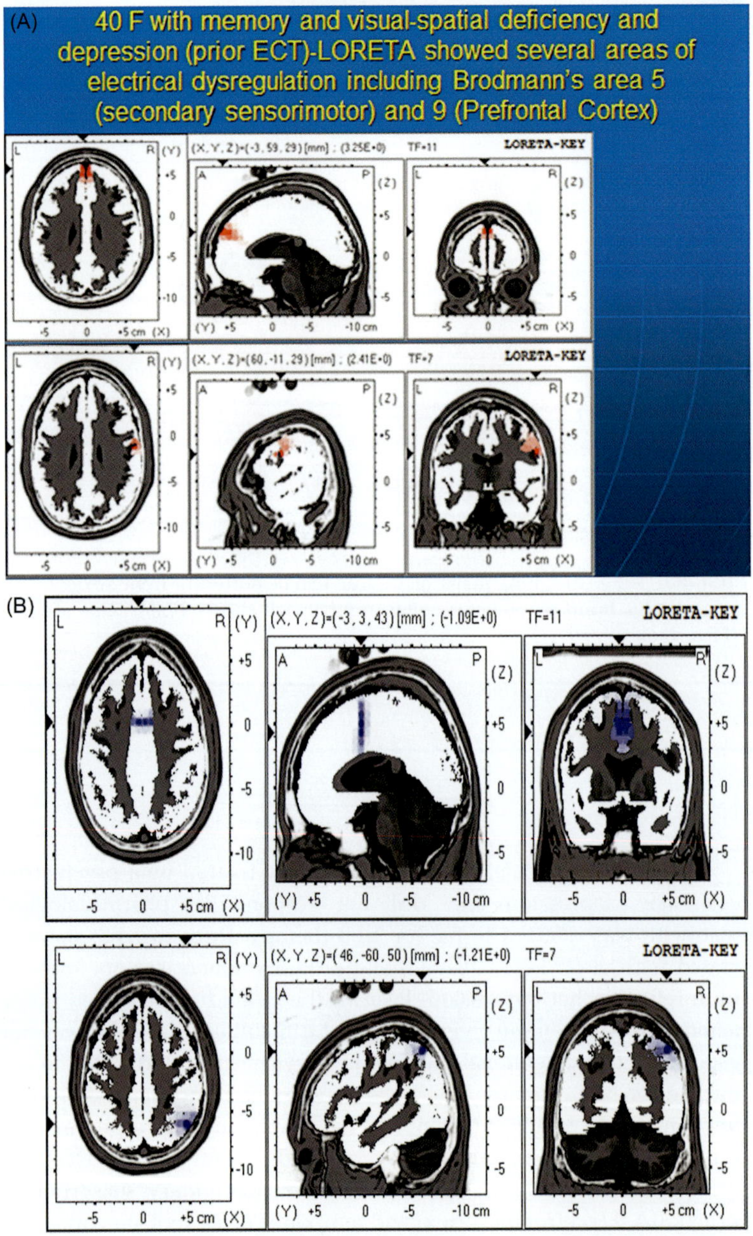

FIGURE 5.3 (A) Pre-NFB LORETA of 40-year-old female diagnosed with depression associated with cognitive dysfunction. Areas of cortical dysregulation are shown in red. (B) 40-year-old female LORETA after NFB shows resolution of previously electrically dysregulated BA-5 and -9.

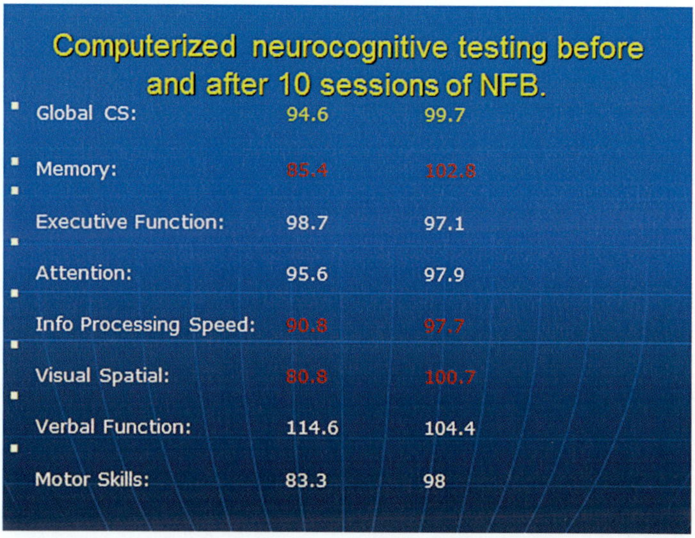

FIGURE 5.4 First vertical row shows scores from computerized cognitive testing before NFB. Second vertical row shows scores after 10 sessions of NFB. Computerized cognitive testing (Neurotrax Corp, Bellaire, TX) shows data based on comparison to age and education matched controls. Expected average score is 100 with one standard deviation being 15.

After 10 sessions of Z-score LORETA NFB, the patient reported major improvement in her mood (as well as mild memory improvement). Repeated computerized cognitive testing revealed marked improvement of previously deficient cognitive domains (Figure 5.4). Memory score increased from 85.4 to 102.8, information processing speed rose from 90.8 to 97.7, and visual–spatial domain went up from 80.8 to 100.7. In addition, post-NFB LORETA showed an improvement of previously identified electrical dysregulation (Figure 5.3B). After successful NFB therapy, the patient was also able to come back to gainful employment in the medical field (after a few years of being unemployed).

CASE 3

A 58-year-old female was referred by her psychiatrist and primary care physician for evaluation of chronic pain associated with depression. She reported a long-standing history of spinal pain (over 20 years) with two prior surgeries and multiple pain management visits.

continued

CASE 3 *(cont'd)*

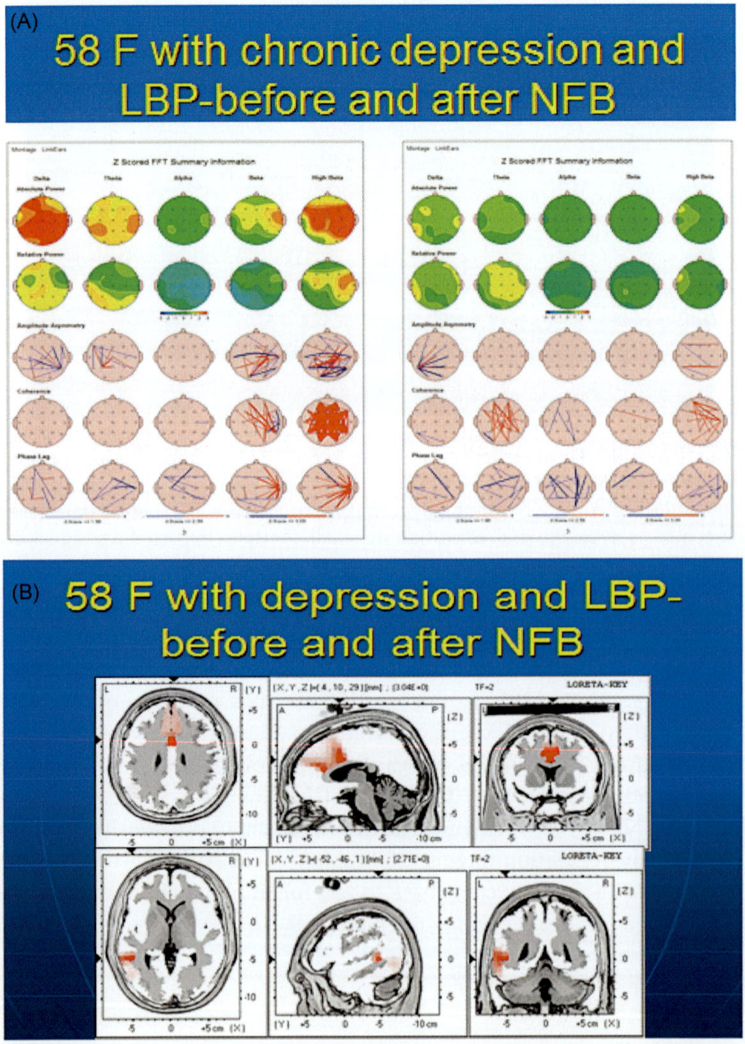

FIGURE 5.5 (A) QEEG brain maps of 58-year-old female suffering from pain and depression before NFB (left image) and after completion of 10 sessions of NFB (right image). There is noticeable reduction of previously (pre-NFB) increased delta, theta, and beta activity in post-NFB pictures (reduction of red color). (B) LORETA images of 58-year-old female suffering from pain and depression before NFB (upper image) and after completion of 10 sessions of NFB (lower image).

This patient had been on multiple medications including narcotics (MS Contin®) and was treated with spinal stimulator placement, with poor pain control. She reported associated headaches and being depressed, and was on two antidepressant medications, and she reported having memory problems. QEEG, before NFB initiation, showed major increase in frontal and central delta and beta power, as well as an area of dysregulation in the AC cortex on LORETA imaging (Figures 5.5A and B). Increase in bilateral temporal theta power was recorded, likely corresponding to her memory problems. The computerized neurocognitive testing showed a low memory score of 53, which is over three standard deviations below the mean. After initiation of NFB, the patient reported marked improvement of all symptoms after just two sessions of Z-score LORETA NFB and continuous improvement in the following sessions. After LORETA NFB, the QEEG showed marked improvement in frontal delta and beta overexpression, and the resolution of the cingulate cortex dysregulation (see Figures 5.5A and B). In addition, bilateral theta power overexpression improved with NFB therapy which was associated with a subjective improvement of memory. She completed a total number of 25 sessions. Unfortunately, the patient sustained another fall/injury to her spine and did not follow up with NFB thereafter due to her inability to drive. No follow-up computerized neurocognitive testing was obtained.

CASE 4

A 58-year-old university professor was seen in my office due to major depression associated with anxiety and memory problems. She noticed problems with teaching due to possible cognitive dysfunction. Figure 5.6 shows her LORETA imaging before NFB, which identified several areas of electrical dysregulation including the cingulate cortex and left temporal region.

The computerized cognitive testing completed before NFB identified deficiency of memory and executive function. Blood work was negative for B12 deficiency.

After 10 sessions of NFB, major improvement in memory (from 42.8 to 107.1) was recorded on neurocognitive Neurotrax testing (Figure 5.7).

continued

CASE 4 (*cont'd*)

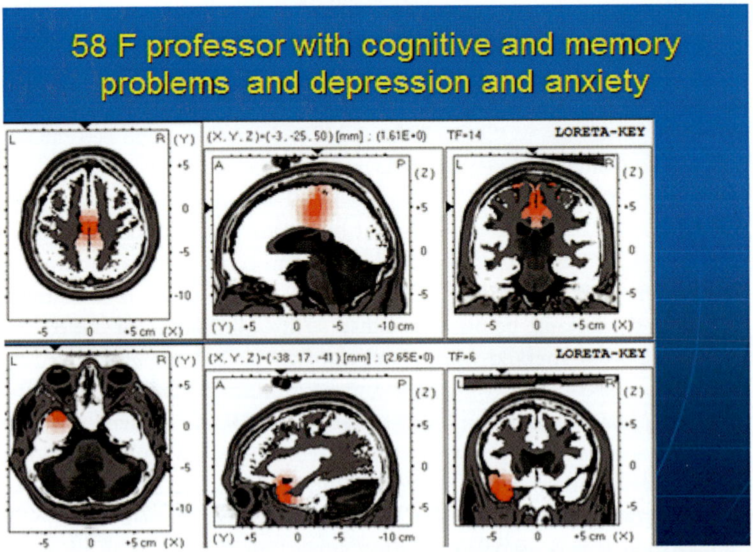

FIGURE 5.6 A 58-year-old female LORETA imaging before NFB shows two areas of electrical dysregulation (in red) including the cingulate cortex and left temporal region.

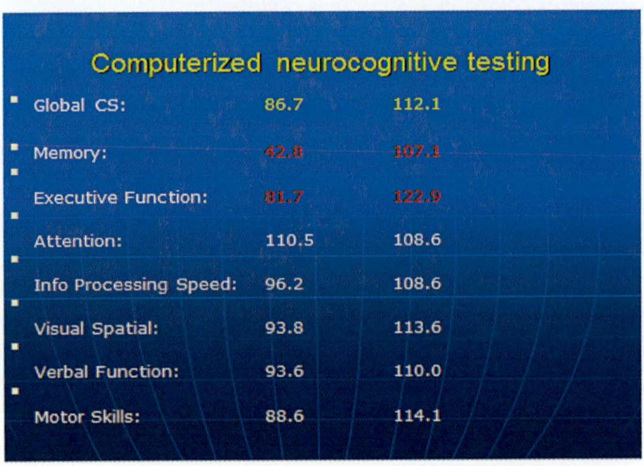

Computerized neurocognitive testing

Global CS:	86.7	112.1
Memory:	42.8	107.1
Executive Function:	81.7	122.9
Attention:	110.5	108.6
Info Processing Speed:	96.2	108.6
Visual Spatial:	93.8	113.6
Verbal Function:	93.6	110.0
Motor Skills:	88.6	114.1

FIGURE 5.7 A 58-year-old female cognitive testing results before (left column) and after (right column) 10 sessions of NFB. Expected score is 100 with one standard deviation being 15.

In addition, marked improvement in the patient's mood and anxiety was reported. Post-NFB LORETA imaging confirmed an improvement in electrical dysregulation of previously identified regions (picture not shown). Patient also reported better performance in her academic settings.

CASE 5

A 34-year-old male presented to my office due to major anxiety and overlapping alcohol (ETOH) addiction. His initial LORETA showed area of electrical dysregulation (Figure 5.8) in the AC and prefrontal cortex (BA-10 and -32).

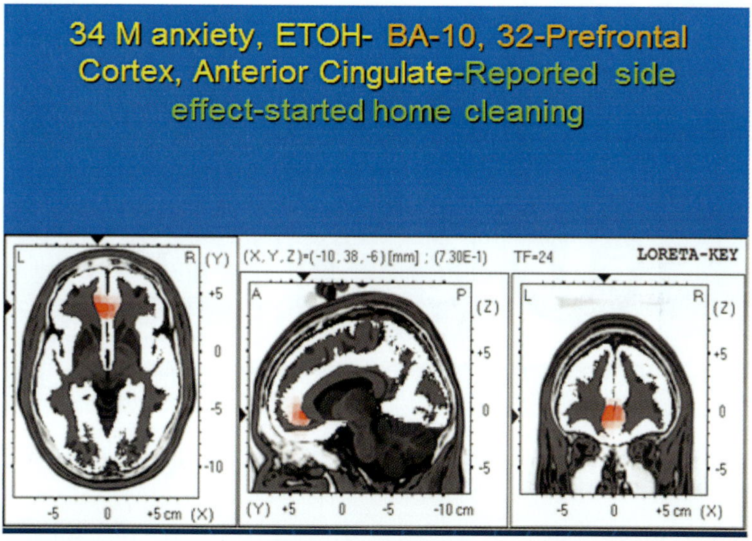

FIGURE 5.8 A 34-year-old male with anxiety and ETOH abuse. LORETA imaging before NFB initiation showed area of electrical dysregulation in BA-10 and -32 (in red).

After several sessions of NFB, this patient also reported change in his personality, describing a new found focus with keeping his home cleaned. He previously labeled himself as messy, not able to keep up with cleaning. In addition, he was able to reduce his alcoholic beverage consumption.

CASE 6

A 41-year-old female was referred to my office by a local psychiatrist due to major depression and anxiety resistant to medications.

continued

CASE 6 (*cont'd*)

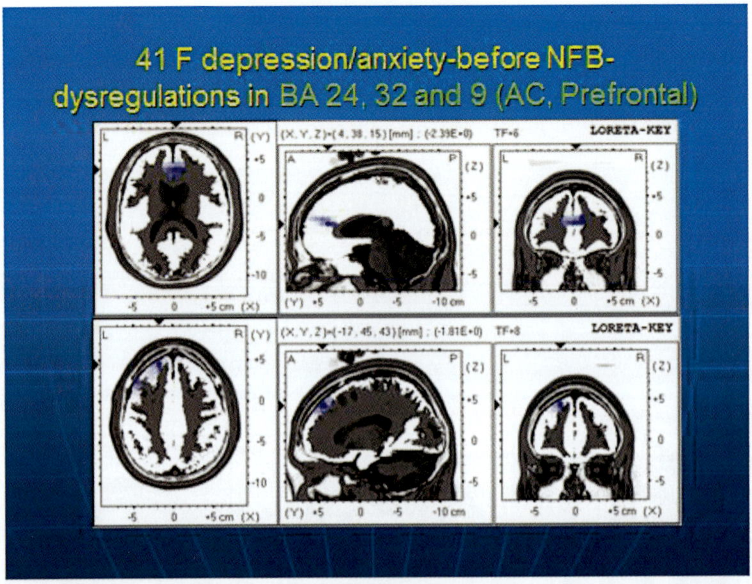

FIGURE 5.9 A 41-year-old female with depression and anxiety. LORETA showed areas of electrical dysregulation in BA-9, -24, and -32 (in blue).

Her LORETA imaging revealed areas of electrical dysregulation (Figure 5.9) in the AC and prefrontal cortex (BA-24, -32, and -9). Following 10 NFB sessions, marked improvement in her mood and electrical dysregulation was noted (data not shown).

CASE 7

A 59-year-old male was referred by his psychiatrist for NFB due to medication resistant depression and anxiety. LORETA imaging showed (Figure 5.10) areas of electrical dysregulations in the posterior cingulate and frontal area (BA-31 and -47). After several sessions of NFB, his mood improved. In addition, his brain maps also exhibited marked correction of previously elevated frontal and temporal beta activity. He was also able to reduce the dosing frequency of his medications for pain.

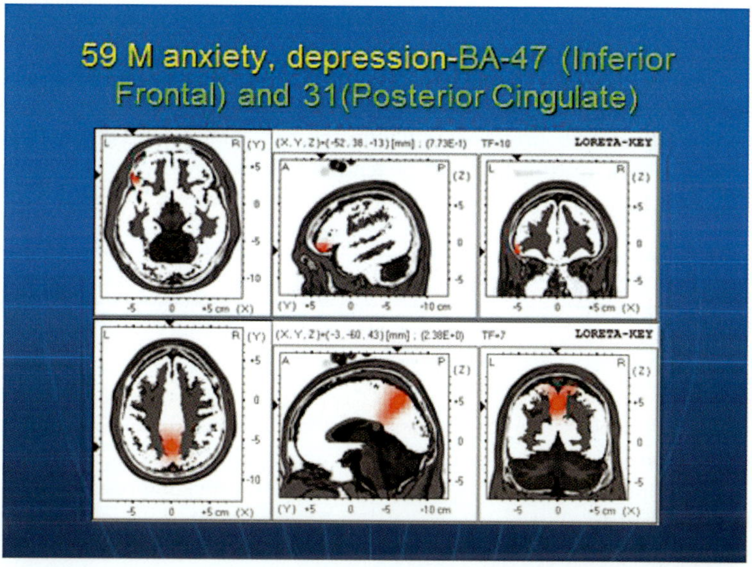

FIGURE 5.10 A 59-year-old male with depression and anxiety. LORETA showed areas of electrical dysregulation in BA-31 and -47 (in red).

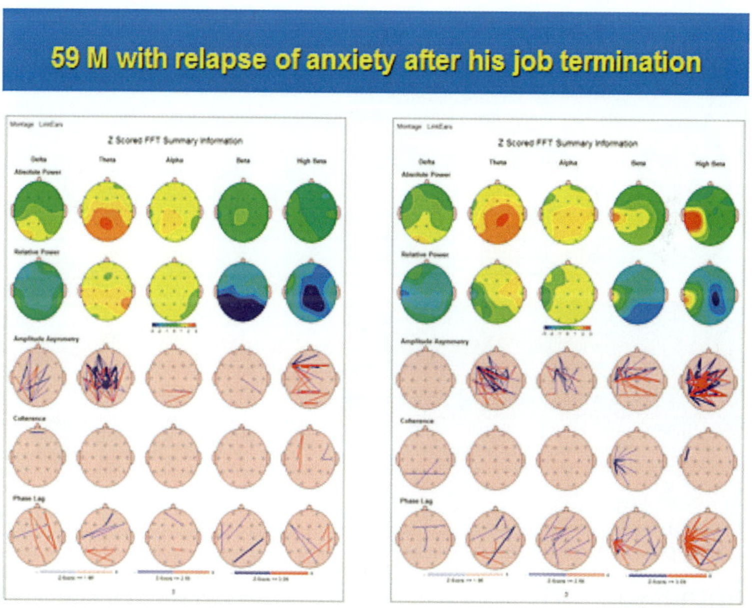

FIGURE 5.11 QEEG brain maps before (left) and after (right) a job termination. A major increase in temporal high beta power can be seen (right) after his job termination.

continued

CASE 7 (*cont'd*)

This patient was doing well for several months on maintenance once a week NFB protocol, until the moment of his job termination, after which a drastic increase of temporal beta power was recorded (Figure 5.11) and worsening of his anxiety was observed.

CASE 8

A 63-year-old nurse practitioner presented for consultation with major depression and anxiety. Her QEEG maps were typical for many depressed patients (increased frontal alpha power). LORETA imaging revealed posterior cingulate electrical dysregulation (Figure 5.12). Subsequent NFB therapy produced major improvement of her symptoms and correction of electrical dysregulation.

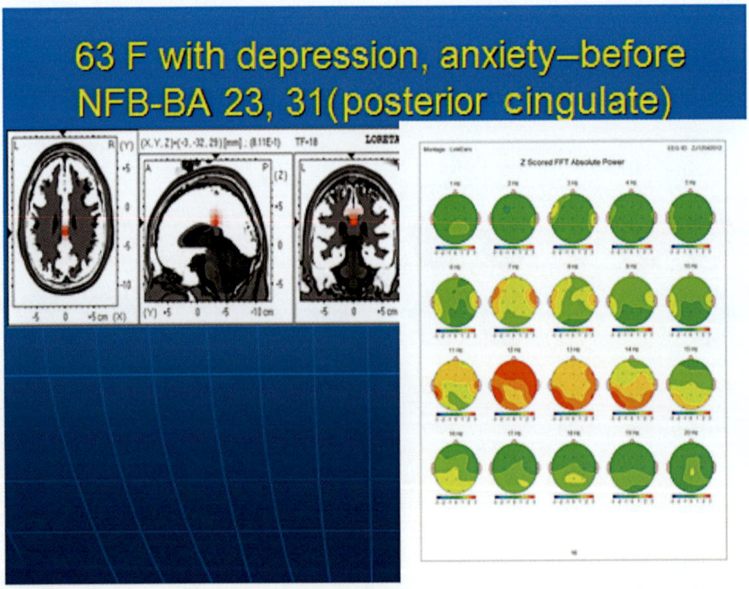

FIGURE 5.12 QEEG maps and LORETA. Marked increase in frontal alpha power and occipital beta power is noted and area of electrical dysregulation (in red) of posterior cingulate.

CASE 9

A 27-year-old law student presented as a self-referral for NFB therapy regarding his cognitive dysfunction, mainly memory. He graduated from law school but was unable to study for bar exams due to problems with retaining previously read information. His QEEG brain maps showed mild increase in occipital beta power, temporal delta, and theta power (Figure 5.13).

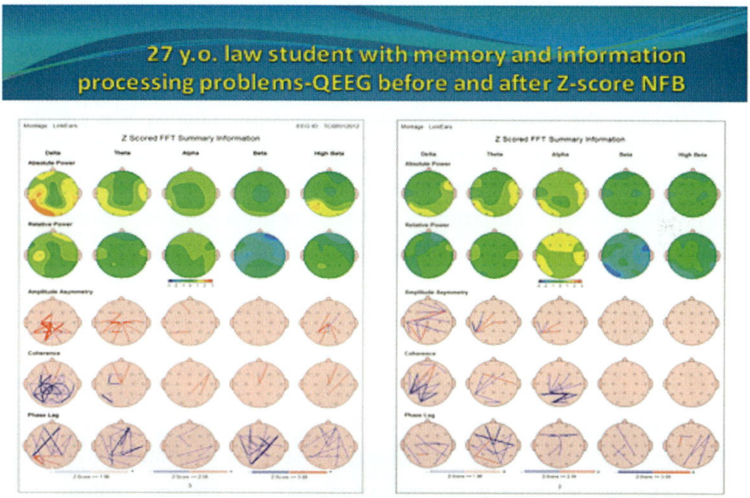

FIGURE 5.13 QEEG maps showed increased bilateral temporal delta and theta power, as well as occipital beta power (left). Marked improvement in the previously dysregulated areas was noted (right) after NFB.

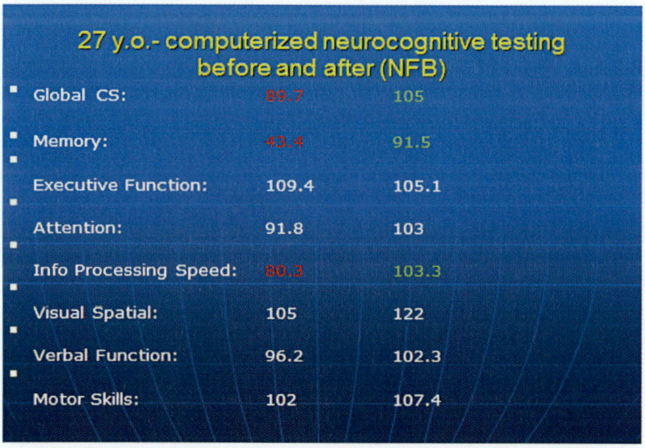

FIGURE 5.14 Computerized cognitive testing before (left) and after (right) NFB.

continued

CASE 9 (*cont'd*)

The neurocognitive testing before NFB showed low memory and information processing speed (Figure 5.14). After 10 NFB sessions, marked improvement in subjective and objective memory was noted (Figure 5.14).

CASE 10

A 19-year-old male was brought for appointment by his adoptive parents indicating problems with cognition, mostly executive function and information processing speed dysfunction. After completing a QEEG and before initiation of NFB, neurocognitive testing was

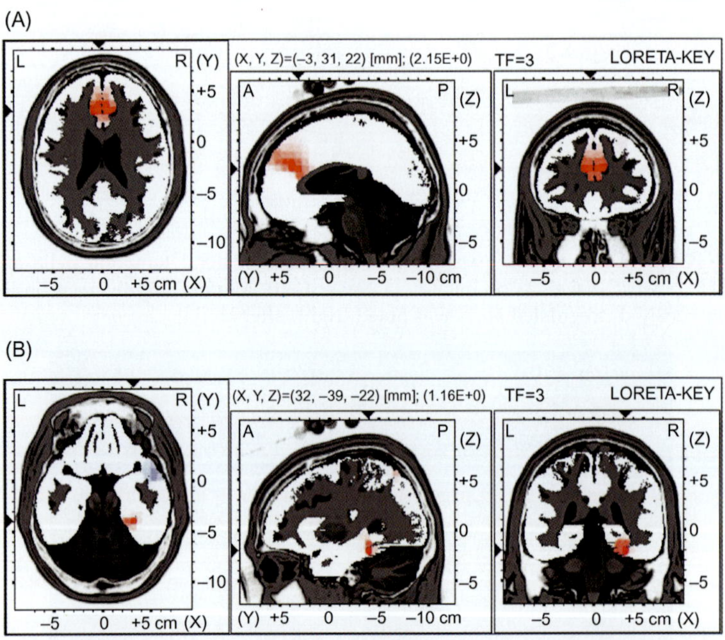

FIGURE 5.15 (A) A-LORETA imaging of 19-year-old patient showing area of electrical dysregulation of AC region BA-32 (in red). (B) Resolution of AC dysregulation after 20 sessions of NFB.

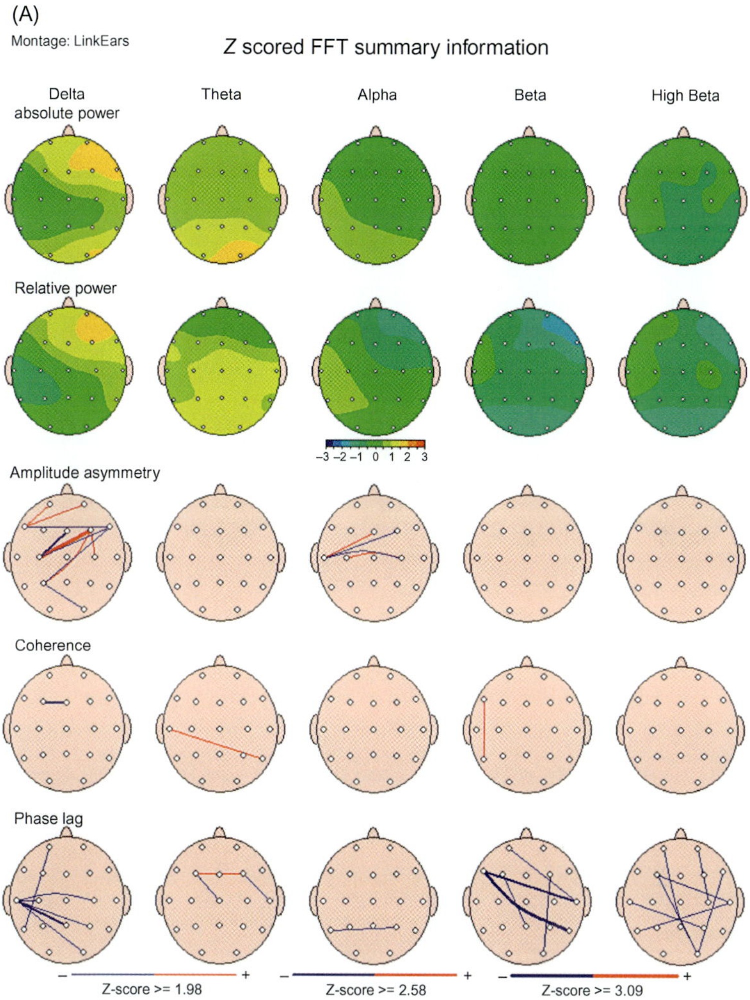

FIGURE 5.16 QEEG of 19-year-old with cognitive problems before initiation of NFB (A) and after course of NFB sessions (B). (A) QEEG before NFB noticeable area of frontal increase in delta power.

completed in March 2013; results showed low cognitive score—global cognitive score 80.2 with low executive function 87.2, and a very low information processing speed of 52.1. His LORETA and QEEG showed evidence of AC electrical dysregulation and increased frontal delta-power (Figures 5.15A and 5.16A). After the first 10 sessions of NFB, his executive function improved to 89.9, and with each round of NFB,

continued

CASE 10 (*cont'd*)

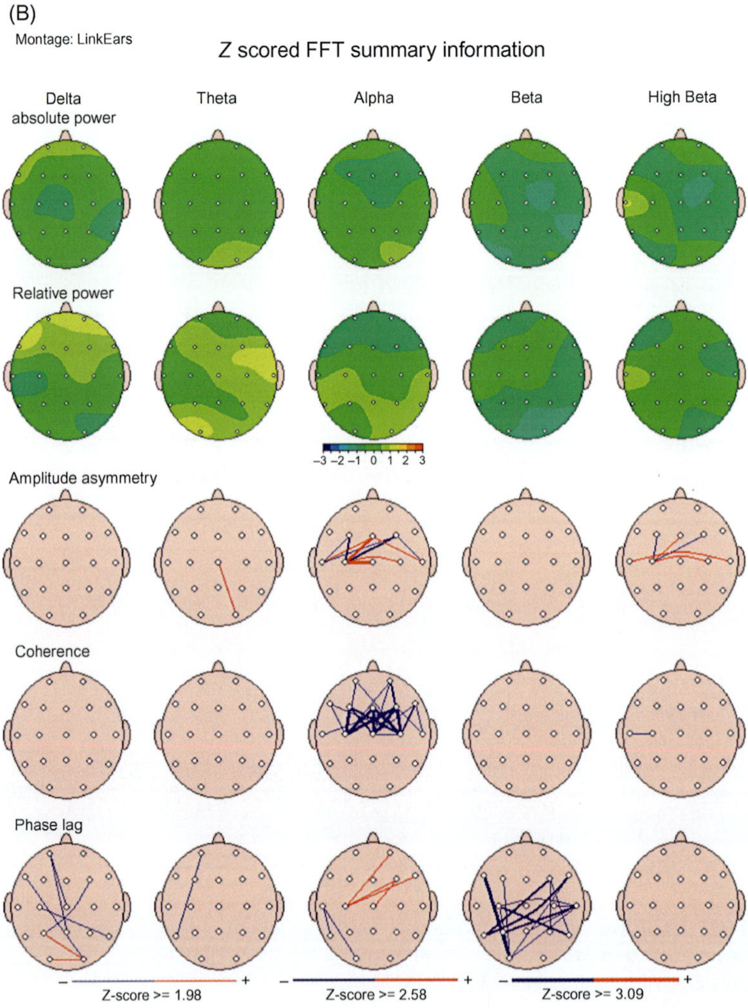

FIGURE 5.16 (B) QEEG after NFB—an improvement in previously overexpressed frontal delta power is recorded.

repeated cognitive testing was giving better results with executive function (subsequently 92 and 97; see Figure 5.17). Also previously electrically dysregulated AC area and frontal delta power overexpression

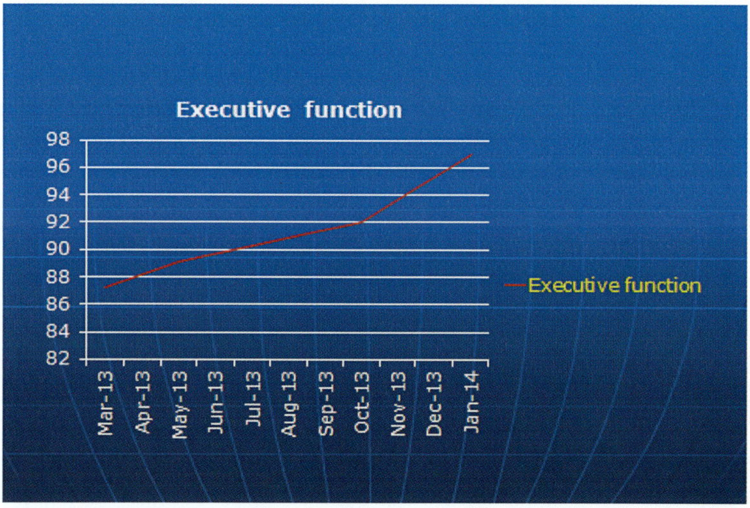

FIGURE 5.17 Executive testing (Neurotrax) before NFB (March 2013) and after each round of 10 sessions of NFB (in May 2013, October 2013, and January 2014) gradual increase in executive function was recorded.

became normalized (Figures 5.15B and 5.16B). In addition to QEEG and cognitive testing, his parents noted a tremendous improvement in social and cognitive performance at home and work.

Our group has already reported evidence of successful cognitive enhancement (Koberda, 2012; Koberda, Moses, Koberda, & Koberda, 2012) with LORETA Z-score NFB. One case report included an individual with Asperger's syndrome (Koberda, 2012) associated with speech expressive dysfunction; another one described a student with low information processing speed and decreased memory (Koberda et al., 2012). Subsequently we have conducted a larger case series report where 35 consecutive patients complaining of cognitive dysfunction were subjected to LORETA Z-score NFB therapy (Koberda, Moses, Koberda, & Winslow, 2014). Before NFB initiation, these patients were evaluated with computerized neurocognitive testing in order to document and confirm any cognitive dysfunction reported in the chief complaint. Many patients underwent brain imaging and laboratory testing to rule out any treatable condition which could have contributed to the patient's symptoms. Electrical imaging with QEEG/LORETA localization was also completed in order to visualize any area of cortical electrical dysregulation which could have been potentially responsible for the patient's symptoms (with specific Brodmann's areas). The NFB protocol was based either on the patient's symptoms, the area of cortical dysregulation, or both. After 10 sessions of surface/LORETA Z-score NFB, the computerized cognitive testing and QEEG were repeated in order to see if any increase in cognitive score and/or reduction in QEEG abnormalities was achieved. In addition, the patient's subjective response was recorded as to whether or not they felt that the therapy was beneficial. Twenty-five patients (71%) were identified as having a significant objective improvement (on average 10 points) in cognitive testing. In addition, subjective cognitive improvement and an objective reduction of QEEG abnormalities with NFB were also achieved in most of the patients. These results are very promising and indicate good effectiveness of LORETA Z-score NFB in cognitive enhancement.

This clinical data illustrates the high effectiveness of Z-score LORETA NFB therapy in complex neuropsychiatric patients, where an improvement of depression/anxiety and other associated cognitive domains can be achieved in most of the patients within just 10 treatment sessions. However, many patients requested to continue NFB for a longer period of time in order to continue benefits of this therapy. Some patients were also treated with additional NFB (5–10 sessions) in case of reoccurrence of the symptoms.

Based on our encouraging data, we recommend implementation of QEEG/LORETA brain mapping testing in all patients suffering from depression, anxiety, and cognitive dysfunction.

Given its potential effectiveness, noninvasive nature, and the likelihood that NFB is relatively free of unwanted side effects, it should be considered on a par with other modalities as a treatment of first choice.

SPECIAL NOTES

Since Dr. Koberda's work presented in this chapter was not supported by any grant and reflects the way he practices NFB, there are no control groups included in this report.

- Neurotrax (MindStreams) computerized cognitive testing has been previously extensively tested for reliability. To minimize learning across sessions, three alternate forms of MindStreams cognitive tests were developed with identical psychometric properties but different items. Equivalence for all three alternate forms was demonstrated to have an acceptable test–retest reliability coefficients as well as the alternate form reliability coefficients.

Acknowledgment

I would like to give a special thanks to Dr. Eric Harris who contributed in editing of this chapter.

References

Alonzo, A., Chan, G., Martin, D., Mitchell, P. B., & Loo, C. (2013). Transcranial direct current stimulation (tDCS) for depression: Analysis of response using a three-factor structure of the Montgomery–Åsberg depression rating scale. *Journal of Affective Disorders, 150*(1), 91–95.

Andersen, I., Thielen, K., Bech, P., Nygaard, E., & Diderichsen, F. (2011). Increasing prevalence of depression from 2000 to 2006. *Scandinavian Journal of Public Health, 39*, 857–863.

Choi, S. W., Chi, S. E., Chung, S. Y., Kim, J. W., Ahn, C. Y., & Kim, H. T. (2011). Is alpha wave neurofeedback effective with randomized clinical trials in depression? A pilot study. *Neuropsychobiology, 63*(1), 45–51.

Kessler, R. C., Chiu, W. T., Demler, O., Merikangas, K. R., & Walters, E. E. (2005). Prevalence, severity, and comorbidity of 12-month DSM-IV disorders in the National Comorbidity Survey Replication. *Archives of General Psychiatry, 62*, 617–627.

Koberda, J. L. (2012). Autistic spectrum disorder (ASD) as a potential target of Z-score LORETA neurofeedback. *The Neuroconnection* 24 [winter 2012, edition (ISNR)].

Koberda, J. L., Koberda, P., Bienkiewicz, A., Moses, A., & Koberda, L. (2013). Pain management using 19-electrode Z-score LORETA neurofeedback. *Journal of Neurotherapy, 17*(3), 179–190.

Koberda, J. L., Moses, A., Koberda, L., & Koberda, P. (2012). Cognitive enhancement using 19-electrode Z-score neurofeedback. *Journal of Neurotherapy, 3*, 224–230.

Koberda, J. L., Moses, A., Koberda, P., Winslow J. Cognitive enhancement with LORETA Z-score neurofeedback. *AAPB meeting*, 2014.

Pittenger, C. (2013). Disorders of memory and plasticity in psychiatric disease. *Dialogues in Clinical Neuroscience, 15*(4), 455–463.

Riva-Posse, P., Holtzheimer, P. E., Garlow, S. J., & Mayberg, H. S. (2013). Practical considerations in the development and refinement of subcallosal cingulate white matter deep brain stimulation for treatment-resistant depression. *World Neurosurgery, 80*. (3–4)S27. e25–34.

Schlaepfer, T. E., & Bewernick, B. H. (2013). Deep brain stimulation for major depression. *Handbook of Clinical Neurology, 116*, 235–243. Available from: http://dx.doi.org/doi:10.1016/B978-0-444-53497-2.00018-8.

Stevens, E. (2014). In Cantor, & Evans (Eds.), *Treating mood disorders—clinical neurotherapy—applications and techniques for treatment*. London, UK: Elsevier.

Thatcher, R. W. (2013). Latest developments in live z-score training: Symptom checklist, phase reset, and LORETA z-score biofeedback. *Journal of Neurotherapy, 17*, 69–87.

Williams, N. R., & Okun, M. S. (2013). Deep brain stimulation (DBS) at the interface of neurology and psychiatry. *The Journal of Clinical Investigation, 123*(11), 4546–4556.

World Health Organization. *Information on mental disorders management: Depression*. Geneva: World Health Organization. Available from <http://www.who.int/mental_health/management/depression/definition/en/index.html>.

CHAPTER

6

LORETA Z-Score Neurofeedback in Chronic Pain and Headaches

J. Lucas Koberda, MD, PhD

Tallahassee NeuroBalance Center, Tallahassee, FL, USA

The International Association for the Study of Pain (http://www.iasp-pain.org) has defined pain as "an unpleasant sensory and emotional experience arising from actual or potential tissue damage."

The neural substrates of pain perception have been intensively explored with neuroimaging techniques (Hanakawa, 2012), such as functional magnetic resonance imaging (fMRI) and positron emission tomography (PET). Many imaging studies have consistently revealed a set of brain regions as substrates of pain perception (Moisset & Bouhassira, 2007). These regions include the anterior cingulate cortex, the insula, and the parietal operculum including the second somatosensory cortex (S2), and the thalamus, which are collectively called the pain matrix.

Headaches are one of the most common complaints in the general population, as well as among children and adolescents. Among different type of headaches, migrainous headaches and tension headaches are the most frequent.

Current treatments for chronic pain are varied in both their approach and efficacy. Pharmacologic therapies used in the treatment of chronic pain include opioids, anticonvulsants, and antidepressants (Finnerup, Sindrup, & Jensen, 2010). These medications modify brain function, but their lack of specificity can lead to side effects that negatively impact the quality of life for the patient. Psychosocial approaches to pain management include cognitive behavioral therapy

Z Score Neurofeedback.
DOI: http://dx.doi.org/10.1016/B978-0-12-801291-8.00006-6

(CBT), hypnosis, emotional disclosure, acceptance-based therapies, and partner-based therapies (Williams, Keefe, & Vlaeyen, 2010). In case of back pain, physical therapy has proven to be an effective form of therapy (Calvo-Muñoz, Gómez-Conesa, & Sánchez-Meca, 2013).

Biofeedback has been found to be beneficial in the rehabilitation of headache (Nestoriuc, Martin, Rief, & Andrasik, 2008) and, in some studies, of chronic back pain (Altmaier, Lehmann, Russell, Weinstein, & Kao, 1992; Glombiewski, Hartwich-Tersek, & Rief, 2010; Keefe, Schapira, & Williams, 1981) and several other pain disorders, for example, temporomandibular joint disorders (Mora, Bleichhardt, Weber, Neff, & Rief, 2010; Orlando, Manfredini, Salvetti, & Bosco, 2007).

A number of methods and therapies have been developed to manipulate brain systems including transcranial magnetic stimulation (TMS), deep brain stimulation (DBS), and neurofeedback (NFB). Each of these methods has strengths and weaknesses. Some success has been reported with the use of direct stimulation of cortical and subcortical areas using TMS and DBS. DBS of the periaqueductal gray (PAG), internal capsule, and sensory thalamus has been shown to be an effective long-term treatment for chronic pain in selected groups of patients (Bittar et al., 2005). However, the invasive nature of DBS is an obvious drawback, especially considering that it is not effective in all patients (Bittar et al., 2005). TMS has shown potential as a short-term treatment for the alleviation of chronic neuropathic pain (Lefaucheur, Drouot, Keravel, & Nguyen, 2001; Lima & Fregni, 2008), but there is no evidence that there are lasting benefits (Lefaucheur, 2006). NFB has been used as a method of noninvasive central modulatory control for the treatment of pain for a number of years with mixed success (Jensen, Hakimian, Sherlin, & Fregni, 2008; Jessup, Neufeld, & Merskey, 1979; Nestoriuc et al., 2008).

Sawamoto et al. (2000) showed that the anterior cingulate cortex and parietal operculum/insula area are activated during painful stimulus. Most pain conditions produce an elevation of beta power on quantitative EEG (QEEG) as a response to painful stimulation (Stern, Jeanmonod & Sarnthein, 2006; Walker, 2011).

NFB is becoming an increasingly popular modality of therapy utilized for reduction of this beta activity and potential pain amelioration (Walker, 2011). In addition to localized beta activity reduction by a standard 1 to 2 electrode NFB, a more specific NFB method called Low Resolution Electromagnetic Tomography (LORETA) capable of targeting specific pain matrix anatomical structures may help in diminishing pain (Koberda, Moses, Koberda, & Koberda, 2012; Thatcher, 2013). For example, the insular cortex and anterior cingulate have been identified as potential targets of NFB for pain control (Moisset & Bouhassira, 2007). An additional enhancement in specificity is the use of a comparison to an age-matched normative database using "live" or real-time Z scores (Thatcher, 1999, 2000). The recent introduction of 19-electrode Z-score LORETA NFB equipment has generated hopes for an improvement of NFB efficiency (Koberda et al., 2012; Thatcher, 2010, 2013).

Previous reports from my clinic described high effectiveness of LORETA Z-score NFB in the treatment of many neuropsychiatric disorders (Koberda, 2012; Koberda, Moses, & Koberda, 2012; Koberda et al., 2012).

In Z-score NFB, a real-time comparison to an age-matched population of healthy subjects simplifies protocol generation and allows clinicians to target modules and hubs that indicate dysregulation and instability in networks related to symptoms (Thatcher, 2013). Z-score NFB increases specificity in operant conditioning, and provides a guide by which extreme Z-score outliers are linked to symptoms, and then reinforced toward states of greater homeostasis and stability. The goal is increased efficiency of information processing in brain networks related to the patient's symptoms (Thatcher, 2013).

In our clinic more than 235 patients suffering from variety of neuropsychiatric disorders have completed Z-score LORETA NFB therapy and many of them presented also with chronic pain.

This chapter describes the treatment of selected pain and headache cases from our neurological clinic using both 19-channel surface Z-score NFB, and 19 channels LORETA Z-score NFB (NF1 and NF2, Neuroguide program-Applied Neuroscience, Inc.). The cases presented include migrainous headache and fibromyalgia (FMS). Migraine is a common, disabling, and often progressive disorder characterized by increased excitability of the central nervous system (Ambrosini, deNoordhout, Sandor, & Schoenen, 2003; Lipton & Bigal, 2005). It occurs in 18% of women and 6% of men in the USA with peak prevalence in individuals between the ages of 25 and 55 (Lipton et al., 2007). FMS is a chronic pain syndrome. The key symptoms of FMS are widespread pain, disturbed sleep, fatigue, and depressed mood (Bennett, 2009; Bennett, Jones, Turk, Russell, & Matallana, 2007). FMS affects 2–7% of the general population and predominantly affects females (Bannwarth et al., 2009).

Protocol selection was based on the patient's symptoms using a "symptom check list," as well as QEEG/LORETA characteristics. Patients with defined pain matrix LORETA dysregulations were frequently subjected to specifically targeted LORETA NFB therapy if they were resistant to the "symptom check list" treatment. Mostly anterior cingulate and insular cortex were targeted. The most frequently applied symptoms for programming from the "symptom check list" were chronic pain, FMS, headache, anxiety, and depression. Neuropathic pain, musculoskeletal pain, and intrinsic connectivity network (ICN) 4 were also used for achieving best results (Thatcher, 2010). Patient's sessions were frequently alternated between surface NFB and LORETA NFB, depending on the degree of elevated beta power or the degree of LORETA pain matrix dysregulation before a particular session.

A commercially available computerized neurocognitive testing was used for the initial assessment of two patients (NeuroTrax Corp, Bellaire, TX). Neurotrax Corp. cognitive testing is a computerized neuropsychological assessment where a patient is compared to aged and education-matched healthy controls where mean = 100 with 1 standard deviation (SD) = 15. QEEG analysis was completed using commercially available Neuroguide software (Applied Neuroscience, Inc.) and previously recorded 19-channel digital electroencephalogram (EEG).

Approximately 1–3 min of artifact free-closed eyes EEG segments were selected after previously recording EEG with the Deymed, Truscan 32, (Deymed Diagnostic, Payette, ID) and subjected to further QEEG analysis.

NFB therapy consisted of 30-min sessions once or twice a week using mostly auditory feedback.

CASE 1

A 59-year-old physician developed neuropathic pain in his groin after a urological procedure. The pain was reported as burning in character and lasting all day. The patient was treated with multiple antipain medications including narcotics. He was also treated with pain management using multiple nerve blocks with no significant improvement. Due to overlapping resistance to the antidepression medications, he was treated with electroconvulsive therapy (ECT), which subsequently may have contributed to his possible cognitive problems. Computerized neurocognitive testing was grossly unremarkable with only mildly below expected memory score (expected 100). Based on the patient report, ECT did not result in any mood improvement.

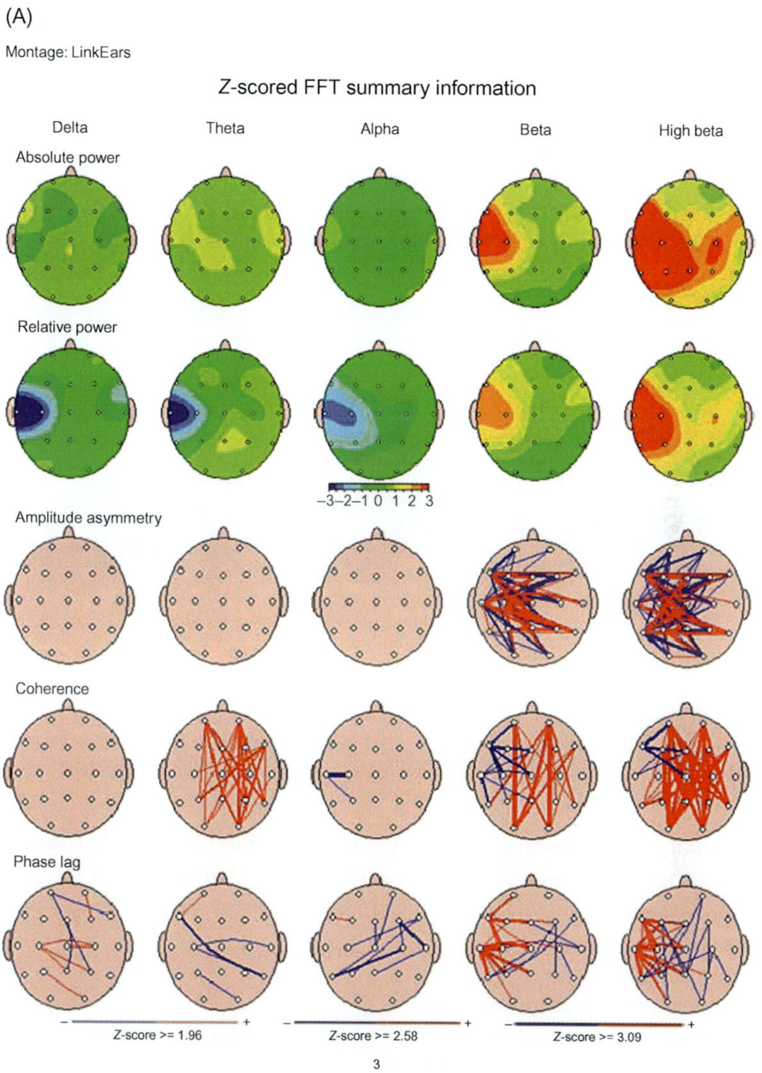

FIGURE 6.1 (A) QEEG before NFB of 59-year-old male with chronic neuropathic pain-marked increase in frontal and temporal beta power was recorded. QEEG compares the data to normal controls with color coding based on SD—green color indicates regions where values of power were between 0–1 SD above database mean; yellow color between 1–2 SD; red color values of power between 2–3 SD.

continued

CASE 1 *(cont'd)*

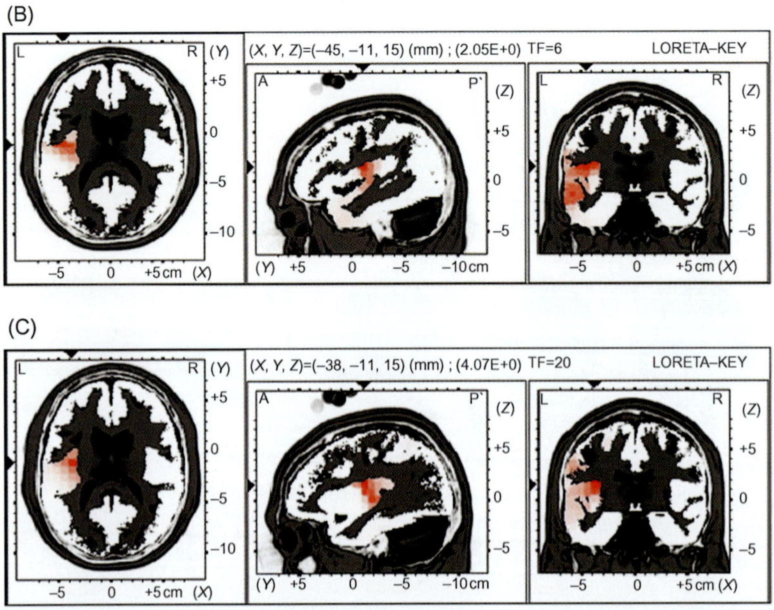

FIGURE 6.1 (B and C) LORETA before NFB -59-year-old patient with chronic neuropathic pain. B shows the left insular area (in red) of dysregulation in theta frequency. C shows the left insular area of dysregulation in beta frequency.

This patient was referred to me by a local psychiatrist for NFB therapy due to refractory to conventional medical treatment pain and depression. His initial QEEG maps showed marked elevation of temporal beta power (Figure 6.1A).

The LORETA showed an increase in the left insular cortex of theta and beta activity (Figure 6.1B and C).

After just four sessions of Z-score LORETA NFB, the patient reported major improvements of his symptoms—80% of neuropathic pain reduction as well as marked improvement of his depression (self-reported). Subsequent QEEG showed major reduction of temporal beta power and LORETA demonstrated resolution of the left insular cortex theta and beta dysregulation (Figure 6.2A and B).

Unfortunately, due to reoccurring symptoms (which is always associated with elevated beta activity on EEG), this patient frequently comes back for more NFB sessions. He has completed 65 sessions so far. Overall, the improvement rate reported by the patient has plateaued at 50% for both pain and depression.

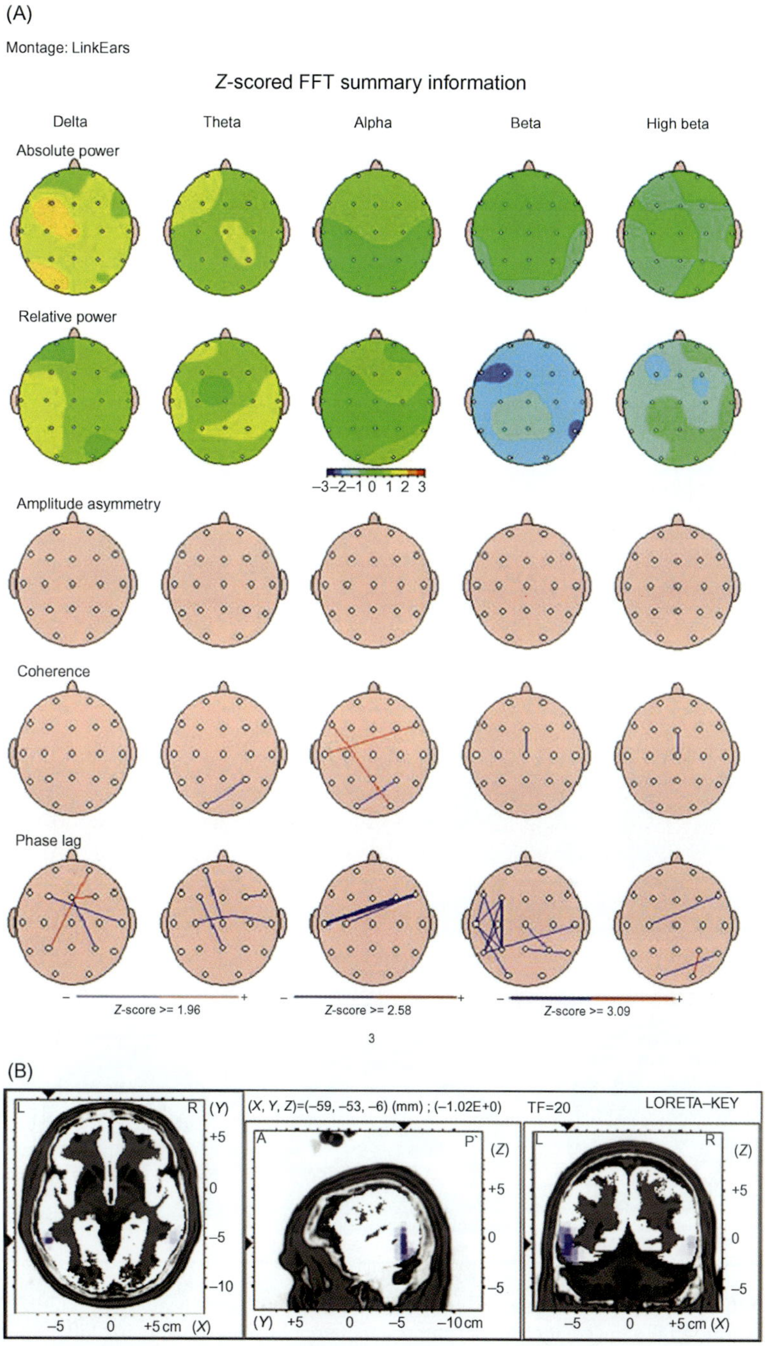

FIGURE 6.2 (A) QEEG of 59-year-old patient with chronic pain showed, after initiation of NFB, resolution of previously elevated beta power. (B) LORETA of 59-year-old patient after the initiation of NFB showed a resolution of dysregulation of insular cortex.

CASE 2

Fifty-eight-year-old female with long-standing history of chronic tension and migrainous headaches, FMS, restless legs syndrome, and peripheral neuropathy expressed interest in NFB. She has been already on multiple medications and followed by pain management.

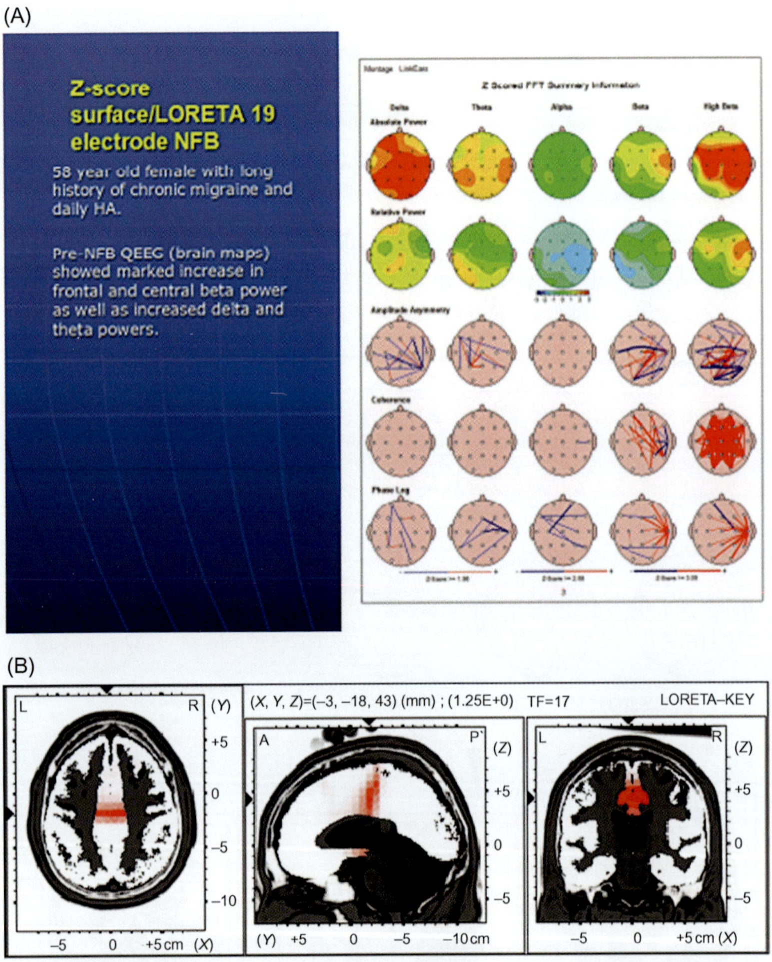

FIGURE 6.3 (A) Fifty-eight-year-old female with chronic headaches–LORETA before NFB showed increased central and temporal beta power. (B) Fifty-eight-year-old female with chronic headaches–LORETA showed area of electrical dysregulation in the cingulate gyrus-Brodmann's area (BA) 24 (area in red).

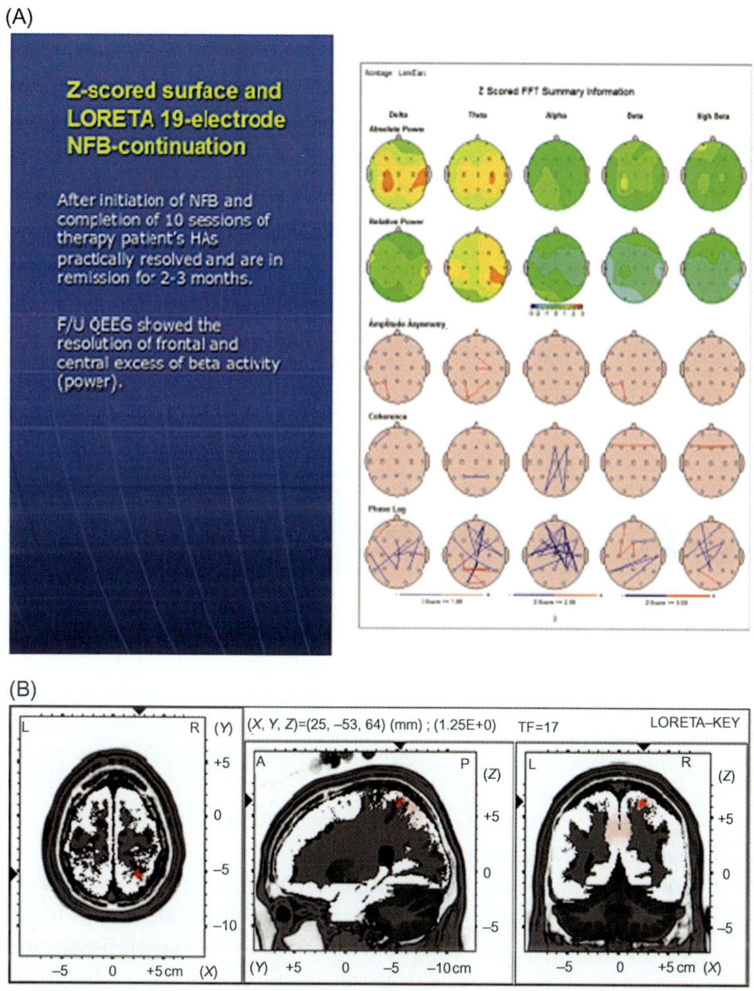

FIGURE 6.4 (A) Fifty-eight-year-old female with chronic headaches–QEEG after the course of NFB resolution of the previously elevated beta power is noted. (B) Fifty-eight-year-old female with chronic headaches after the course of NFB resolution of the dysregulated cingulate electrical activity.

Her QEEG showed marked elevation of central beta power as well as increased delta and theta powers (Figure 6.3A). LORETA imaging indicated electrical dysregulation in the cingulate cortex-BA-24 (Figure 6.3B). After two sessions of LORETA Z-score NFB she reported marked improvement of her chronic pain and headaches and decided not to

continued

CASE 2 (*cont'd*)

continue visits with pain management since her symptoms were resolving. Repeated QEEG during the pain improvement period was completed and showed marked improvement of previously elevated beta power (Figure 6.4A) as well as resolution of BA-24 electrical dysregulation (Figure 6.4B). She completed a total of 20 NFB sessions and has been in remission for 3 months when some exacerbation of symptoms were noted. Subsequently, more NFB sessions were needed to maintain pain control. Exacerbation of pain was always associated with increase in beta activity on EEG.

CASE 3

A sixty-eight male developed shingles, leading to numbness and a burning sensation in both legs. He was subsequently diagnosed with postherpetic neuropathy and sensory-motor polyneuropathy. He was placed on multiple medications including pregabalin (Lyrica) and nortryptyline. His QEEG before NFB showed marked increase in frontal delta power, as well as bilateral temporal beta power (Figure 6.5A).

In addition, the left insular dysregulation was identified on LORETA imaging (Figure 6.5B).

Patient reported mild improvement of pain after the fourth NFB Z-score LORETA session and major improvement after the fifth session. He reported that he could wear shoes again (before NFB was only able to wear sandals due to neuropathic pain). Patient completed initial 12 NFB sessions after which he reported around 60% pain reduction when compared to before NFB. Three months later, the patient came for additional NFB therapy, reporting 50% pain reduction. Subsequent NFB sessions have given him approximately 75% pain reduction when compared to previous NFB period. QEEG completed during the period of pain improvement showed marked decrease of delta and beta overexpression, as well as resolution of the insular dysregulation (Figure 6.6A and B).

Patient still continues NFB with a total of 45 sessions completed so far.

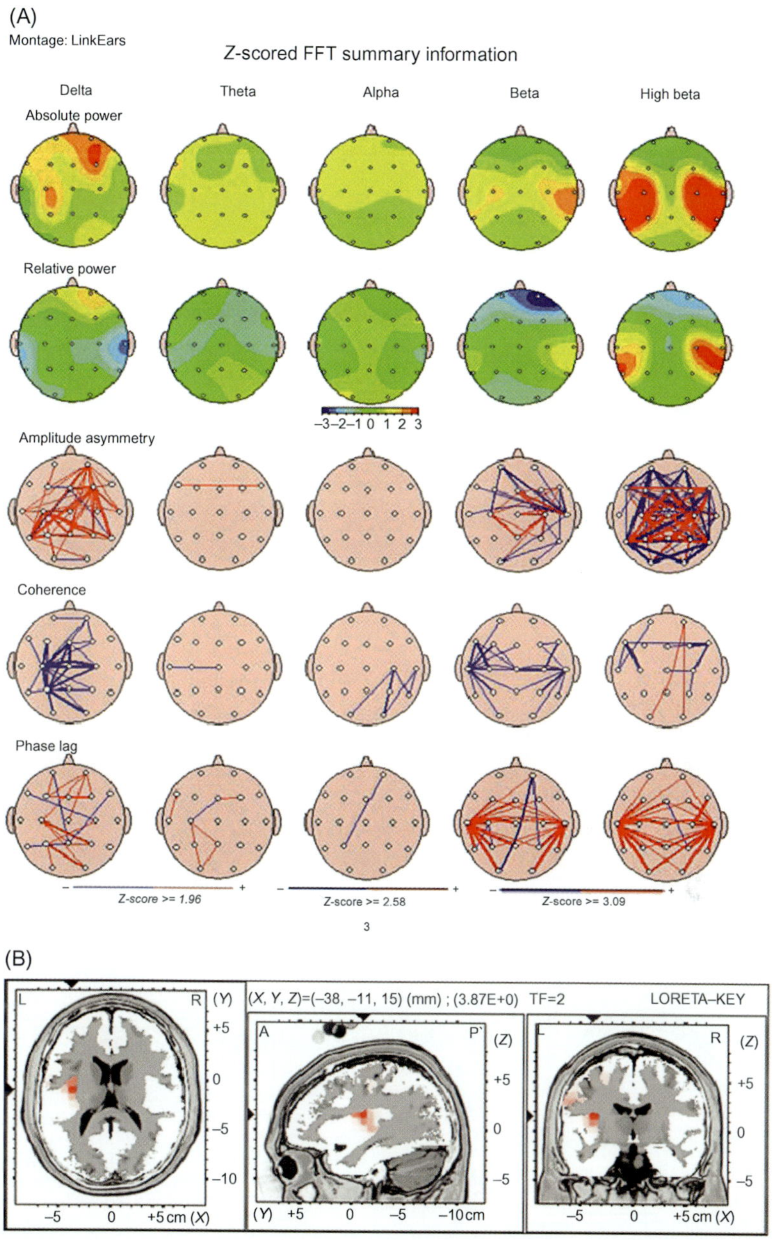

FIGURE 6.5 (A) Sixty-eight-year old male with chronic peripheral neuropathy. QEEG showed bilateral temporal increase of beta power and frontal increase of delta power. (B) Before NFB initiation LORETA showed the left insular cortex dysregulation (in red).

continued

CASE 3 *(cont'd)*

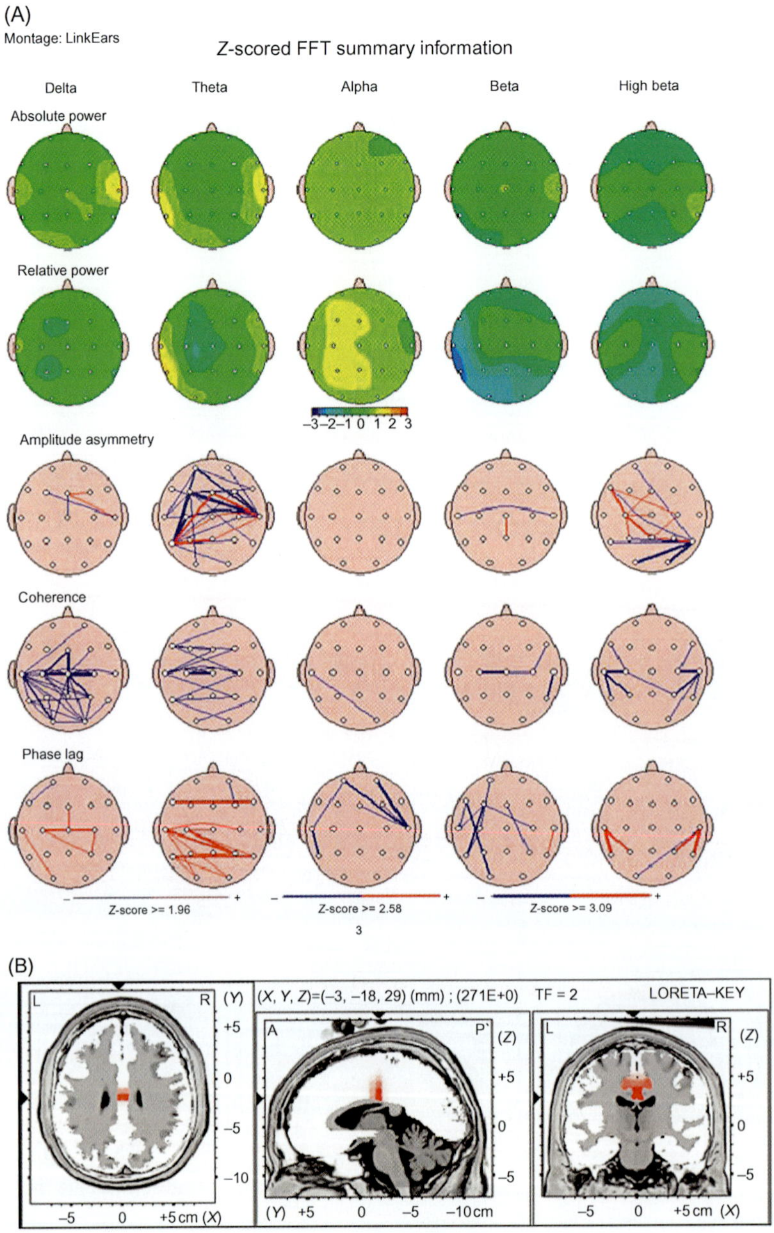

FIGURE 6.6 (A) QEEG after NFB initiation and marked pain reduction showed major improvement in delta and beta power overexpression. (B) After NFB initiation and marked pain reduction LORETA showed the resolution of the left insular cortex dysregulation.

CASE 4

This is a 46-year-old female with 18 months history of the right trigeminal neuralgia. Patient has been taking pregabalin (Lyrica) 100 mg PO twice a day (BID) for neuralgic pain and duloxetine (Cymbalta) for depression and pain. Patient reported that despite taking an increased dose of Lyrica

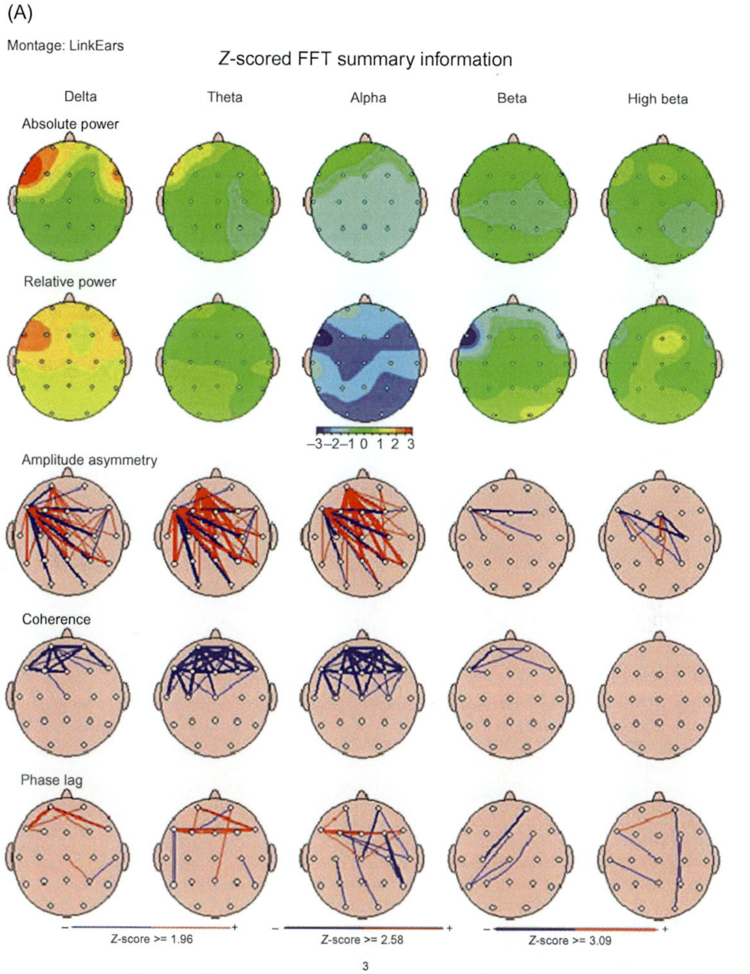

FIGURE 6.7 (A) Forty-six-year-old with chronic pain caused by trigeminal neuralgia. QEEG showed marked increase in frontotemporal delta power and mild elevation of frontocentral beta power.

continued

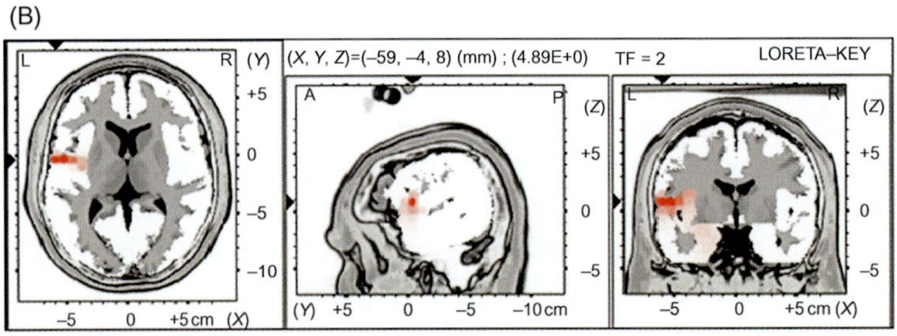

FIGURE 6.7 (B) Before initiation of NFB-LORETA showing area of dysregulation of the left insular cortex (in red).

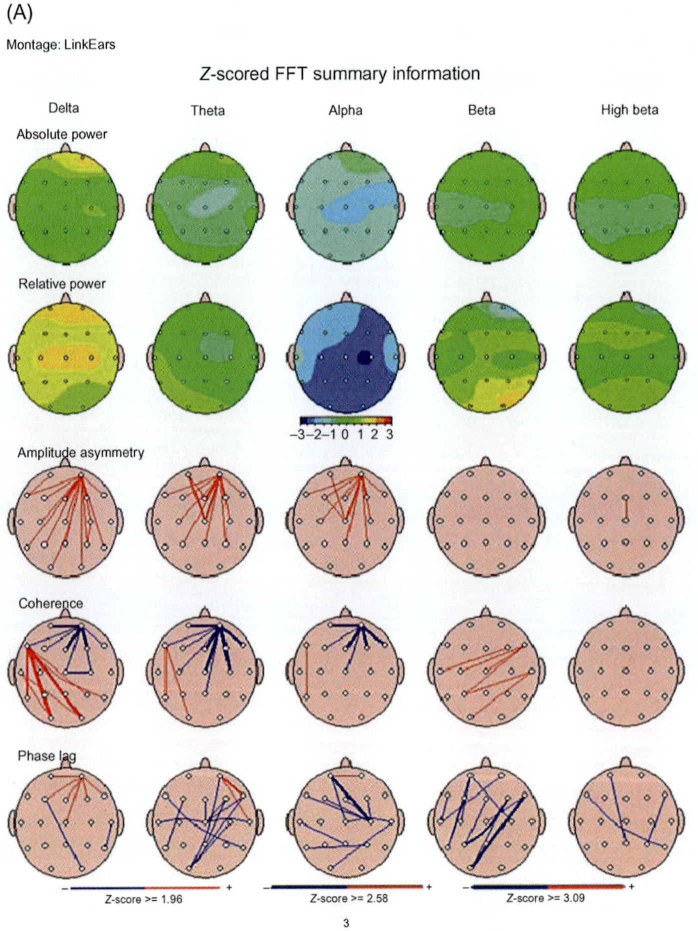

FIGURE 6.8 (A) After NFB initiation and pain resolution QEEG showed marked improvement in both delta and beta overexpression.

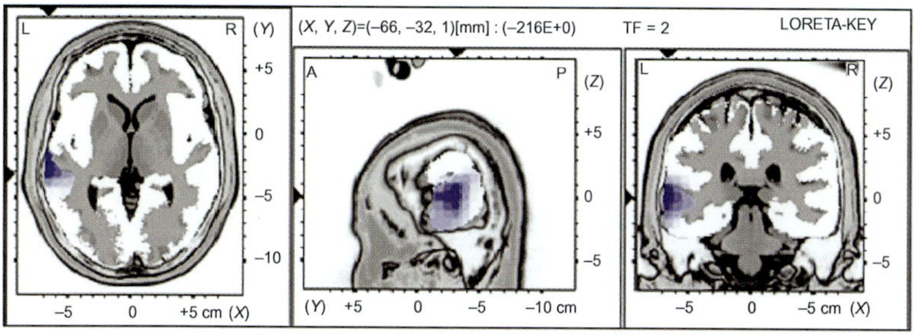

FIGURE 6.8 (B) After NFB initiation and resolution of the pain LORETA showed no more evidence of the left insular cortex dysregulation.

(previously was on 50 mg BID), the pain was not improving and she gained a lot of weight (her weight exceeded over 300 lb). Patient was interested in trying an alternative modality of therapy, exhibiting interest with starting Z-score LORETA NFB. Her initial QEEG showed elevation of frontotemporal delta and theta power, as well as frontal beta power (Figure 6.7A).

In addition, LORETA analysis showed an area of dysregulation in the left insular cortex (Figure 6.7B). She reported marked pain improvement after the first session of NFB, and was able to reduce the dose of Lyrica after the second session and discontinue Lyrica completely after the fourth session. Patient completed 10 sessions of NFB and has been in remission for over 4 months period. QEEG completed after total pain resolution showed an improvement in frontal delta, theta, and beta power, as well as a resolution of insular cortex dysregulation (Figure 6.8A and B).

CASE 5

Fifty-three-year-old female was referred to our clinic due to a 2-year history of neuropathic pain in lower extremities. Patient was previously tried on medications including gabapentin and Cymbalta with minimal improvement of symptoms. QEEG maps completed before NFB showed central area of increased beta power (Figure 6.9A) and

continued

CASE 5 (*cont'd*)

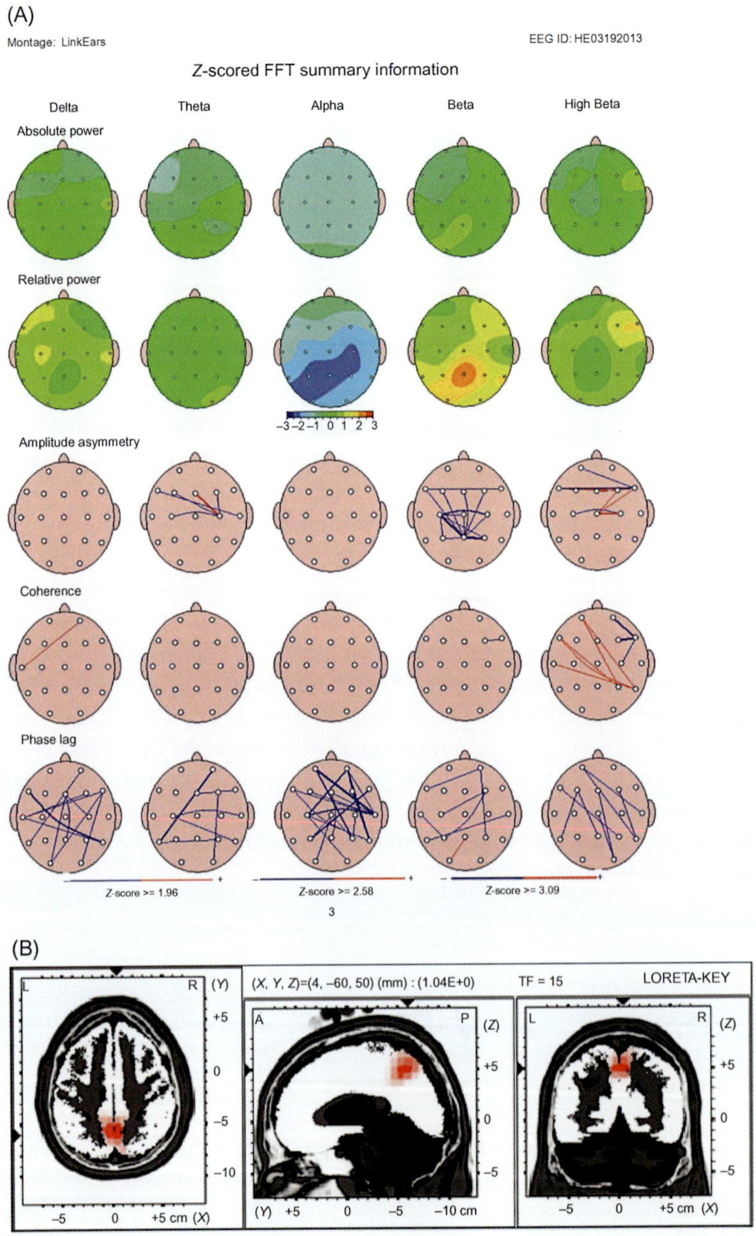

FIGURE 6.9 (A) Fifty-three-year-old female with neuropathic pain before NFB shows area of increased central and occipital beta power. (B) Fifty-three-year-old female with neuropathic pain before NFB-LORETA shows area of electrical dysregulation-B-7 (in red).

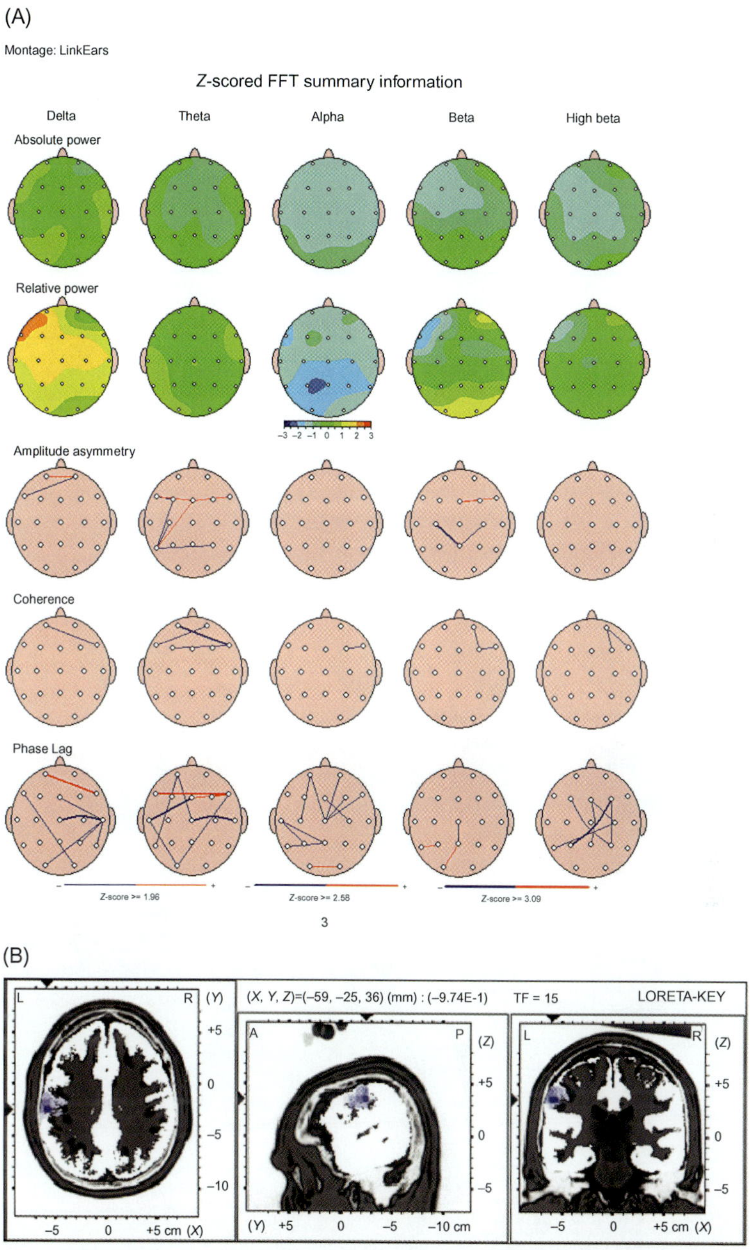

FIGURE 6.10 (A) Fifty-three-year-old female with neuropathic pain QEEG after NFB resolution of previously elevated beta power. (B) Fifty-three-year-old female with neuropathic pain LORETA after NFB resolution of previously dysregulated BA-7 cortical dysregulation.

continued

CASE 5 (*cont'd*)

LORETA imaging indicated BA-7 (secondary sensory-motor cortex) electrical dysregulation (Figure 6.9B). After five sessions of NFB, patient reported an improvement of her symptoms and brain mapping/LORETA revealed resolution of previously dysregulated BA-7 region (Figure 6.10A and B). Total 10 NFB sessions so far was completed.

CASE 6

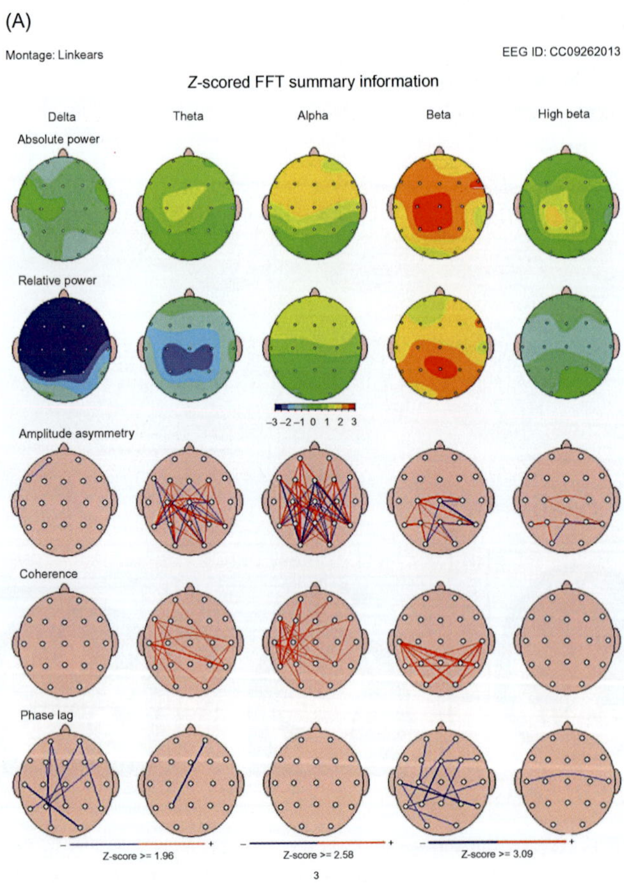

FIGURE 6.11 (A) Sixty-five-year-old male with headaches before NFB-QEEG showed overexpressed frontal and central beta power.

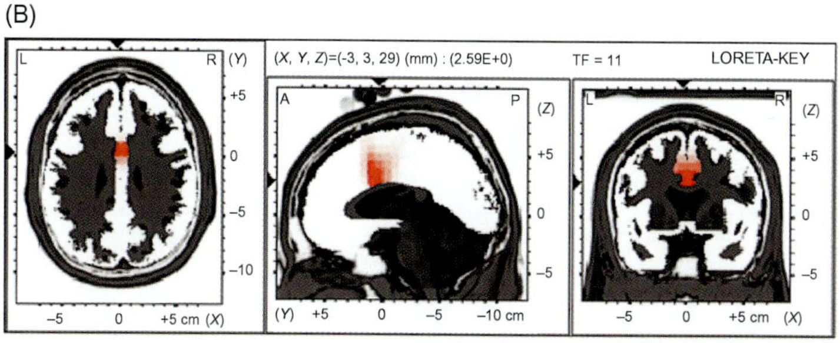

FIGURE 6.11 (B) Sixty-five-year-old male with headaches before NFB-LORETA showed area of cortical dysregulation in the cingulate region-BA-24 (in red).

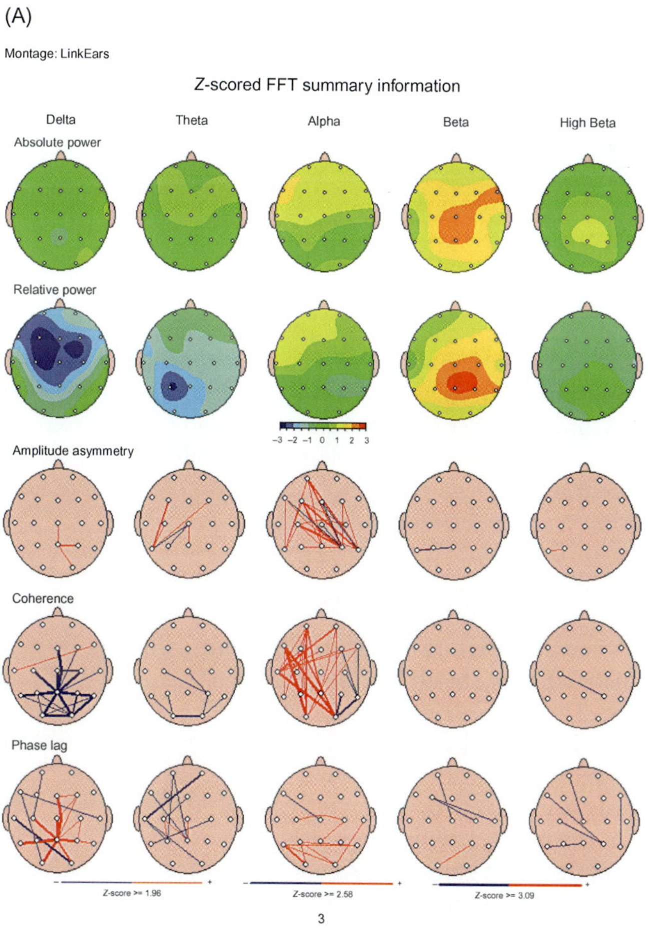

FIGURE 6.12 (A) Sixty-five-year-old male with headaches after NFB-QEEG shows an improvement of previously overexpressed frontal and central beta power.

continued

CASE 6 *(cont'd)*

(B)

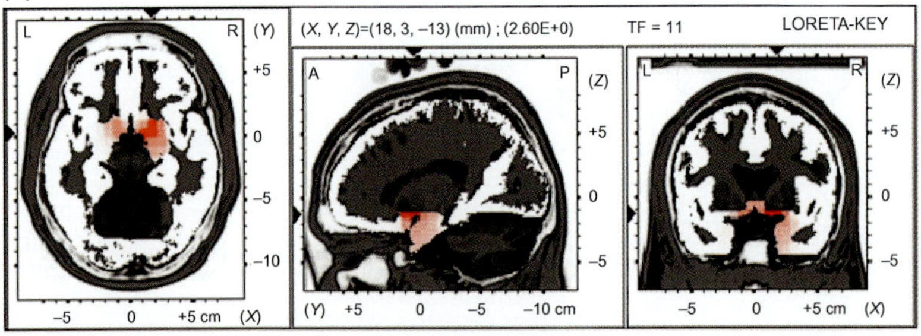

FIGURE 6.12 (B) Sixty-five-year-old male with headaches after NFB-LORETA showed resolution of previously dysregulated BA-24.

This is a 65-year-old male with long-standing history of migrainous and tension headaches frontal in location and sometimes lasting all day. Patient expressed interest in NFB since he noticed an exacerbation in recent headaches with a poor response to medications. His QEEG showed increased frontal and central beta power and LORETA imaging indicated cingulate gyrus (BA-24) electrical dysregulation (Figure 6.11A and B). Initial improvement of his headaches was noted after the first NFB session. After 10 sessions of LORETA Z-score NFB, his headaches markedly improved as well as frontal beta power (Figure 6.12A). LORETA imaging after the course of NFB also showed resolution of previously dysregulated cortical electrical activity (Figure 6.12B). Since this patient recently completed his therapy we are not sure how long his remission will be before possible headaches reoccur.

Table 6.1 contains the summary of 23 patients suffering from headaches who completed Z-score LORETA NFB in my clinic. As we can see most of our patients (22 out of 23) responded very well to NFB therapy with 95% reporting headaches reduction (subjective response). The majority of the patients (17 out of 23) also were found to have an objective improvement (74% improvement of beta power overexpression) on brain mapping reanalysis. Most of the patients noticed an improvement by NFB session #5; however, many of them felt pain improvement just after two to three sessions.

The above cases indicate a remarkable potential of chronic pain reduction by direct cortical regulation using Z-score LORETA NFB. Regardless of the origin of the injury evoking the neuropathic pain, trigeminal or postherpetic neuralgia, peripheral neuropathy, or chronic

TABLE 6.1 Summary of Headache Patients

Patient	Subjective Perception	Objective Reduction of Beta Power	Number of Sessions Needed to Notice Subjective Improvement	Total # NFB Sessions
1. 35, F	Improved	−	2	5
2. 20, F	Improved	+	3	15
3. 53, F	Improved	−	6	7
4. 22, M	Improved	−	2	4
5. 58, F	Improved	+	5	21
6. 50, F	Improved	−	4	10
7. 20, F	Improved	+	3	8
8. 20, F	Improved	+	3	6
9. 44, F	No improvement	−	−	10
10. 24, F	Improved	+	3	26+
11. 52, F	Improved	+	3	10
12. 43, F	Improved	−	4	8
13. 23, F	Improved	+	2	11+
14. 38, F	Improved	+	5	14
15. 36, F TN	Improved	+	2	10
16. 31, M	Improved	+	2	10
17. 49, F	Improved	+	6	7
18. 27, F	Improved	+	3	3
19. 50, F	Improved	+	2	10
20. 57, F	Improved	+	4	26+
21. 38, F	Improved	+	4	10
22. 65, M	Improved	+	1	10
23. 51, M	Improved	+	4	15

TN, trigeminal neuralgia.

spinal pain, similar findings in the cortical dysregulation can be identified. At the same time, very similar therapeutic approaches also can be undertaken in order to ameliorate the above symptoms. Previously, other researchers described efficiency of NFB in pain reduction including headaches, FMS, and other pain syndromes (Stokes & Lappin, 2010;

Walker, 2011). Dr. Stokes reported 70% of migraine patients experienced at least 50% pain reduction. An even better response was reported by Dr. Walker, who found that 54% of patients with recurrent migraines experienced complete headache cessation after completion of NFB, with additional 39% of patients experienced reduction of migraine frequency of greater than 50%. Burning mouth syndrome, complex regional pain syndrome and trigeminal neuralgia are neurological conditions which were also reported to be effectively treated by NFB (Jensen, Greirson, Tracy-Smith, Bacigalupi, & Othmer, 2007; Kenchadze, Iverieli, Okribelashvili, Geladze, & Khachapuridze, 2011; Sime, 2004). Ibric and Dragomirescu (2009) found that of the 74 patients who had been unsuccessfully treated for pain from chronic disease, injury, surgery, or other sources, 68 (92%) reported a clinically significant improvement in their pain following at least 19 sessions of NFB. However, prior reports were usually employing standard 1–2 electrode systems, frequently aiming at reduction of excessive beta cortical activity. The Penfield's sensory homunculus-cortical areas were also described as potential starting NFB targets (Ibric & Dragomirescu, 2009).

Recently Dr. Prinsloo proposed a brain–computer interface as a learning paradigm to augment neuroplasticity for oncological pain management (Prinsloo, Gabel, Lyle, & Cohen, 2013).

The presented chapter reports illustrate marked improvement in pain control after a relatively short course of 19-electrode Z-score LORETA NFB treatments. Our center previously also retrospectively compared Z-score LORETA 19-electrode NFB to traditional one electrode NFB therapy of neuropsychiatric patients, which indicated much more rapid improvement using Z-score 19-electrode NFB training (Koberda et al., 2012). A larger study may be needed to explore the full potential of Z-score 19-electrode NFB for pain modulation, as well as in other medical conditions.

CONCLUSION

Z-score LORETA NFB represents a significant advancement in the field of EEG biofeedback, whereby direct targeting of dysregulated brain structures can be achieved by applying LORETA imaging. The pain cases described above (who have failed prior conventional treatment) are good examples of the effective clinical application of Z-score LORETA NFB in pain management.

Acknowledgment

I would like to give a special thanks to Dr. Eric Harris who contributed in editing of this chapter.

References

Altmaier, E. M., Lehmann, T. R., Russell, D. W., Weinstein, J. N., & Kao, C. F. (1992). The effectiveness of psychological interventions for the rehabilitation of low back pain: A randomized controlled trial evaluation. *Pain, 49*(3), 329–335.

Ambrosini, A., deNoordhout, A. M., Sandor, P. S., & Schoenen, J. (2003). Electrophysiological studies in migraine: A comprehensive review of their interest and limitations. *Cephalalgia, 23*(Suppl. 1), 13–31.

Bannwarth, B., Blotman, F., Lay, K. R., Caubère, J. -P., André, E., & Taïeb, C. (2009). Fibromyalgia syndrome in the general population of France: A prevalence study. *Joint Bone Spine, 76*(2), 184–187.

Bennett, R. M. (2009). Clinical manifestations and diagnosis of fibromyalgia. *Rheumatic Disease Clinics of North America, 35*(2), 215–232.

Bennett, R. M., Jones, J., Turk, D. C., Russell, I. J., & Matallana, L. (2007). An internet survey of 2,596 people with fibromyalgia. *BMC Musculoskeletal Disorders, 8*, 27.

Bittar, R. G., Kar-Purkayastha, I., Owen, S. L., Bear, R. E., Green, A., Wang, S. Y., et al. (2005). Deep brain stimulation for pain relief: A meta-analysis. *Journal of Clinical Neuroscience, 12*, 515–519.

Calvo-Muñoz, I., Gómez-Conesa, A., & Sánchez-Meca, J. (2013). Physical therapy treatments for low back pain in children and adolescents: A meta-analysis. *BMC Musculoskeletal Disorders, 14*, 55.

Caro, X. J., & Winter, E. F. (2011). EEG biofeedback treatment improves certain attention and somatic symptoms in fibromyalgia: A pilot study. *Applied Psychophysiology and Biofeedback, 36*(3), 193–200.

Finnerup, N. B., Sindrup, S. H., & Jensen, T. S. (2010). The evidence for pharmacological treatment of neuropathic pain. *Pain, 150*, 573–581.

Glombiewski, J. A., Hartwich-Tersek, J., & Rief, W. (2010). Two psychological interventions are effective in severely disabled, chronic back pain patients: A randomised controlled trial. *International Journal of Behavioral Medicine, 17*(2), 97–107.

Hanakawa, T. (2012). Neural mechanisms underlying deafferentation pain: A hypothesis from a neuroimaging perspective. *Journal of Orthopaedic Science, 17*(3), 331–335.

Ibric, V. L., & Dragomirescu, L. G. (2009). Neurofeedback in pain management. In T. H. Budzynski, H. K. Budzynski, J. R. Evans, & A. Arbarbanel (Eds.), *Introduction to quantitative EEG and neurofeedback: Advanced theory and applications* (2nd ed., pp. 417–452). Boston, MA: Academic Press.

Jensen, M., Greirson, C., Tracy-Smith, V., Bacigalupi, S., & Othmer, S. (2007). Neurofeedback for treatment of pain associated with complex regional pain syndrome type I: A case series. *Journal of Neurotherapeutics, 11*, 45–53.

Jensen, M. P., Hakimian, S., Sherlin, L. H., & Fregni, F. (2008). New insights into neuromodulatory approaches for the treatment of pain. *Journal of Pain, 9*(3), 193–199.

Jessup, B. A., Neufeld, R. W. J., & Merskey, H. (1979). Biofeedback therapy for headache and other pain: Evaluative review. *Pain, 7*, 225–270.

Kayiran, S., Dursun, E., Dursun, N., Ermutlu, N., & Karamürsel, S. (2010). Neurofeedback intervention in fibromyalgia syndrome: A randomized, controlled, rater blind clinical trial. *Applied Psychophysiology and Biofeedback, 35*(4), 293–302.

Kayiran, S., Dursun, E., Ermutlu, N., Dursun, N., & Karamürsel, S. (2007). Neurofeedback in fibromyalgia syndrome. *Ağrı - The Journal of The Turkish Society of Algology, 19*(3) 47–53.

Keefe, F. J., Schapira, B., & Williams, R. B. (1981). EMG-assisted relaxation training in the management of chronic low back pain. *American Journal of Clinical Biofeedback, 4*(2), 93–103.

Kenchadze, R., Iverieli, M., Okribelashvili, N., Geladze, N., & Khachapuridze, N. (2011). The psychological aspects of burning mouth syndrome. *Georgian Medical News, 194*, 24–28.

Koberda, J. L. (2012). Autistic spectrum disorder (ASD) as a potential target of Z-score LORETA neurofeedback. *NeuroConnections*. edition (ISNR), *4*(winter) 22–24.

Koberda, J. L., Moses, A., & Koberda, P. (2012). Cognitive enhancement using 19-electrode Z-score neurofeedback. *Journal of Neurotherapy, 16*, 224–230.

Koberda J.L., Moses A., Koberda P., & Koberda L. Comparison of the effectiveness of Z-score surface/LORETA 19-electrodes neurofeedback to standard 1-electrode neurofeedback. *Presented during the ISNR meeting in Orlando, FL* 2012.

Lefaucheur, J. P. (2006). New insights into the therapeutic potential of non-invasive transcranial cortical stimulation in chronic neuropathic pain. *Pain, 122*, 11–13.

Lefaucheur, J. P., Drouot, X., Keravel, Y., & Nguyen, J. P. (2001). Pain relief induced by repetitive transcranial magnetic stimulation of precentral cortex. *Neuroreport, 12*, 2963–2965.

Lima, M. C., & Fregni, F. (2008). Motor cortex stimulation for chronic pain: Systematic review and meta-analysis of the literature. *Neurology, 70*, 2329–2337.

Lipton, R., & Bigal, M. (2005). Migraine: Epidemiology, impact and risk factors for progression. *Headache*S3–S13.

Lipton, R., Bigal, M., Diamond, M., Freitag, F., Reed, M. L., & Stewart, W. F. (2007). Migraine prevalence, disease burden, and the need for preventive therapy. *Neurology, 68*(5), 343–349.

Moisset, X., & Bouhassira, D. (2007). Brain imaging of neuropathic pain. *Neuroimage, 37* (Suppl. 1), S80–S88.

Moont, R., Crispel, Y., Lev, R., Pud, D., & Yarnitsky, D. (2012). Temporal changes in cortical activation during distraction from pain: A comparative LORETA study with conditioned pain modulation. *Brain Research, 1435*, 105–117.

Mora, M. C. S., Bleichhardt, G., Weber, D., Neff, A., & Rief, W. (2010). Biofeedback-based cognitive-behavioral treatment for chronic temporomandibular disorders. *Psychotherapeutica, 55*(3), 217–224.

Nestoriuc, Y., Martin, A., Rief, W., & Andrasik, F. (2008). Biofeedback treatment for headache disorders: A comprehensive efficacy review. *Applied Psychophysiology and Biofeedback, 33*, 125–140.

Orlando, B., Manfredini, D., Salvetti, G., & Bosco, M. (2007). Evaluation of the effectiveness of biobehavioral therapy in the treatment of temporomandibular disorders: A literature review. *Behavioral Medicine, 33*(3), 101–118.

Prinsloo, S., Gabel, S., Lyle, R., & Cohen, L. (2013). Neuromodulation of cancer pain. 25 February.

Sawamoto, N., Honda, M., Okada, T., Hanakawa, T., Kanda, M., Fukuyama, H., et al. (2000). Expectation of pain enhances responses to nonpainful somatosensory stimulation in the anterior cingulate cortex and parietal operculum/posterior insula: An event-related functional magnetic resonance imaging study. *Journal of Neuroscience, 1*(20), 7438–7445.

Sime, A. (2004). Case study of trigeminal neuralgia using neurofeedback and peripheral biofeedback. *Journal of Neurotherapeutics, 8*, 59–71.

Stern, J., Jeanmonod, D., & Sarnthein, J. (2006). Persistent EEG overactivation in the cortical pain matrix of neurogenic pain patients. *Neuroimage, 31*(2), 721–731.

Stokes, D. A., & Lappin, M. S. (2010). Neurofeedback and biofeedback with 37 migraineurs: A clinical outcome study. *Behavioral and Brain Functions, 6*, 9.

Thatcher, R. W. (1999). EEG database guided neurotherapy. In J. R. Evans, & A. Abarbanel (Eds.), *Introduction to quantitative EEG and neurofeedback*. San Diego, CA: Academic Press.

Thatcher, R. W. (2000). EEG operant conditioning (biofeedback) and traumatic brain injury. *Clinical EEG, 31*(1), 38–44.

Thatcher, R. W. (2010). LORETA Z-score biofeedback. *Neuroconnections, December*, 9–13.

Thatcher, R. W. (2013). Latest developments in live Z-score training: Symptom check list, Phase reset, and Loreta Z-score biofeedback. (Version of record first published: February 26) *Journal of Neurotherapy*, *17*, 69–87

Walker, J. E. (2011). QEEG-guided neurofeedback for recurrent migraine headaches. *Clinical EEG Neuroscience*, *42*(1), 59–61.

Williams, A. C., Keefe, F., & Vlaeyen, J. W. S. (2010). Pain psychology for non-psychologists. In J. Mogil (Ed.), *Pain 2010—An updated review: Refresher course syllabus* (pp. 161–178). Seattle, WA: IASP Press.

CHAPTER

7

Treating Executive Functioning Disorders Using LORETA Z-Scored EEG Biofeedback

William A. Lambos, PhD and Rebecca A. Williams, BSc

ABF Behavioral Health, Tampa, FL, USA

The frontal lobes perform the most advanced and complex functions in all of the brain, the so-called executive functions. They are linked to intentionality, purposefulness, and complex decision-making. They reach significant development only in humans; arguably, they make us human. The entire human evolution has been termed "the age of the frontal lobes." My teacher, Alexandr Luria, called the frontal lobes "the organ of civilization."

Goldberg, 2009

INTRODUCTION

No aspect of the human brain so distinguishes it—and us—from our animal ancestors more than the prefrontal cortex. Twice the size of the same area in our nearest evolutionary relative, the chimpanzee, the human frontal lobes are characterized by the densest proliferation of neurons in the brain. The interconnections among nerve cells are also staggering in depth and complexity, and the field of cognitive neuroscience has a great deal yet to understand about this most complex and singular of structures.

One of the realities closely intertwined with this state of affairs is that the diagnostic nosology upon which the majority of mental health is based, the DSM, contains no diagnosis corresponding to "executive functioning disorder." In DSM-IV-TR, the only diagnosis available to practitioners was "cognitive disorder NOS." In DSM 5, an effort was

Z Score Neurofeedback.
DOI: http://dx.doi.org/10.1016/B978-0-12-801291-8.00007-8

made to include a chapter on "Neurocognitive Disorders," and a new diagnosis, "Major or Mild Neurocognitive Disorder" is available. However, in nearly every example given, it must be related to etiology, whether it is neurodegenerative disease (e.g., Alzheimer's dementia), genetic abnormality (e.g., Wilson's disease), or traumatic brain injury (as evidenced via neuroimaging such as an MRI scan).

This does not, however, conform to the reality we experience in our own clinic, nor to that we discuss with experienced colleagues who practice in our area. For example, a large number of children and adolescents referred to us with prior diagnoses of AD/HD, oppositional defiant disorder, Asperger's syndrome, and unspecified neurodevelopmental disorder do not, upon careful assessment, turn out to meet the criteria for these conditions. AD/HD in particular seems to be misdiagnosed in more than half the cases referred to us. We believe this because, when we assess these individuals using both qEEG and normed neuropsychological assessments, they show neither brain patterns nor neurocognitive deficits typical of inattention and/or hyperactivity. For example, more than half of the individuals labeled as AD/HD can score significantly above the norms for nonclinical individuals on a continuous performance test or a test of complex attention. Moreover, many of these patients do not respond well to stimulant pharmacotherapy. Although there may have been some decrease in activity level that has been associated with fewer disruptions in the classroom, it is often also the case that grades and study habits have not improved. Side effects for many of these patients are worrisome as well and include a loss of appetite and body weight, insomnia, a turn away from previous social interaction patterns, and other unwelcomed personality changes. Even more worrisome, there is growing evidence that children exposed to stimulant pharmacotherapy are significantly more likely than their nonmedicated peers to experience issues later in life with substance abuse and dependence disorders.

Assessing these clients is further complicated by the unfortunate reality that even where we suspect the underlying issue is one of executive dysfunction, there are very few (if any) performance-based tests which offer the sensitivity and specificity necessary to support the hypothesis. In fact, as a student of Elkhonen Goldberg during postdoctoral certification in clinical neuropsychology, one of us (Lambos) became very attuned to the deficiencies of existing tests of executive functioning. The reasons for this are hypothesized in the following sections.

THE DOMAINS OF EXECUTIVE DYSFUNCTION

Although it is somewhat of an oversimplification, there are essentially six areas that are said to characterize executive functioning, sorted into two broad domains (Goldberg, 2009). Those associated with the dorsolateral prefrontal cortex (DLPFC), sometimes called the *frontal convexity*, comprise Brodmann areas 6, 9, 10, 44, 45 46, and 68. These areas seem to mediate an individual's ability to engage in situation or task appropriate planning activity, organization of the cognitive process, goal-directed behavior, and critical judgment. Temporal sequencing seems also to be associated with this large area of the PFC. It is clear that if any of these capabilities are disrupted by disease, lesion, trauma, or other insult to the brain, attention will most likely also be impaired.

The second major area of the prefrontal cortex is the orbitofrontal prefrontal cortex, which is comprised of Brodmann areas 11, 12, and 47 (Fuster, 1997). This area, sometimes referred to as the *frontal concavity*, is associated with the abilities to control one's impulses, to understand the consequences of one's actions, and the ability to look at the world from another person's point of view—known as *Theory of Mind*.[1]

In our opinion, it is not surprising that dysregulations of either of these areas of the frontal lobes are often characterized as problems of attention and/or problems of hyperactivity, and subsequently labeled as AD/HD. But they are *not* examples of a disorder of attention *per se*. Rather, they reflect deficits in executive functioning as described above. We make this assertion based on thorough assessments of such patients, both biometric and neuropsychological, and on their response to various interventions. We examine the first of these—assessment—in the following section.

THE ASSESSMENT OF EXECUTIVE FUNCTIONING DISORDER PATIENTS

As with every patient we assess, the process begins with a lengthy diagnostic interview. Individuals, whether children or adults, who have been diagnosed with a disorder of attention or of impulse control are asked when the diagnosis was made, by whom, and based on what criteria. In perhaps four out of five cases, no objective criteria have been offered to support the diagnosis. More typically, either a teacher has expressed an opinion to the parents that their child has attention deficit disorder, or a pediatrician or neurologist has supplied the diagnosis

[1]The dorsolateral and orbitofrontal areas hardly comprise the entire PFC. There are well-documented syndromes associated with the medial (or mesial) PFC, as well as many areas associated with motor functions, including speech. However, they are either treated as separate clinical issues (as with expressive aphasia) or much less frequently seen in clinical practice—at least in ours—and so are considered beyond the scope of this chapter.

based on patient or parental description of behavior lasting <20 min. When asked about the typical day for such patients during our own interview, we are more likely to hear evidence of poor organizational skills, lack of planning, insensitivity to the consequences of their choice of behaviors (i.e., not learning from past mistakes), emotional outbursts, and other signs more typical of frontal lobe dysfunction than of AD/HD.

Moreover, we use various assessment instruments with the purpose of differentiating focal disorders of attention from broader problems with executive functioning. These include continuous performance tests (such as the Conners CPT-II), the CNS-VS neurocognitive screening battery, and for younger clients, behavior scales such as the Connors Behavioral Rating Scales (CBRS) and more recently, a well-designed inventory of executive functioning called the Comprehensive Executive Functioning Inventory (CEFI). A qEEG is administered to every client as well.

Looking over our data for the past several years, it is apparent that many patients who have been diagnosed as AD/HD can perform at or above the nonclinical norms on continuous performance tasks. Many can also do well on complex attention tests. This is hard to square with a diagnosis of AD/HD. On the other hand, they may perform poorly on tests better designed to isolate issues with frontal lobe functioning such as the Wisconsin Card Sort (a test of mental flexibility), planning (the Tower of London task), or show consistency across raters as having impulse control issues or poor organization and/or planning skills.

Also worth discussing is whether or not a disorder of attention should be considered an executive functioning problem in its own right. Nearly every test or scale of executive functioning includes some assessment of attention. And especially with respect to complex attention tasks, which involve assessing one aspect of a stimulus over another (such as the Stroop task), it is not clear whether poor performance on complex attention tests should be characterized as a disorder of attention or of executive functioning.

Another issue of importance to the practitioner treating frontal lobe disorders is the complication of *compensatory dysregulations*. The complexity of the PFC, and the importance of its role in guiding global behaviors and choices necessary to meet one's needs—the issue of *agency*—has given rise to a large set of possible compensatory mechanisms that the cortical network can bring to bear when executive functioning is difficult for the impacted individual. For example, dysregulations of the precuneus, an area in the parietal lobe, are quite often seen on qEEG maps of individuals with executive functioning disorders. We believe these dysregulations are, as a rule, compensatory in nature to frontal lobe dysfunction, and hence in such cases it is counterproductive to "chase" such dysregulations as targets of EEG biofeedback. More often than not, the patient reports a worsening of symptoms when one follows that strategy. We have found it far more productive to match symptoms to locations in the cortex associated with the symptomatic difficulties, establish the primacy of the executive dysregulation using independent normed neuropsychological tests, and then follow the best matches between the symptom checklist (SCL) for the presenting problem to choose a protocol. In follow-up qEEG maps, the secondary or compensatory dysregulations resolve themselves in nearly every case as the brain finds a more direct mechanism through which to exert control and restore normative executive functioning.

Our approach to these issues has been both pragmatic and, we believe, scientific. For individuals who appear to have issues that are singularly associated with attention, such as poor performance on the CPT-II but otherwise appear to have intact frontal lobe functioning, we diagnose and typically treat for a disorder of attention. Others, who may suffer from attention deficits in combination with poor working memory, below average mental flexibility, or other attributes of frontal lobe functioning, we consider to have an executive functioning disorder. qEEG brain maps are also used to support one diagnosis over the other. In addition to the dictum of diagnosing dysregulation of qEEG maps based on "location, location, location" (Thatcher, 2012), the comparative matches or mismatches on the SCL in Neuroguide for different symptoms are relied on to guide our diagnostic decisions. Above all else, we never attempt to train are area of the cortex that shows dysregulation if is not part of one of the underlying network nodes or connections for the presenting problem—i.e., we do not "chase dysregulation" just because they are out of the normative range of Z-scores.

Ultimately, diagnoses are merely labels. Patients want help in overcoming their own or their children's academic, social, and emotional difficulties. But as we hope the case studies we present in the chapter will demonstrate, it can make a significant difference what label is used to characterize a functional behavioral health problem. In particular, we have found that the *broader the impact on overall executive functioning* determined in the assessment process, the *less likely* the individual is to benefit from stimulant pharmacotherapy. Further, *the protocols selected in treating with Z-scored LORETA biofeedback for attention deficits or oppositional behavior may be poor choices for treating patients whom are better characterized as suffering from more general problems with executive functioning.*

In general, our experience has led us to believe that if AD/HD (the inattentive type in particular) is defined as a focal deficit in the ability to sustain focus to a repetitive or uninteresting task over a brief period of time (perhaps 15–20 min), then it is a much rarer disorder than published prevalence rates would suggest. On the other hand, disorders of attention that are part of a broader pattern of problems with executive functioning, either of the orbitofrontal or dorsolateral variety, then a majority of individuals, and children in particular, are misdiagnosed as "having" AD/HD when in fact they suffer from more intricate issues with frontal lobe functioning and, hence, are better diagnosed as meeting the criteria for a deficit of executive functioning, however, it may be coded in the DSM.

Finally, and as stated earlier, AD/HD is not the only condition mistaken for disorders of executive functioning. The same or a parallel analysis can be made for a number of other conditions which impact academic and social functioning but which are mischaracterized as personality disorders, reactive attachment disorder, oppositional defiant behavior disorder, and so forth. The case studies that follow are intended to make these points in as salient a manner as possible.

EXECUTIVE DYSFUNCTION CASE STUDIES

Case 1 is a 13-year-old, nonmedicated, male who presented with great difficulties in his ability to organize and plan. His ability to self-direct for projects and long-term assignments was poor, but he was able to do above average work in school with a great deal of support from his mother and his teachers. His mother brought him in for assessment because she was unsure of his capacity to function the following year, when he would be attending high school, and the support from the teachers and school became more difficult to arrange and for the school to sustain.

The assessment revealed poor scores on several areas of frontal lobe functioning, but a nonclinical classification on the Conners CPT-II. The areas in which he showed the largest deficits on the CNS-VS were working memory and cognitive flexibility. Both simple and complex attention scores were within the norm for his age, but he had been diagnosed twice as having attention deficit disorder (once by his physician, a general practitioner, and once by the school psychologist). His parents were very reluctant to place him on stimulants and came to us for alternative treatment.

Following treatment with 19-channel LORETA neurofeedback, Case 1 reported having an increase in his ability to organize and plan his assignments. Both his mother and his teachers reported Case 1 not needing as much support to accomplish his projects on time. Additionally, Case 1 reported an increase in his self-pride because of his newfound independence.

Figure 7.1 shows the pretreatment and post 10 session absolute power maps in the Laplacian montage for the eyes closed condition. The pretreatment maps show significant excess frontal excess power in nearly every frequency, as is expected with DLPFC deficits. Additionally, there

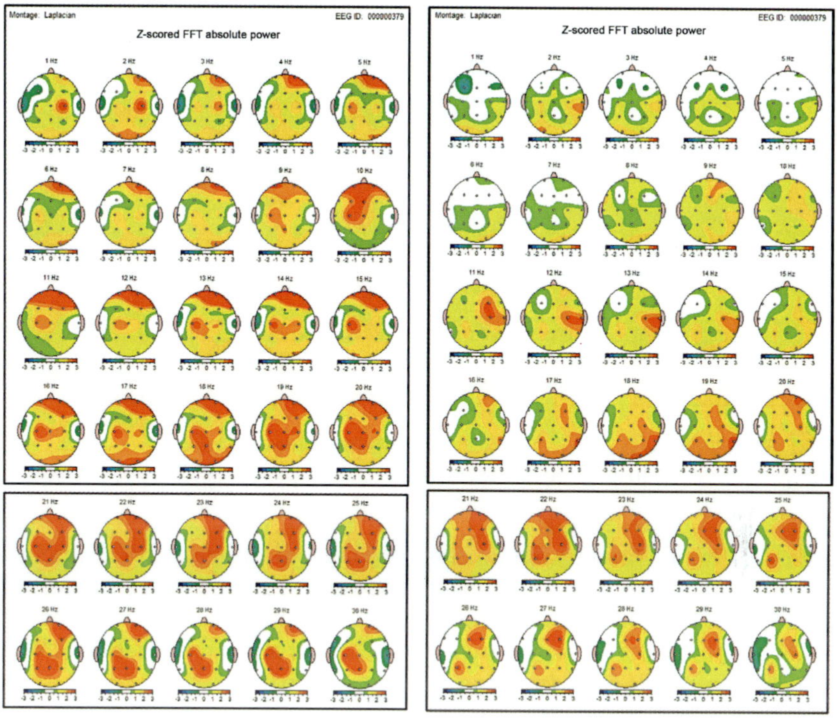

FIGURE 7.1 Case 1, Z-scored FFT absolute power for eyes closed in the Laplacian montage. Pretreatment (left) compared to post 10 sessions (right), symptom driven 19-channel LORETA neurofeedback using protocols associated with executive functioning deficits.

is notable excess power in central and posterior sites in the beta frequency range. Following 10 sessions of symptom driven 19-channel LORETA neurofeedback with the "executive functioning" symptom protocol, there are noteworthy reductions in the excess frontal power in the lower frequencies and to a notable degree a reduction in power dysregulation in central and posterior sites in the beta frequency range.

Figure 7.2 shows LORETA phase lag dysregulation between Brodmann area 9 and Brodmann areas 10, 44, and 45 of the DLPFC. As the hypothesis suggests, executive function deficits that involve planning, organization, and attention are associated with aberrant activity in and between these cortical areas. After 10 LORETA neurofeedback sessions, normalization can be seen in the phase lag metric between these Brodmann areas.

Figure 7.3 shows dysregulations in current source density measures of the DLPFC region at more than three standard deviations, pretreatment. These findings are consistent with symptoms associated with deficits in executive functioning, such as planning, attention, and

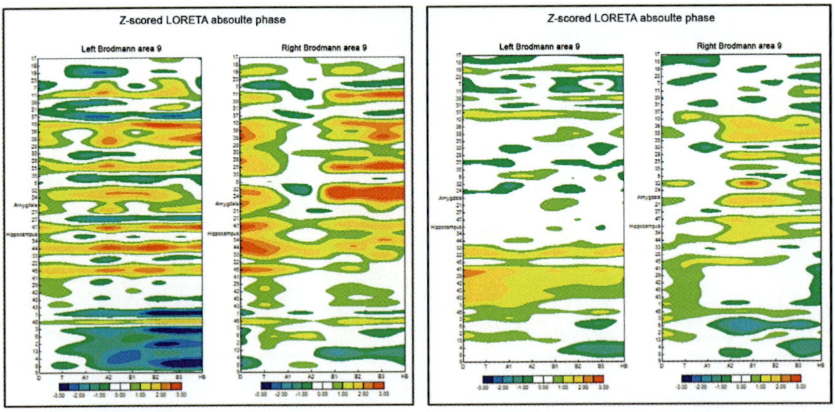

FIGURE 7.2 Case 2, Z-scored LORETA absolute phase measures in the eyes closed condition, pretreatment (left) and post 10 sessions (right) of 19-channel LORETA neurofeedback.

organization. Following 10 sessions of symptom driven LORETA neurofeedback, the current source density measures are normalized to within neurotypical range and client feedback is positive with an increase in his ability to carry out assignment instructions and meet deadlines with little to no outside help from his teachers and parents.

Case 2 is a 15-year-old male prescribed with Concerta (27.0 mg) who presents with poor participation in class and the inability to follow directions. He is described as having insensitivity to others' feelings, and exhibiting poor decision making, inefficient planning, and disorganization. Following 30 sessions of 19-channel symptom driven LORETA neurofeedback in which 3 different SCL matches were established over the course of training and remapping, Case 2 was able to come off of his medication completely and is reported to have improved significantly in his behavior and organizational abilities. Additionally, his theory of mind was reported to improve, and his friendships at school improved significantly.

The Z-scored absolute power measures, seen in Figure 7.4, show frontal power measures of beta frequencies between 12 and 21 Hz are above three standard deviations from the reference population. This finding is consistent with the hypothesis in that there is frontal lobe dysregulation. Following 30 sessions of 19-channel LORETA neurofeedback targeted for symptoms of executive function, a significant reduction in the frontal lobe excess power is evinced. Measures in these frequencies are now within normative limits.

The LORETA phase maps seen in Figure 7.5 show significant dysregulation in connectivity between Brodmann area 9 and a large portion of the cortex. With respect to frontal lobe function, the relationship

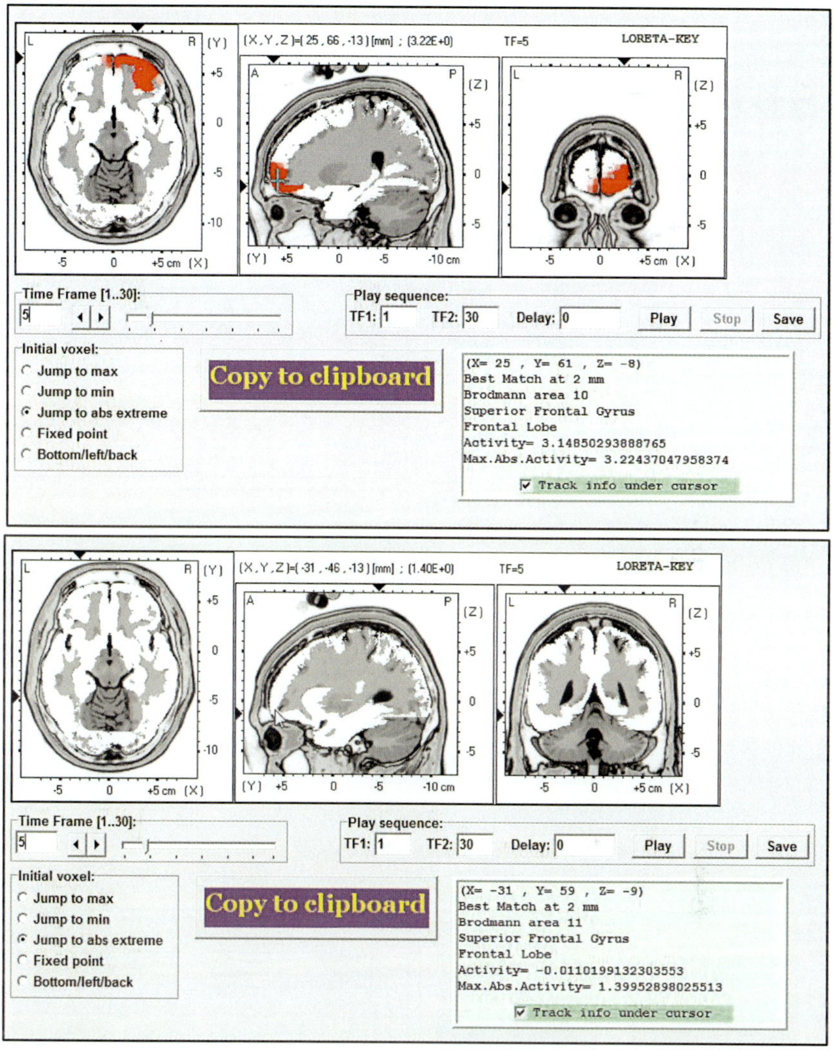

FIGURE 7.3 Case 1, eyes closed LORETA current source density dysregulation in the pretreatment (top) measures on the frontal gyri in the DLPFC. Post 10 19-channel LORETA neurofeedback (bottom) DLPFC measures.

between Brodmann area 9 and Brodmann areas 47 (orbital frontal) and 45 (DLPFC) and the hippocampus and amygdala is important. The pretreatment shows noteworthy aberrations in phase connectivity between the DLPFC regions, contributing to this individual's deficits with organization and attention as well as with theory of mind. LORETA neurofeedback successfully improved phase measures in these areas and

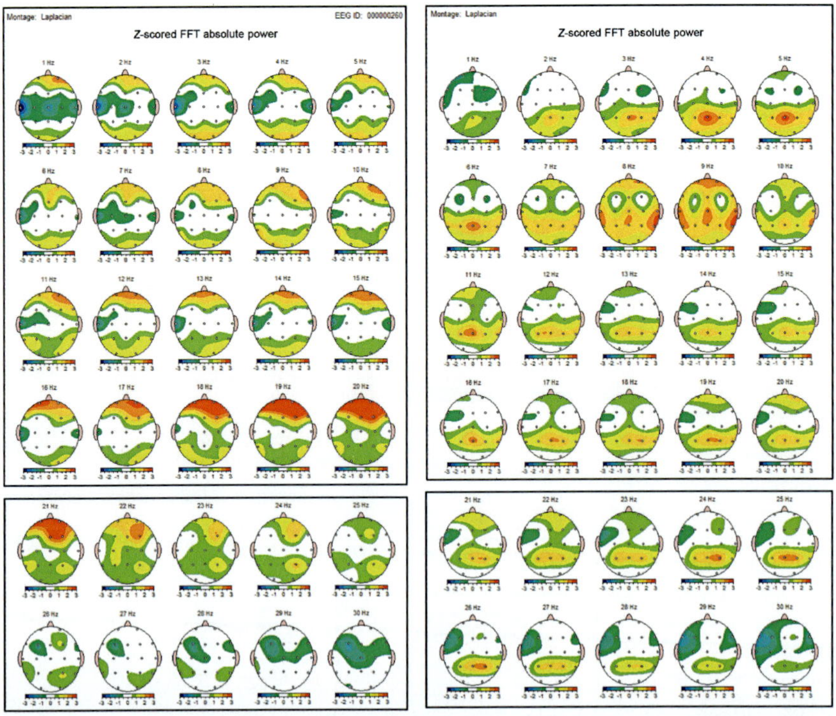

FIGURE 7.4 Case 2, Z-scored FFT absolute power for the eyes closed condition in the Laplacian montage. Pretreatment (left) compared to post 30 sessions of 19-channel LORETA neurofeedback (right).

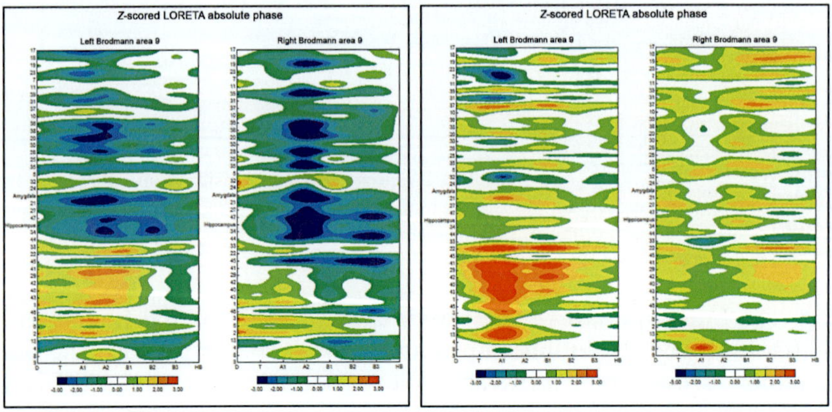

FIGURE 7.5 Case 2, pretreatment Z-scored LORETA absolute phase (left) compared to post 30 sessions of 19-channel LORETA neurofeedback (right), eyes closed.

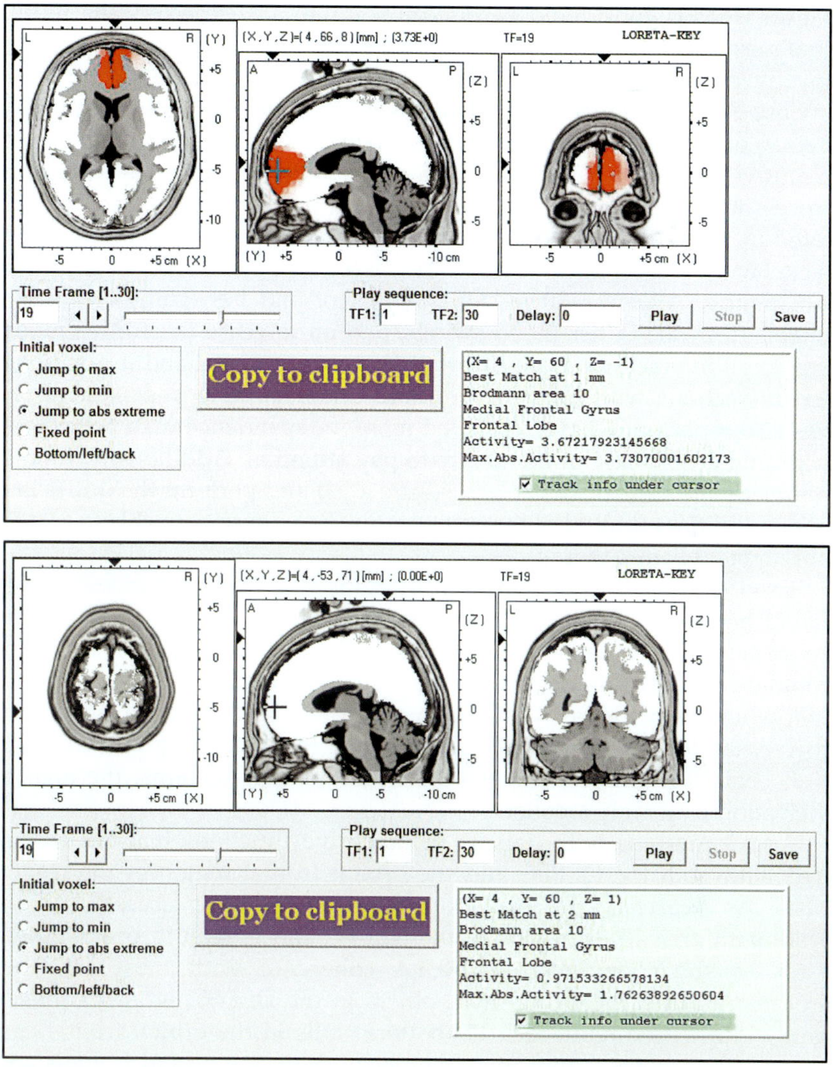

FIGURE 7.6 Case 2, current source density measures pretreatment (top) and following 30 sessions of LORETA neurofeedback (bottom), eyes closed.

improving Case 2's attention and organizational abilities as well as his theory of mind.

Figure 7.6 shows the current source density measures in the DLPFC above three standard deviations from the reference population, pretreatment. This area is, as mentioned previously, directly involved with planning, organization, sequencing, and attention. Post 30 sessions of LORETA neurofeedback, current source density measures are well within what is considered neurotypical limits. As expected, the individual's executive functioning, as reported by self, parents and teachers, improved markedly.

Case 3 is an 18-year-old female who presents with poor empathy, theory of mind, and disinhibition. Aside from these orbital frontal executive functions, Case 3 also presents with attention and auditory processing deficits, poor social interactions, and anxiety. Case 3 participated in 30 sessions of symptom driven 19-channel LORETA neurofeedback, with a focus on symptoms associated with poor executive functioning. After the 30 sessions, the client and her family reported a notable decrease in her mood swings, and an increase in positive mood. Her social interactions were reported to have improved and it was noted her interactions with others were more understanding and patient. She was also reported to have displayed more independence with her schoolwork and an increase in her ability to pay attention. Additionally, following treatment, Case 3 was able to secure a job and perform the duties and responsibilities required of the position. She had never been able to sustain employment before therapy.

Based on Case 3's presenting conditions it is expected excess power would be seen in the frontal lobe region (Figure 7.7). Power is, in some frequencies, more than three standard deviations from the reference population. This dysregulation is seen in every frequency band. Following 30 sessions of LORETA neurofeedback, the excess frontal power has largely normalized throughout the frequency spectrum. In high beta frequencies, where some dysregulation remains, the area of aberration is notably smaller.

Case 3 presents with deficits in executive functions that are associated with both the DLPFC and the orbital frontal region of the frontal lobes. As expected, dysregulations in the Brodmann areas are seen. Brodmann area 10 (top) falls in the DLPFC and is seen in pretreatment maps to show significant LORETA coherence with most all other Brodmann areas, including those others in the DLPFC, in all frequency bandwidths. Brodmann area 11 (bottom) falls in the orbital frontal cortex and also shows significant coherence within the orbital frontals and the DLPFC and other Brodmann areas across the entire cortex. After 30 sessions of LORETA neurofeedback with a focus on executive function deficits, coherence aberrations are nearly normalized in all between Brodmann 10 and 11 and all other areas in most frequencies. As reported by the client, executive functioning showed noteworthy improvements as well as other cognitive functions, such as math abilities and auditory processing functions (Figure 7.8).

Figure 7.9 shows excess current source density in Brodmann area 38 at nearly four standard deviations above the normative database. This area is responsible for executive functions, such as theory of mind,

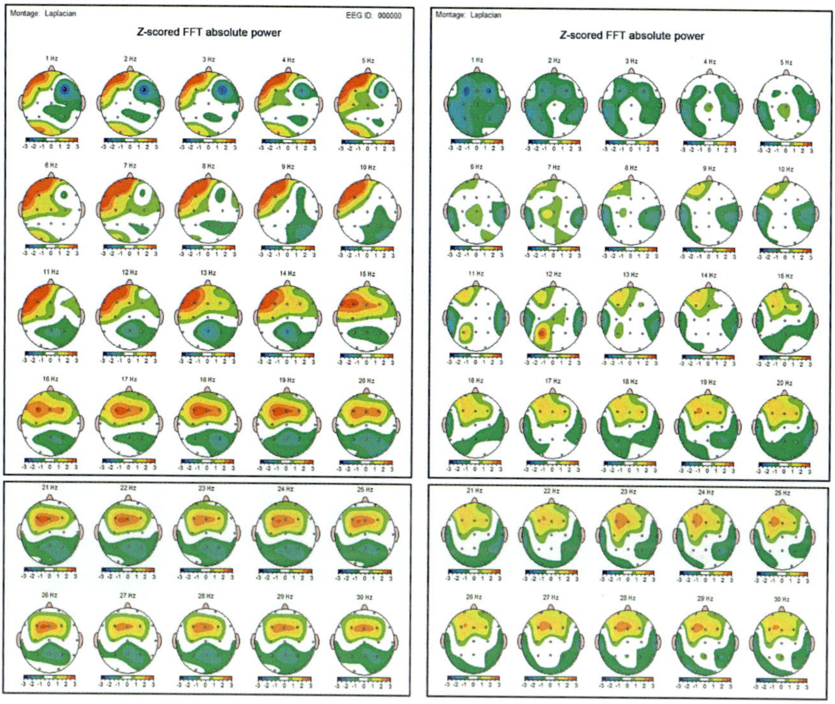

FIGURE 7.7 Case 3, Z-scored FFT absolute power for the eyes open condition in the Laplacian montage. Pretreatment (left) compared to post 30 sessions of 19-channel LORETA neurofeedback (right).

inhibition, and empathy. Figure 7.10 shows dysregulation in current source density measures in Brodmann area 9, a structure involved in executive function tasks such as organization, planning, and attention. Similarly, the dysregulation is above three standard deviations from the reference population. After 30 sessions of LORETA neurofeedback focused on executive function symptoms, there is normalization in the frontal lobes. Likewise, the reported symptoms associated with these areas have improved significantly.

CONCLUSION

Executive functioning represents what are probably the most complex set of cortical interrelationships in the brain. The goals of using previous learning and memories, knowledge of causal relationships, the ability to project and assess the impact of each choice of action at every point along the path of daily commerce of the environment are

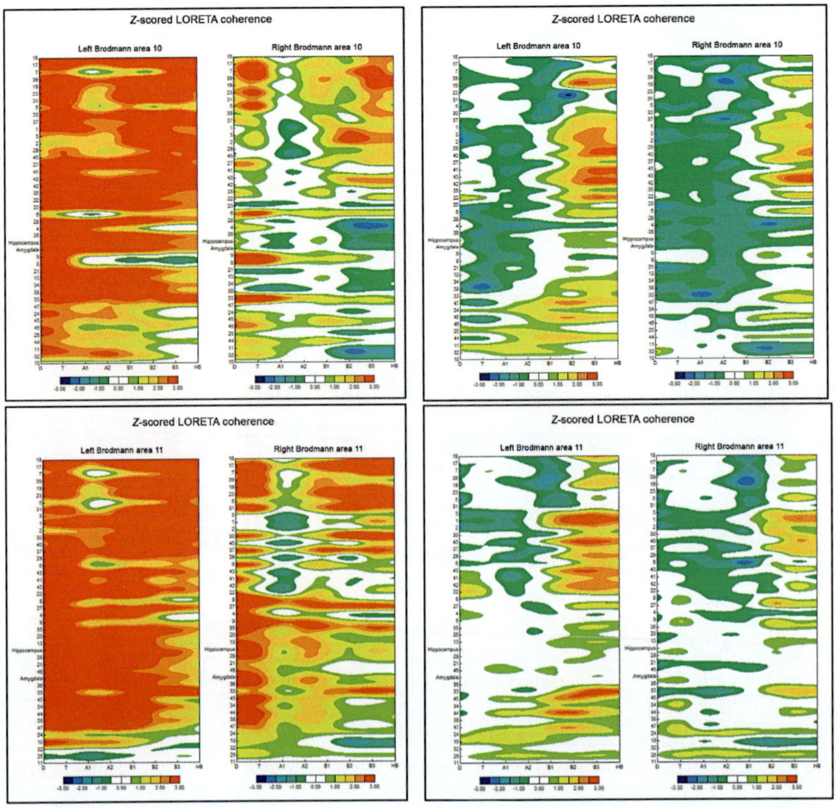

FIGURE 7.8 Case 3, pretreatment Z-scored LORETA coherence (left) compared to post 30 sessions of 19-channel LORETA neurofeedback (right), eyes open.

staggeringly complex. It must, by necessity, involve creating multiple possible future realities and comparing each against the criteria of how well it meets the ongoing needs of the individual without resulting in unwanted impacts on others. Always of importance is maintaining equanimity and as positive a possible view of the individual as perceived by his or her peers.

Given the complexity and subtlety of the task of successful executive functioning, it is really not surprising that it has been overlooked as a unitary phenomenon in our prevailing mental health nosology, the DSM. It has been easier to identify local dysregulations and attempt to normalize them in hopes that the patient will improve. But chasing dysregulations for the patient who suffers from a disorder of one or more aspects of executive functioning is among the poorest choices of treatments for such people.

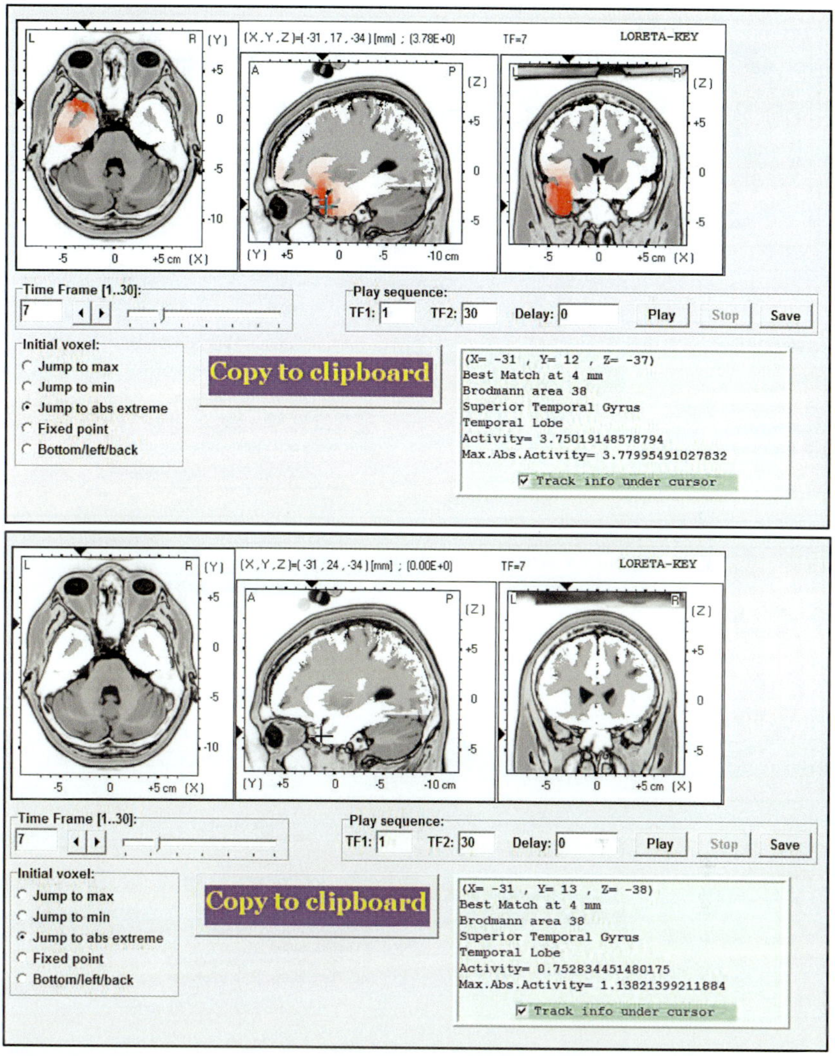

FIGURE 7.9 Case 3, current source density measures pretreatment (top) and following 30 sessions of LORETA neurofeedback (bottom), eyes open.

Rather, following the strategy we have outlined in this chapter, we hope to have demonstrated that if a careful and accurate assessment is achieved, and the feedback protocols are guided by choice of symptom and location matching, such patients can be helped as readily as most others with less complex dysregulations. Finally, since so few of the professionals who refer these patients for treatment have likely

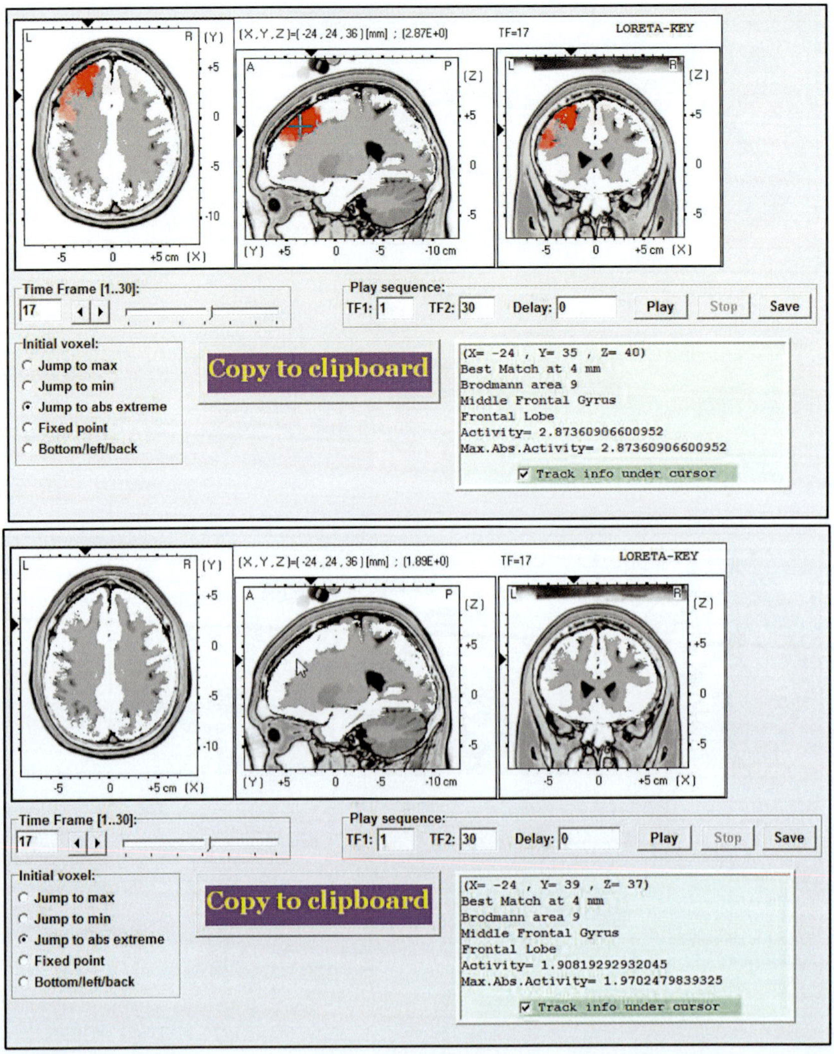

FIGURE 7.10 Case 3, current source density measures pretreatment (top) and following 30 sessions of LORETA neurofeedback (bottom), eyes open.

misdiagnosed them, one can never assume the accuracy of a preexisting diagnosis.

Fortunately, symptom guided LORETA biofeedback on such patients, once properly assessed, offers a very successful potential interventional strategy for these patients. It is, as of this writing, perhaps the only intervention currently available that can quickly and efficiently help patients with executive functioning disorders.

References

Fuster, J. M. (1997). *The prefrontal cortex: Anatomy, physiology, and neuropsychology of the frontal lobe* (3rd ed.). Philadelphia, PA: Lippincott-Raven.

Goldberg, E. (2009). *The new executive brain: Frontal lobes in a complex world* (Kindle Locations 110–112). Kindle Edition.

Thatcher, R. W. (2012). *Handbook of quantitative electroencephalography and EEG biofeedback.* St. Petersburg, FL: ANI Publishing Co.

CHAPTER

8

Combining LORETA Z-Score Neurofeedback with Heart Rate Variability Training

Michael Thompson, Lynda Thompson and Andrea Reid-Chung

ADD Centre & Biofeedback Institute of Toronto, Mississauga, ON, Canada

INTRODUCTION

This chapter focuses on using low-resolution electromagnetic tomography (LORETA) neurofeedback (LNFB) in clinical practice. It will address three areas: (i) appropriate assessment and treatment planning, (ii) intervention that combines LNFB with heart rate variability (HRV) training, and (iii) how to explain to patients, parents, and referring physicians the rationale for the combined intervention, citing the relevant neuroanatomy and neurophysiology using simple terminology.

Experienced clinicians typically use a multimodal approach to help their clients. At the ADD Centre and Biofeedback Institute of Toronto, a combination of neurofeedback (NFB; single channel, two channel, and LORETA Z-score NFB, as appropriate), biofeedback (BFB, especially HRV training but also electromyogram (EMG), temperature and electrodermal response (EDR; when needed), educational approaches (metacognitive strategies during sessions), and counseling are all used on a regular basis. Other modalities that include transcranial direct current stimulation (tDCS), passive infrared hemoencephalography (pIR HEG), audiovisual stimulation (AVS), and Cogmed (computer exercises for home use to improve attention and memory) may additionally be used in selected patients. There is always discussion of diet, sleep, and exercise, too, with encouragement to optimize these variables. NFB and HRV training are the core components that reliably produce

Z Score Neurofeedback.
DOI: http://dx.doi.org/10.1016/B978-0-12-801291-8.00008-X

long-lasting results. Both approaches train oscillatory systems and they are complementary because they influence many of the same structures in the nervous system due to heart–brain links, as discussed in detail later in this chapter. Since our clinical experience has been that regular single channel NFB is enhanced by the addition of HRV training, we continue to use the combined approach when using LNFB. This latter combination is increasingly being applied for adolescents and adults who are complex cases. The outline of the chapter is as follows:

Assessment: Data from the initial assessment is used to make decisions regarding the use of LNFB rather than single or two channel NFB. We mention when there might be advantages to using single channel NFB. This section additionally provides an overview of decision making regarding how to choose relevant Brodmann areas (BAs) for LNFB training. (See Thompson, Thompson, & Wenqing, 2008 for an explication of BAs, their primary functions, and their relationship to 10–20 sites.)

Intervention: This section explains why and how LNFB is combined with HRV training in clinical practice.

HRV measurements: This section provides an overview of how HRV training is carried out.

Neuroanatomical connections: This section provides the neuroanatomical and neurophysiological rationale for combining HRV training with LNFB by explaining heart–brain connections.

Case examples: Three case examples are given to illustrate particular points regarding how to combine LNFB and HRV.

ASSESSMENT

The first part of the initial assessment takes a half day (about 3.5 h) and includes completion of questionnaires, clinical interview, two continuous performance tests (the T.O.V.A., Test of Variables of Attention, and the IVA, Integrated Visual and Auditory Continuous Performance Test), and a single channel quantitative electroencephalogram (QEEG) recording at Cz. A sample NFB + HRV training session is then carried out. Statistics for relevant parameters are graphed across five eyes open conditions: 3-min (eyes open) baseline with a raw EEG screen (no feedback), 3-min HRV training screen (visual feedback showing lines for respiration and heart rate (HR) changes, which the client tries to get "in sync"), then three 2-min segments using training screens for NFB. The NFB provides visual feedback in the form of animations plus audio feedback (music) and both are activated when brainwave amplitudes for selected frequency bands change in the correct direction; for example, decrease 4–8 Hz to reduce tuning out, increase 13–15 Hz for a calm and alert mental state, keep 52–58 Hz very low to minimize muscle artifact. The five segments of the practice training session are graphed to show a learning curve. The patient's EEG sample from the baseline condition is artifacted and then graphed as a spectral array showing the magnitude (mean amplitude) for each frequency from 2 to 40 Hz. The learning curve and this graph, plus important ratios that were tracked, such as the theta/beta power ratio for investigating attention-deficit/hyperactivity disorder (ADHD) (Monastra et al., 1999) are discussed with the client and their parents or spouse, as applicable. If the person is an appropriate candidate for an NFB intervention, goals for training are also discussed.

At the end of the initial assessment, three decisions are made. The first is whether the assessor deems the person to be an appropriate candidate for training. (Exclusions might be because of severe family dysfunction, in which case family therapy or marital therapy might be recommended as a first step, with a BFB intervention held in reserve for future consideration.) A second decision concerns whether psychoeducational testing should be booked to assess learning strengths and weaknesses where this information would help guide the metacognitive strategies component of training. Increasingly, to save the client time and money, we are having adolescents and adults complete an online neuropsychological test battery available through a company called CNS Vital Signs. With students who might have a learning disability (LD), we will do full intellectual and academic testing. The third decision concerns whether a 19 channel QEEG assessment including LORETA analysis should be carried out. The 19 channel ("full cap") assessment at our center includes not only EEG data collection (eyes open and eyes closed) but also data collection for evoked potentials (event related potentials, ERPs) done during a continuous performance test, and HRV data collection.

This decision regarding who goes on for 19 channel assessment is based on the clinical presentation and on the Principle of Parsimony, which suggests that the least invasive, least disruptive, and least costly assessment that provides sufficient information to guide appropriate treatment should be done. A child presenting with ADHD without complications, such as LDs or behavioral problems or a medical history of head injuries, for example, likely does not need a 19 channel assessment because an appropriate intervention can be based on single channel assessment. He/she can be trained to self-regulate attention using a basic treatment combination of single channel NFB at the central location (Cz) accompanied by HRV training (or just belly breathing in a young child who might fidget with the sensors used for HRV) and coaching in metacognitive strategies ("learning to learn") with that part of each session done "on task." On the other hand, a patient who has a more complex presentation, such as a history of traumatic brain injury (TBI), should have the 19 channel QEEG. More complex presentations include, but are not limited to, patients with severe LDs, autistic spectrum disorder (ASD, including Asperger's syndrome) if they can tolerate having a cap on, affect disorders, or TBI/concussions.

Mild TBI is a good example of a condition which requires the more comprehensive approach of 19 channel QEEG and LORETA clients who present with postconcussion symptoms even many years after they have suffered from one or more concussions or whiplash injuries are found to have deviations from database norms (DBNs) involving different areas of the brain and different neural networks that match with their symptoms. No two clients will be exactly alike but virtually all of these clients with postconcussion syndrome complain about cognitive and memory impairments. The majority also have symptoms related to affect networks, including depression, anxiety, irritability ("short fuse"), and less resiliency in the face of stress (Thompson, Thompson, Thompson, & Hagedorn, 2011). In some, the injury appears to have resulted in abnormal EEG findings similar to those found in people with Asperger's syndrome, with less activation in the right temporal–parietal junction, the posterior cingulate, and the left orbital frontal cortex. These patients show changes in their ability to correctly interpret social interactions (Thompson, Thompson, & Reid, 2010). In a number of people a combination of networks is affected, resulting in significant personality changes to the degree that other family members state that the patient is no longer the person they knew. When there are postconcussion symptoms, one almost invariably finds QEEG, ERP, CPT (continuous performance task), HRV, and neuropsychological testing findings that differ from normal.

Postconcussion the ERP data often demonstrate decreased amplitude and longer latency ("low and slow") of the P3a and P3b components and may show similar changes in N1 and P2 components as well. (P3a refers to the P300 response—a positive wave that occurs around 300 ms or later after the stimulus, measured at Cz. It reflects brain speed related mainly to attention and vigilance. P3b is the response measured at Pz that reflects working memory and information processing. N1 and P2 responses are automatic and indicate the brain has registered that the stimulus occurred, even though the person is not yet consciously aware of the stimulus.) The CPT involves clicking when a large blue circle appears but not clicking for a smaller blue circle or for a visual distracter (a checkerboard image) or a sound. CPT scores may show differences from DBNs in errors of omission, errors of commission, reaction time, and reaction time variability. QEEG, ERP, and HRV data are recorded at our offices using a set 20-min recording procedure done eyes open, eyes closed, and on task doing the CPT, and analysis is done by Evoke Neuroscience in New York (Evoke Neuroscience. DJ Technologies, 1133 Broadway, Suite #412, New York, NY). We additionally do our own QEEG analysis using Neuroguide (NG). We also do our own analysis of HRV data using Thought Technology Infiniti equipment for data collection and their CardioPro software to generate the internationally approved statistics used in HRV research. Even in young athletic clients, we observe differences in standard deviation (SD) of the normalized (N) R-R interval (SDNN). It should be above 70 ms, yet it is often <30 ms after a concussion. In addition, these patients demonstrate a decrease in total power, which should be >2000 ms^2, to <500 ms^2. The QEEG, when also analyzed using LORETA Z-scores, most often demonstrates multiple sites with differences of >2 SD from the DBNs. Norms are available in a number of commonly used databases, including WinEEG, NG, and SKIL (Sterman–Kaiser Imaging Labs). For patients with postconcussion syndrome, although we have had excellent results using single channel NFB in the past by sequentially training the various sites and parameters (amplitude, coherence) that were outside DBNs, we now include sessions of LNFB with a goal of being more efficient by simultaneously training more sites and more parameters at the same time, while also being able to target areas deeper in the cortex, such as the cingulate cortex.

LNFB is an attractive option when there are multiple midline and ventral structures involved as source locations and when sites have a number of parameters (amplitude, coherence, and phase measurements) outside DBNs. When looking at brain maps, it is often not clear what structures in the cortex we are actually dealing with. Surface sites on brain maps that show deviations from DBNs may be quite distant from the principle BA that is the source of the deviation. That source is identified through LORETA mathematics, as developed by Roberto Pasqual-Marqui. For example, BA 25 is a deep, ventral, midline structure located in the subgenual area ("below the knee" of the cingulated gyrus) and it is often localized as the source for observed deviations in the brain map seen at F3 and/or F4 and Fz on the surface. On the other hand, we feel compelled to note that we have often observed the deviation and the affect symptoms in such cases, to be normalized using single channel NFB at FCz plus HRV. We now hope for faster results when we use LNFB. We posit that HRV training may additionally increase the effectiveness and the speed with which results are attained. For example, in Affect network disorders the cingulate gyrus, BA 25, and the insula all have direct connections from the solitary nucleus in the medulla. It is the key nucleus for afferents from the baroreceptors that are important in HRV training and we observe very quick emotional control and patient satisfaction when we use HRV training combined with NFB.

The advantage of LORETA Z-score NFB over traditional NFB is increased specificity of the training and the possibility to train activity at locations not otherwise identifiable by conventional surface EEG and, in addition, there is the possibility to train up to 24 targeted areas (BAs) at the same time. A disadvantage is that this procedure takes more time to set up and clean up at each session. In addition, we feel it should only be done by experienced clinicians who have a good working knowledge of neuroanatomy and BA functions. Such people can make reasonable judgments about what parameters are appropriate for training and will be careful not to target areas where Z-scores might be outside DBNs for good, healthy, reasons. Examples of "abnormal" findings that one would not target for change include deviations from DBNs that reflect activation that is a compensatory phenomena or deviations in an area of superior functioning in that individual. If there are findings that are 2 SD outside the DBNs near Wernicke's area in someone who is a gifted speaker and author of an international "bestseller," you do not want to change that any more than you would want to decrease that person's IQ to below 130. Another point to keep in mind is that LNFB is limited by the original databases only going to 30 Hz because the computers used to collect the data when the databases were developed were slower and the sampling rate was only 128 samples per second. Although the range from 0.5 to 30 Hz does cover almost all the spontaneously generated EEG which is used in NFB, it still leaves us using single channel surface NFB for patients who require training at higher frequencies. For example, some patients show beta spindling associated with negative ruminations in the 31–35 Hz range. In addition, some patients benefit from careful enhancement of gamma activity, 39–41 Hz.

What Are We "Targeting?"

Whether we do single channel NFB or LNFB, we are trying to influence neural networks (Thompson et al., 2011). These are interconnected, functionally related groups of neurons that involve various BAs. Brodmann published his work on the human cortex in 1909 showing all the different sections of the cortex with numbers from 1 to 52 based on cytoarchitecture (cell shape/morphology). Starting near the center of the cortex below the central sulcus, he named the area "1." He then gave a new number to each adjoining area that was made up of new cell types. The adage, "structure dictates function," for the most part, is reasonably met by this method of identifying different areas of the cortex. Each BA does appear to have a primary function, however, it is also true that each BA can have a number of other functions and be involved in many different functional networks (Lloyd, 2007). The function of the moment depends on which network is activated.

A BA does not activate in isolation from other brain structures. Each BA represents just one area out of many that are involved in one or more neural networks that involve cortical–subcortical connections (Thompson & Thompson, 2007). Behavior requires coordinated activity involving many functionally related cortical areas. This may be one reason why practitioners have obtained good results when doing NFB over a single site such as Cz (Thompson & Thompson, 2010). Approximately 50% of the EEG amplitude at any single site, such as Cz, arises from neurons directly beneath the electrode (with electrode diameter of 0.5–1.0 cm) and 95% arises from an area with a radius of 6 cm measured from the center of the recording electrode (Thatcher, 2012 (pp. 35, 37, 51) after Nunez, 1981, 1995). However, training at central midline sites such as Cz, Fz, and Pz likely influences not just that small area of the cortex directly under that electrode but also key areas lying beneath that bit of cortex, such as the cingulate gyrus, that are involved in many networks. A network serves to synchronize the functions of groups of neurons in many different but functionally related sections of the cerebral cortex. The cingulate gyrus is one central area that is involved in the functioning of the executive, affect, salience, and default networks (Seeley et al., 2007; Supekar et al., 2010; Thompson et al., 2011). In addition to subcortical connections to the basal ganglia and brainstem, it is, through the cingulum, directly connected to the frontal, parietal, and temporal lobes.

Hypothetically, affecting the activity of the cingulate gyrus may be assumed to have indirect effects on many deeper structures even though the NFB operant conditioning of brainwave activity is done at a site on the surface of the scalp. Strong support for this hypothesis comes from research done in Montreal, Canada, concerning children with ADHD who received NFB training with electrode placement at Cz. Using fMRI as the pre-post measure, the experimental group, as compared to the control group, showed increased activation in a number of cortical and subcortical areas. Specifically, during a counting Stroop task, there were changes in activation in the left substantia nigra and left caudate, right anterior cingulate gyrus, and left superior parietal area. During a GO/NO GO task, there was again increased activation in left substantia nigra, left caudate, and right anterior cingulate gyrus, plus changes in left thalamus, right and left lateral frontal areas (Beauregard & Levesque, 2006).

A grouping of deeper areas in the cortex has been referred to as central midline structures (CMSs) (Northoff et al., 2006). Most of these areas can be seen in Figure 8.5. Thus EEG BFB training to influence these areas can be done either by Cz, FCz, CPz, single channel NFB combined with appropriate cognitive exercises to activate different mental states and influence appropriate neural networks that the client wishes to alter or, alternatively, one can have a more direct effect by using LORETA NFB to influence these areas. The latter approach should be more efficient.

When doing NFB, the professional is assuming that the targeted site(s) influences a particular network of neurons while inhibiting all other networks that are not involved with the targeted functions. This goal can be achieved by virtue of loops that go from cortex to basal ganglia to thalamus to functionally related areas of the cortex. This is why the thalamus is so central in producing rhythmic activity. When a particular nucleus within the thalamus is activated, it is like opening that particular thalamic gateway so that "messages" are sent to all functionally related areas of the cortex (Kropotov, 2009). This may intensify a selected program of action that involves many, often widely separated, areas of the cortex. We think of these functionally related areas as a "neural network."

A Theoretical Dilemma

The authors postulate that it may be possible that single channel NFB training in some instances could have a theoretical advantage over training that involves multiple sites. By having an effect on a network from a single central site, single channel NFB may allow the brain to balance the degree to which other affected sites within that network are changed. NFB at one site avoids making incorrect decisions about the degree to which multiple sites are being "normalized" when we use Z-score directed LNFB. It could be argued that single channel NFB might be a more "balanced" or natural approach to changing the brain and does not have the theoretical danger of adversely affecting a site that is outside DBNs due to genius or due to compensatory changes. This theoretical dilemma can only be resolved by years of data collection and research.

However, to counter the forgoing concern, in LNFB the program takes the patient's key symptoms and "matches" them with BAs known to subsume these same symptoms. BAs that are outside the DBNs but do NOT match will not be involved in the Z-score normalization training. The practitioner can make changes in selected BAs and frequency bands even after this "matching" process is done. For example, one of our patient's did not check off depression (only anxiety) as a problem. However, in his assessment BA 25 was well outside DBNs. It was not included in the "match" by the program. We therefore entered it. (*Note*: If the patient had ranked depression as a major symptom, it would have been included in the first place.)

When the matching process is completed, the patient then sits in front of the computer monitor and receives visual and auditory feedback. It is operant conditioning. It is possible to train 168 measurements at one time. Importantly, the clinician has the option of changing the feedback criteria from the 85% of scores within a defined limit to 100%.

That would mean that all targeted variables at all targeted BAs would have to be met in order to get positive feedback. This option is used when one or two most important areas for a particular patient are well outside the DBNs but will not be influenced if the 85% default setting is used. This forces the client to move all the training parameters into the chosen Z-score window in order to receive feedback. Case example #2 below addresses this.

Intervention: Adding HRV Training to Training Done with LNFB

Repeatedly, at the ADD Centre, our adult and even our adolescent clients have told us early in training that doing their HRV breathing techniques at home and at work absolutely correlated with gaining immediate control over situations that, in the past, had been overwhelmingly stressful. Others stated that, although they did not consider themselves to be anxious or overly stressed, the HRV technique improved their focus, concentration, and work efficiency. For most clients, it was a relatively simple addition to our program to teach the client to relax their muscles, warm their hands, and gain some control over HRV. For many of these clients, an initial 20-min stress test demonstrated to them that physiological variables such as skin conduction, skin temperature, muscle tension, HR, and breathing rate, depth, and regularity, all change markedly with even a minor stress. They also observed that they were capable of controlling these variables. For the trainer, it demonstrated which of these variables altered the most with stress and therefore might be useful to train with BFB.

Stress Test

For a stress assessment sensors include a blood volume photoplethysmographic (BVP) on a finger or thumb of the nondominant (left) hand to detect the pulse. The temperature sensor is placed on the pulp of the client's right little finger. The skin conduction/electrodermal (EDR) sensors are usually placed on the right index and ring fingers. A stretch receptor belt is put around the waist to detect diaphragmatic breathing. Muscle tension is demonstrated by EMG recording. This may be carried out using a head band with sensors over the forehead. However, we prefer to use an EMG sensor over a trapezius (shoulder) muscle. This placement of the EMG sensor will show us when a patient is using shoulder and thoracic tension to inhale (Figure 8.1). This shoulder placement of an EMG sensor allows the patient to relax muscle tension and learn diaphragmatic breathing at the same time (Thompson & Thompson, 2003, 2007).

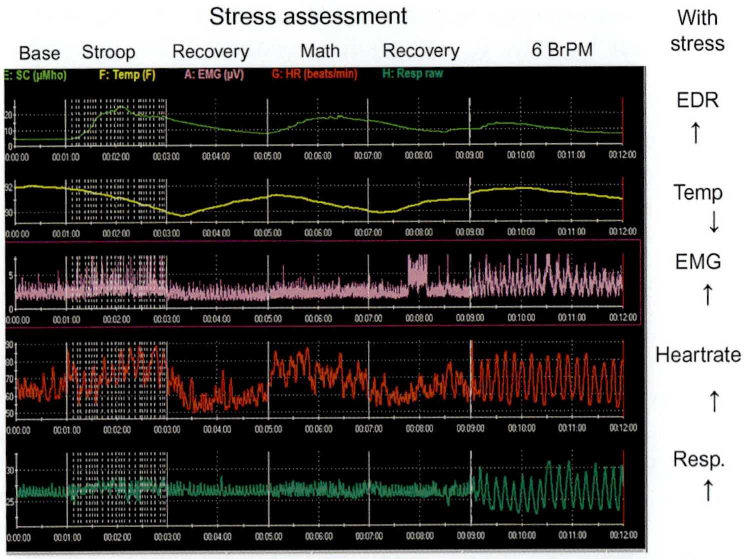

FIGURE 8.1 Stress assessment profile. Observe that in the final segment, when breathing at 6 BrPM, this client used their shoulder (and presumably their thoracic) muscles (EMG) when breathing. This was noted and they learned to relax their muscles and breathe diaphragmatically. *Screen from Thompson & Thompson, using Thought Technology Biograph Infiniti Instrumentation.*

The HR is measured using the plethysmograph which measures red light reflected from blood vessels in a finger or thumb. Instead of measuring R-R intervals with electrocardiogram (EKG) leads (which is done during the 19 channel EEG assessment) we are measuring pulse to pulse time, which gives the same figures at rest (though may not do so during tasks) for the SD of the R-R intervals with artifacts "corrected" called SDNN (Giardino, Lehrer, & Edelberg, 2002). SDNN and spectral power are calculated after the session using the CardioPro program from Thought Technology. This program was developed to provide the statistics that are used internationally for HRV measures.

In our stress test, there are just two mild stressors but they have been very effective in producing sufficient stress in hundreds of clients. After a 1-min baseline, the first stressor, in this version of a stress test, is a Stroop Color Test. On each list of words stating a color (red, green, blue, etc.), the client is instructed to say the color that the word is printed in and to NOT read the word. Thus the word "red" may be printed in "green" ink and the client must say "green." The second stressor, in this version of a stress test, is a math problem (e.g., serial 7s). Although we have not found artifacts to be a problem for our purposes, to obtain data without artifact produced by speech, the trainer may just have the client rest their hand on the table and point to a color or, in the math test, print one number as an answer. Alternatively, the client can just point to one of five alternative answers. The client whose data is summarized in Figure 8.1 showed a typical reaction to stress and recovery. Typically with stress, skin conduction increases, skin temperature decreases, and this is shown in Figure 8.1. Muscle tension, as measured by the EMG, increases, HR increases, and respiration may show one or more changes and become rapid, shallow, and/or irregular. After each stressor, the client is given a 2-min recovery time and the reader will notice that after the stroop test in the 2 min allowed for recovery, skin conduction decreased, skin temperature rose, muscle tension decreased, HR decreased, respiration became regular. Everyone will react to stress, the important factor is how rapidly they recover. The reader will also note that after the 2 min postmath test recovery, we do a final 3-min section in which the clinician leads the patient in diaphragmatic, approximately 6 breaths per minute (BrPM), breathing. In this last segment, while following the instructor's breathing, most patients are able to note how their HR synchronizes with their breathing in a beautiful sine wave pattern. Indeed, this can be seen in Figure 8.2. We have found that it is highly motivating for the patient to

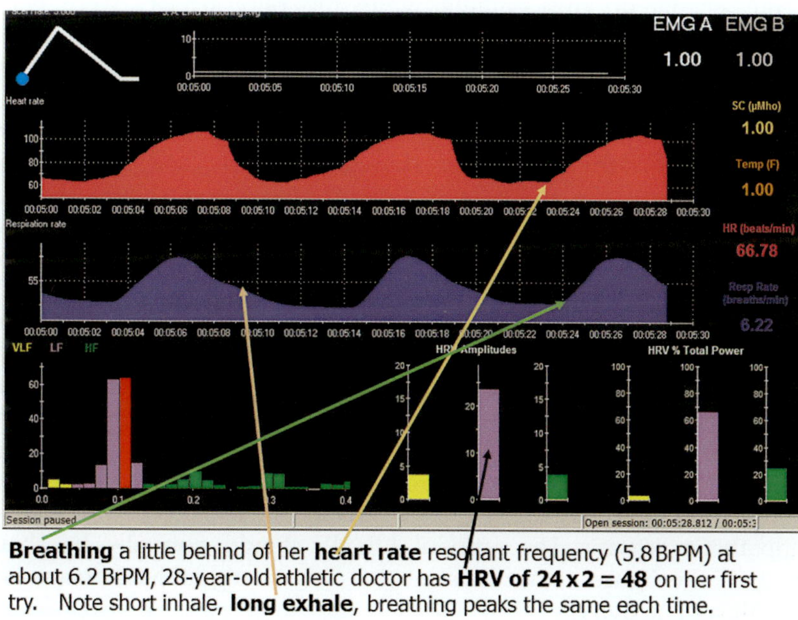

FIGURE 8.2 HRV feedback screen. *Figure from Thompson and Thompson, 2003.*

see the effects of stress on their physiology and then see this vivid demonstration of how they can self-regulate and control their own physiology. Clients who have experienced chronic stress may demonstrate an atypical pattern. With stress their skin temperature may increase rather than decrease and/or their skin conduction (EDR) may be a flat line rather than show a typical increase.

The screen in Figure 8.1 shows changes in each of the measurements with stress followed by some recovery when the first stress stopped but somewhat less ability to recover after the second (math) stressor. In the last 3-min section, the client breathes slowly with the trainer at 6 BrPM with expiration longer than inspiration. The client usually feels a little stressed when they are told to follow the trainers breathing and this may be reflected by a small rise in skin conduction and a slight drop in skin temperature as shown in Figure 8.2. It is possible to also look at EEG changes (usually at Cz) for each section but this is not shown in this summary.

HRV Training Method

Clinically, for the control of stress and anxiety, and to attain a calm focused concentration during the session, the most effective BFB training appeared at our Centre to be HRV. It was also very easy to have all our clients do this training while the EEG sensors were being applied at the beginning of each session and during the EEG NFB sessions. The most commonly used screen by our clients is shown in Figure 8.2.

This doctor during the demonstration was not using other BFB variables such as skin conduction, skin temperature, and EMG. These variables are on the right hand side of the screen should they be required. In the spectrum in the lower left corner the *x*-axis is frequency. She is breathing at 6 BrPM and her HR is following this and showing 6 variations per minute. The international statistics for HRV (Task Force, 1996) define very low (VLF), low (LF), and high (HF) frequency for HR. LF 0.04–0.15 Hz is *purple* in the feedback screen. This is what usually should have the highest power and it is what we are encouraging in HRV training. It is said to reflect a balance of sympathetic and parasympathetic activity. VLF is *yellow* <0.04 Hz and may reflect sympathetic activity and other variables but this is not agreed upon at this time. HF is *green*, 0.15–0.4 Hz. HF is said to reflect parasympathetic activity. The ratio of LF/HF should normally be about 1.5–2. In the figure, it can be seen that this young athletic doctor has very high LF activity.

At the ADD Centre, clients are asked to find a breathing rate, usually between 5.5 and 6.5 BrPM, that results in an even amplitude of both breathing and HR changes with synchrony of their HR changes and their BrPM. To accomplish this, they are asked to make inspiration shorter than expiration and to have each of the blue and red "*mountains*" all exactly the same height and shape (Figure 8.2). Some clients initially count to themselves saying: inhale, 1, 2, 3, exhale, 4, 5, 6, 7, 8, hold, 9, 10, inhale... When this synchrony is difficult to achieve rapidly, the staff will use the methodology described by Lehrer (2013), beginning at 7.5 BrPM and decreasing in 0.5 s steps to 4.5 BrPM to find the frequency at which the amplitude of HR variations is maximal in order to establish the resonant HR frequency for that particular client. The single and two channel NFB training screens at the ADD Centre have a double line graph (red for HR overlapping blue for respiration rate) on each screen so that the client can follow their attainment of synchrony between HR and respiration while they do their NFB (Thompson, Thompson, Thompson, Reid, & Hagedorn, 2013). With LNFB, a separate computer and monitor are used for the HRV feedback while the patient is doing LNFB.

Heart Rate Variability

Definitions

- HRV is the variation in interval (R-R) between heart beats.
- RSA (respiratory sinus arrhythmia) is the naturally occurring variation in HR that occurs during the breathing cycle. It is directly proportional to HRV.
- HRV training includes monitoring RSA and adjusting breathing patterns to increase HRV.

HRV refers to the constant variations in HR that may be observed in healthy individuals. These variations may be measured in terms of the interbeat intervals (IBIs). These are the intervals between heart beats. This interval is measured between the R waves in the adjacent EKG QRS complexes. The SD of these IBIs is called SDRR and when computed after all artifacts have been "corrected" is called SDNN. "N" stands for "normal." The interbeat, R1–R2, and R2–R3 (IBI 1) intervals are shown as examples in Figure 8.3. One cannot have artifacts in assessment data (Peper, Shaffer, & Lin, 2010). The reader will note that unlike artifact removal from an EEG, in an EKG record time sections must not be removed. Experts can "correct" the artifacts manually but fortunately the CardioPro program can rapidly do this for regular practitioners. Briefly, this program normalizes the IBI data by adding small IBI values together and splitting large ones into two or more IBIs. Pairs of IBI values where one is short and the other long are averaged. It is important to understand that the beat time information (i.e., the

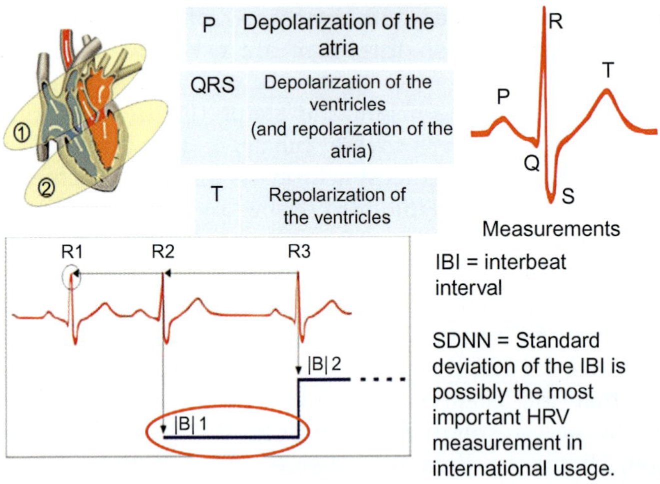

FIGURE 8.3 EKG origin and the standard measurement SDNN. *Figure with permission from Thought Technology. Procomp Infiniti and CardioPro Programs. Thought Technology, Montreal, Canada.*

moment of each beat) needs to be maintained for the HRV analysis to be valid and the program does this for us.

Figure 8.3 shows the QRS wave of the EKG and the IBIs, R1–R2, and R2–R3. Interbeat (R-R) interval (IBI) is the basis for most HRV statistics. *RR interval becomes NN after artifacts are "corrected" in the record.*

Heart–Brain Connections Produce Oscillations

The reader will note that most of our BFB measurements, such as skin temperature, EDR, and EMG, involve only the sympathetic portion of the autonomic nervous system (ANS). They are "tonic" measurements. HRV is a completely different phenomenon. It is an oscillating and not a tonic measurement (Lehrer & Eddie, 2013). It is said to be the only means we have to obtain a simple measurement of the parasympathetic portion of the ANS.

The Heart as an Oscillating System

The healthy beating heart is the principle component of an oscillating system called the cardiovascular system (CVS). A healthy heart is constantly changing its rate. Every person's heart has its own unique resonant frequency. This is often close to 6 variations per minute. However, it will be less for men than women and less for tall persons than those who are shorter because it is partly dependent on total blood volume. It will therefore also be higher for children than adults. When the resonant frequency is achieved, the clinician will note almost perfect synchrony between breathing and HR changes: inspiration and an increase in the HR, expiration and a decrease in HR (Lehrer, 2007a). This was seen in the HRV training screen (Figure 8.2).

GOAL OF TRAINING HRV

Our goal in HRV training is to increase the heart rate variations (HRV). When this is achieved, we will see an increase in the amplitude of these variations and an increase in SDNN. The maximum change will occur when the client breathes at the resonant frequency of their own heart. When any resonant system (such as the heart) is rhythmically stimulated at its resonant frequency, the external stimulation magnifies the persistent oscillations, thus greatly increasing total variability. Think of pushing a child on a swing. You know that if you push the swing just as the child has reached the height of the swing's oscillation, then the swing will go higher and higher as you push until it reaches its maximum arc. In this case, the maximum depends on the length of the rope holding the seat of the swing. In the case of the heart, the HRV will increase with training to a maximum for that patient. Breathing diaphragmatically at this resonant frequency will usually be observed to result in the highest amplitude of HRV for that person.

VAGAL CONTROL OF HRV

Without parasympathetic control, the innate rhythm of the sinoatrial (SA) node (about 100 bpm (beats per minute)) would drive HR. Health is tightly related to oscillatory systems (Lehrer & Eddie, 2013). Oscillations in vagal input are the main system for controlling oscillations in the HR. The right vagus nerve primarily innervates the SA node. The left vagus primarily innervates the atrial–ventricular (AV) node. However, there is significant overlap in this anatomical distribution. Atrial muscle is also innervated by vagal efferents, whereas the ventricular myocardium is only sparsely innervated by vagal efferents. Sympathetic efferent nerves are found throughout the atria (especially in the SA node) and ventricles (Klabunde, 2013). Figure 8.4 shows the carotid and the aortic arch baroreceptors. These baroreceptors are mechano receptors that respond to blood pressure (BP). When the BP rises, the resulting expansion of these baroreceptors sends afferent signals to the nucleus of the solitary tract in the medulla. This nucleus sends signals to many areas in the brain but the final result for HR is that in the brainstem the dorsal nucleus of the vagus and the nucleus

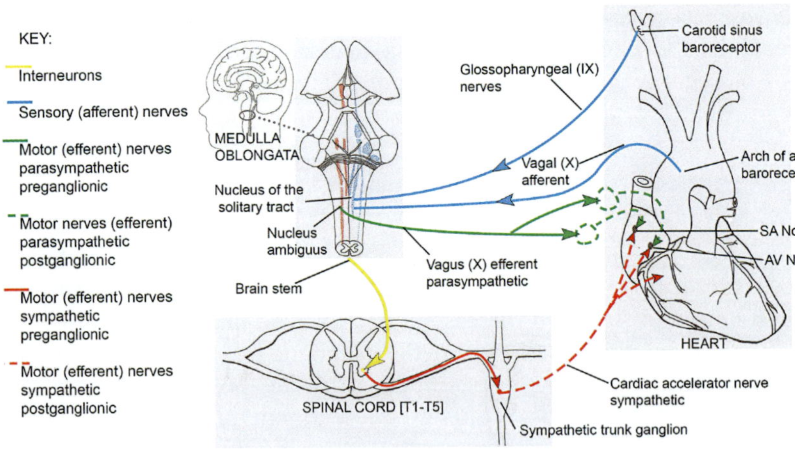

FIGURE 8.4 Afferent and efferent ANS connections between the brainstem and the CVS. *Drawing by Maya Berenkey from Thompson and Thompson, 2003.*

ambiguous send parasympathetic vagal efferents to the heart that slow the HR, resulting in a decrease in BP. Vice versa, when BP falls the opposite will occur, parasympathetic drive decreases and HR will increase.

GOAL OF TRAINING HRV AND WHY WE COMBINE IT WITH NFB

Our goal in HRV training is to increase the heart rate variations (HRV). When any resonant system (such as the heart) is rhythmically stimulated at its resonant frequency, the external stimulation magnifies the persistent oscillations, thus greatly increasing total variability. Diaphragmatically breathing at your resonant frequency will usually be observed to result in the highest amplitude of HRV. Training HRV is important for the majority of clients seen at the ADD Centre. HRV training is known to reduce anxiety and stress (Mikosch et al., 2010; Reiner, 2008). It can also improve cognitive functioning in stressful conditions (Prinsloo et al., 2011).

As a result of HRV training alone, researchers have demonstrated improvements in mental processing (Thayer, Hansen, Saus-Rose, & Johnson, 2009) and emotional stability (Applehans & Lueken, 2006). HRV training has been investigated in the treatment of emotional disorders, such as depression (Grippo & Johnson, 2009; Hassett et al., 2007) and anxiety (Karavidas et al., 2007). HRV training has also been shown to benefit physical conditions, such as asthma (Lehrer et al., 2006, 2008), hypertension (Lin et al., 2012), and cardiac functioning (Lehrer & Vaschillo, 2008). There are many heart–brain connections and at our Centre, we have documented evidence of improved brainwave patterns being found in conjunction with HRV training, namely, an increase in the amplitude of sensorimotor rhythm (12–15 Hz) activity (Reid, Nihon, Thompson, & Thompson, 2013). Given the multitude of conditions helped when a person increases the variations in the time between their heart beats, it made sense to add this intervention when working with clients who were appropriate for NFB training.

All of our 19 channel QEEG assessments include EKG. The observation that TBI impairs cardiac function has become increasingly apparent through work with clients who have had vehicular accidents (car, motorcycle, bicycle) and concussions in sports (Baguley, Heriseanu, Felmingham, & Cameron, 2006; Thompson & Hagedorn, 2012). As previously noted, at the Biofeedback Institute of Toronto we have observed large deviations from expected normal values for different measurements of HRV in relatively young and otherwise healthy athletes who have suffered a head injury. This has been documented by others investigating the effects of concussion in athletes (Thompson & Hagedorn, 2012). Thompson and Hagedorn demonstrated that, after a concussion, even an otherwise healthy athlete can show major cardiac changes. The amplitude of the variations in HR and the SDs of the HR variations after the effects of artifacts have been removed (SDNN) are both lower than would be expected in a person of similar age and health.

We have also noted lower than expected HRV measurements, such as SDNN and total power, in patients who present with affect disorders. This observation is supported in the literature (Grippo & Johnson, 2009). Grippo et al. have reviewed the effects of stress and depression on HRV. They reported that it can impair cardiac functioning and, in particular, HRV variables (Grippo & Johnson, 2009).

Thus the very patients that we wish to have use LNFB are the same patients who can benefit from HRV training.

What Are the Links that Underlie These Clinical Observations?

The literature reveals that some of the connections between HRV and brain functioning are being elucidated by investigating the effects of brain damage on cardiac functions. In many of our TBI assessments, LORETA indicates involvement of the insulae (BA 13) and this area has been one of the "targets" in our work using LNFB. Interestingly, research has demonstrated that injury, as from a stroke, to the right insula has dramatic effects on autonomic balance and heart functioning

(Nagai, Hoshide, & Kario, 2010; Shah, Klumpp, Angstadt, Nathan, & Phan, 2009). Stroke affecting the right insula can result in low values for SD of the artifacted R-R interval (SDNN). It can also result in higher values for the ratio of the amplitude of LF/HF spectral power, in addition to findings of nonsustained ventricular tachycardia, and premature ventricular contractions. There is an increase in nocturnal BP and higher norepinephrine levels. Patients with left insular cortex involvement have a decrease in baroreceptor sensitivity (BRS) (Sykora, Diedler, Rupp, Turcani, & Steiner, 2009). BRS an index of baroreflex function is based on the quantification of RR interval changes related to BP changes and is measured in ms/mm Hg (La Rovere, Pinna, & Raczak, 2008; Lehrer, 2013; Zöllei, Paprika, & Rudas, 2003).

The insula is an important regulator of autonomic balance. The right insula predominately affects the sympathetic and the left the parasympathetic system, in part through connections to the nucleus accumbens, which has a role in balancing the sympathetic and parasympathetic systems (Nagai et al., 2010). The insular cortex has reciprocal connections with the anterior cingulate gyrus, amygdala, entorhinal cortex, orbitofrontal cortex, and temporal pole which are all involved in the affect and default networks and may also be implicated in executive functioning. It has afferent connections with hippocampus formation. Additionally, the insular cortex has dense reciprocal connections with subcortical autonomic core centers including the hypothalamic paraventriculi nuclei. The paraventricular nuclei can control the hypothalamic–pituitary–adrenal axis (HPA) and both parasympathetic and sympathetic aspects of the ANS. These nuclei also have important connections to the lateral hypothalamic area (sympathetic system), nucleus tractus solitarius (HRV control), and parabrachial nucleus (respiratory control), and all of these centers are also reciprocally connected to each other.

In a similar vein, Baguley et al. compared HRV data on 16 TBI age-matched subjects with and without dysautonomia (eight subjects in each group) and 16 noninjured controls. The subject's average age was 32 ± 12 years. There were more male subjects in the TBI group. Mode of injury included eight motor vehicle accidents, four assaults, two falls, and two sport accidents. The average days post injury was 81 ± 58. The TBI group revealed significant differences in HRV parameters compared to controls. The TBI group were a mean of 77 days post injury and had a significantly higher mean HR than controls (89.5 vs. 67.6 bpm, $p < 0.001$). Fourier analysis of HRV demonstrated lower total power in the TBI group compared to controls. The mean SDNN (ms) for the control group was 60.2 with an SD of 26.9 while the mean SDNN (ms) for the TBI group was 40.6 with an SD of 16.4. They concluded that the TBI group's value was significantly lower than controls. The total power (ms^2) of the controls was 4065 (SD 4082) and in the TBI group only 1656

(SD 1237). The LF power (ms^2) of the controls was 1304 (SD 1484) and in the TBI group only 189 (SD 152) (Baguley et al., 2006). Thus TBI does appear to lead to changes in HRV.

There have been similar findings in depressed patients. Depressed patients show changes in autonomic regulation of the heart. In an extensive review by Grippo and Johnson (2009), it is noted that there is activation of sympathetic drive and a decrease in vagal tone with a resulting increase in HR, decrease in HRV, and reduced baroreceptor reflex function. This review goes on to note that similar autonomic changes can also be associated with hypertension, increased body mass index, and increased blood glucose level and that these autonomic changes are observed in both acute and chronic cardiovascular conditions. These changes can be predisposing factors for ventricular fibrillation. Important for our work is that HRV has been shown to be reduced in depressed patients both with and without cardiovascular disease and HRV may be lower in more severely depressed patients (Grippo & Johnson, 2009). We have been emphasizing LNFB plus HRV training. However, there is excellent research to demonstrate that clinicians should also counsel their patients concerning the importance of integrating appropriate diet, sleep, and exercise habits into their training program (Beniamini, Rubenstein, Zaichkowsky, & Crim, 1997; Zoeller, 2007).

Neuroanatomical Links Between HRV Training and NFB Training

We have already noted that the healthy beating heart is the principle component of an oscillating system called the CVS (Lehrer & Eddie, 2013). When the resonant frequency is achieved during HRV training, the clinician will note almost perfect synchrony between inspiration and an increase in the HR and between expiration and a decrease in HR.

At the ADD Centre some years ago, the question arose as to whether we could go beyond clinical observation and explain why both NFB combined with BFB could be expected to help patients who had complex presentations more than either modality alone. In simple terms, could we show that the areas of the brain that subsume these different systems and networks are neuroanatomically linked and that the manner in which they are linked might reasonably be expected to respond to a combination of NFB plus HRV training? Could training to simultaneously improve HRV *and* EEG variables improve the patient's thinking, feeling, and behavior? We concluded that the answer is yes, in theory, and yes, in practice.

The field of combined EEG NFB and peripheral BFB has its foundations in functional neuroanatomy and neurophysiology. QEEG is a means of quantifying EEG data using high speed computers in order to distinguish, both with statistics and images, patterns that are outside normal, average population, database figures. LORETA allows the practitioner to find the source of different frequencies deep within the cortex. The data from QEEG and LORETA when combined with the practitioner's knowledge of the dominant functions of different BAs and their relationship to neural networks (Thompson and Thompson, 2003; Thatcher, 2012; Thompson et al., 2007; Thompson et al., 2011) can assist the practitioner in deciding whether a specific frequency at that site may correlate with a patient's symptoms. This data can help the clinician decide whether or not a pattern correlates to a cognitive, motor, sensory, or affect problem for a specific patient.

NFB + HRV can then be used to give almost instantaneous visual, auditory, and/or tactile feedback to inform the client as to whether or not they are meeting their objectives for moving their EEG patterns and their HRV to a more optimal level for their functioning. The reader will note the deliberate omission in this discussion of the word "abnormal." What might be an optimal change for one client may not be the best for another.

Using QEEG and LORETA, clients who present with affect disorders, LDs, ASDs, or TBI (even a number of years after they have suffered from one or more concussions) are found at the ADD Centre to have a large number of symptoms that correlate with deviations from DBNs involving different areas of the brain and different neural networks. As noted at the beginning of this chapter, virtually all of the postconcussion (TBI) clients presenting at the Biofeedback Institute of Toronto over the last 20 years have had cognitive impairments, including difficulties that involve memory. The majority also have had symptoms related to affect networks, including depression, anxiety, irritability, and a change in their ability to handle stress. In some, the injury appears to have resulted in abnormal EEG findings similar to those found in Asperger's syndrome, with less activation in the right temporal–parietal junction, the posterior cingulate, and the left orbital frontal cortex. These latter patients show changes in their ability to correctly interpret social interactions (Thompson & Thompson, 2010).

In particular, with these complex clients, we wanted to help our staff go beyond their clinical observations and understand why NFB and HRV training might have effects on the same neural networks and therefore help these patients. In simple terms, could we show that the areas of the brain that subsume these different systems and networks are neuroanatomically linked and that the manner in which they are linked might reasonably be expected to respond to a combination of NFB combined with HRV training? These links are illustrated in Figures 8.5 and 8.6.

Note in Figure 8.6 that the amygdala innervates the hypothalamic nuclei. It also innervates the parabrachial nucleus, which controls respiratory rate and the locus coeruleus, which produces norepinephrine

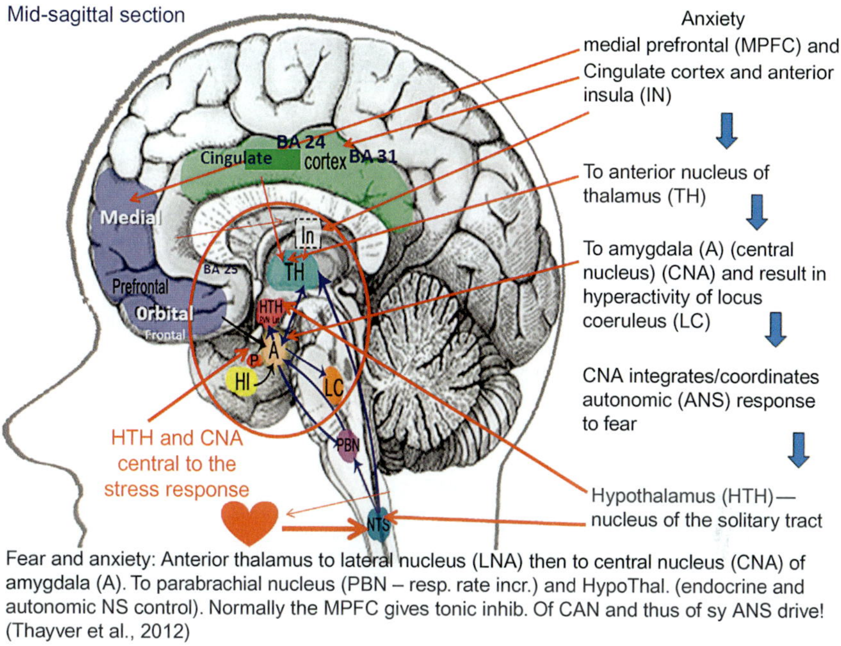

FIGURE 8.5 Central cortical and subcortical structures. Importantly, the paraventricular nucleus projects directly to the dorsal motor nucleus of the vagus and the nucleus ambiguous and thus directly has effects on HRV. It also projects directly on to sympathetic autonomic relay nuclei in the brainstem. TH, Thalamus; CNA, central nucleus amygdala; HI, hippocampus; IN, insula; A, amygdala; PBN, parabrachial nucleus; HTH, hypothalamus; ANS, autonomic nervous system; NTS, nucleus tractus solitarius; P, pituitary; PVN, paraventricular nucleus. *Diagram by Maya Berenkey from Thompson and Thompson, 2003.*

and thus relates to an increase in BP and to fear related behaviors. The amygdala is inhibited by the medial prefrontal cortex (Thayer, Åhs, Fredrikson, Sollers III, & Wager, 2012) and the fusiform and superior temporal areas (Porges, 2007).

How Do You Combine HRV Training with NFB and LNFB?

There are a number of instruments that allow one to simultaneously do BFB and NFB. Our experience has been with the Biograph program and the Infiniti instrument (Thought Technology) which has screens that give feedback for EEG parameters, such as decreasing the amplitude of slow waves (theta) and some HF beta waves while increasing the amplitude of lower frequency fast waves (sensorimotor rhythm (SR) or beta) while also showing when the person has synchrony between their breathing and the changes in their HR. When doing LNFB the

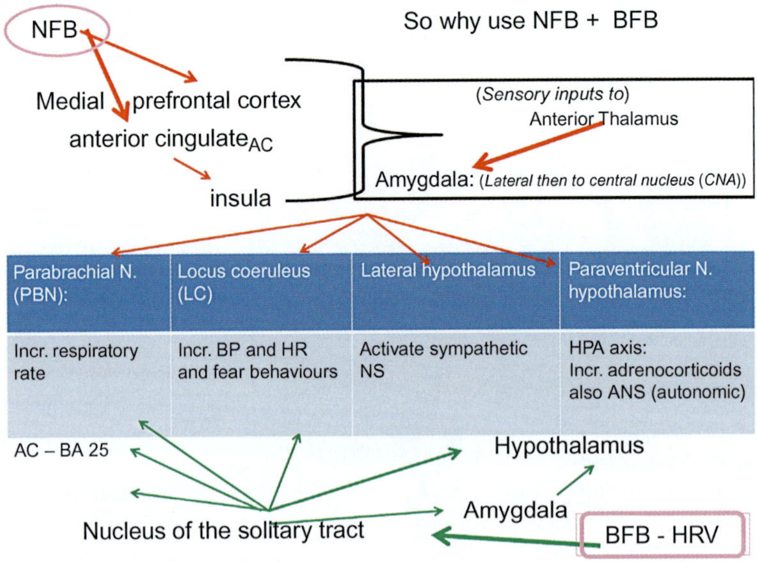

FIGURE 8.6 Illustration of how NFB and HRV training can both affect the same central structures. *Figure from Thompson and Thompson, 2003.*

HRV training is done while the trainer is putting on the 19 channel electrocap, thus making good use of the time it takes to put the cap on and achieve proper impedance values for all the electrodes. Clients appreciate being able to use this time productively and to learn a technique that they can utilize during their session and also in everyday life whenever they need to feel calm. They can also practice effortless diaphragmatic breathing at the rate that achieves the highest variability in their HR, called their resonance frequency (or, sometimes, resonant frequency), on a daily basis. With practice it becomes easier to utilize this diaphragmatic breathing when under stress; for example, when there is a deadline and one needs to be highly focused during a stressful period at work or school. For that matter, getting the cap on can be a bit uncomfortable and constitutes a minor stress, so it helps to give a task to focus on during what can take 5–10 min, and what could be better than a task that recruits the vagal response, which is associated with a person feeling calm and safe (Porges, 2007). It also helps prepare the client mentally and physiologically to get the most out of their LORETA Z-score session. As the client uses the setup time to achieve synchrony between their breathing and HR, they have reported that it helps get them get into the right mindset for training. They will often continue using the breathing as they strive to change their brainwave patterns during their LORETA Z-score session.

Some patients will also do the HRV training while they are doing an LNFB session. Note that the LORETA Z-score (LNFB) session is done using one computer and a second computer is used for the HRV training because it is not advisable to run both programs on a single computer due to the large amount of data processing that is required in these programs. The clinician can be checking impedances on the computer screen that will also give the LNFB while the client is watching the monitor for the HRV training. It also allows for monitoring what is happening regarding the clients breathing and HR during the LNFB, since the clinician could monitor that screen while the client/patient is watching and listening to the feedback concerning their brainwaves. Is your patient getting anxious or frustrated? Switch back to focusing on the HRV screen till they regain good synchrony between respiration and pulse parameters. Researching the effects of combining HRV training and LNFB in different populations, such as those with TBI, learning difficulties, anxiety disorders, or depression symptoms, provides groundbreaking and clinically relevant topics for graduate students because, though it has been applied clinically, the benefits have yet to be researched in a rigorous way.

How Do You Do LORETA NFB + HRV Training for Optimal Learning of the Task of Changing Brainwave and HRV Patterns?

Case Examples

CASE 1

Case 1 demonstrates the rationale for using ALL-OR-NONE training. We have been successful doing training using the *z*-tunes style feedback available on the LORETA Z-score program. Z-tunes enables the client to be rewarded for achieving a certain percent of brainwave patterns below the selected threshold. In some cases, a client may be receiving rewards during the training without shifting the brainwave patterns that have the highest SD from the database mean. These areas that have the highest SDs are also often the areas of greatest concern for the client because they usually relate to the most severe symptoms. With the *z*-tunes method, the client can still be rewarded with feedback even if these important areas remain high as long as a certain percentage of other brainwave patterns are below the threshold. To resolve

continued

CASE 1 *(cont'd)*

this problem, we have been using the all-or-none function provided in the LORETA Z-score NFB program. If we are working on many sites, as in the example below, in addition to using the 100% all-or-none setting, we will pick and use only the top three "matches" (the three areas with the highest SDs that "match" the client's most severe symptoms). In the example below, we reduced the number of sites (BAs) trained in session 11 and then from sessions 12–16 we focused on training only the top 3. During the 12th session, we had an audience (student) and the client performed extremely well under pressure. The following session the values rose and then gradually decreased over the remaining sessions. All this client's presenting symptoms are now in remission (Figure 8.7).

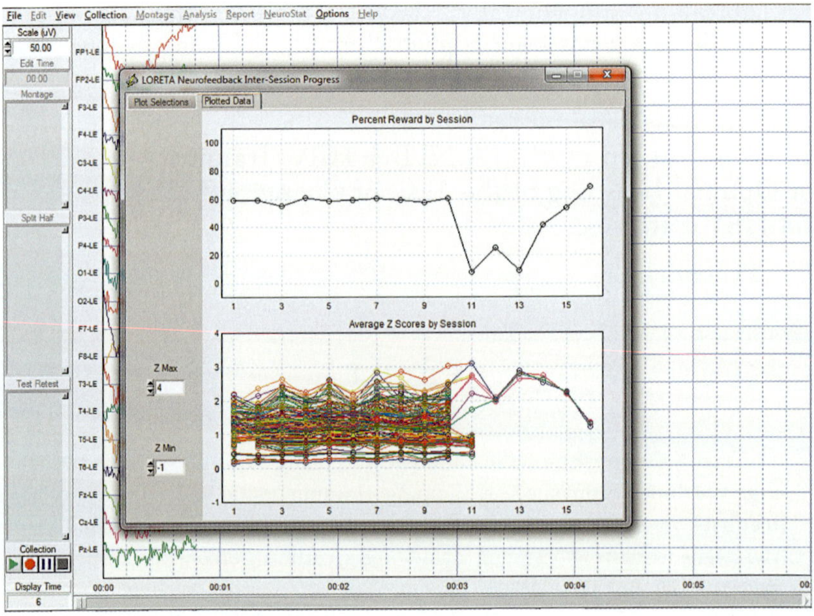

FIGURE 8.7 Progress over 16 LNFB (+HRV) sessions. *Figure from Thompson and Thompson, 2003.*

At session 11, only the 3 BAs with the most extreme Z-score deviations (matching the patient's most severe symptoms) were targeted during the training and "all-or-none" was used. This meant that the client must put all the target areas within the threshold window that was set.

It is important not to stop training immediately when the graph shows SDs to be below 1.5. We have experienced cases who stopped training due to travel and regressed (Thompson, Thompson, Thompson, et al., 2013).

CASE 2

Case 2 demonstrates LNFB within session reward point improvements and HRV changes. Client, (U), presented with panic attacks at night time and anxiety throughout the day. His mind was always busy but often just with negative ruminations. He was obsessed with fear of raising his HR and therefore did no exercise. Following 40 sessions of NFB training and, later, LNFB, both combined with HRV training, his SDNN went from a range of 58–67 ms to a range of 103–149 ms. His scores on the Burns Anxiety Inventory dropped into the mild range. He was swimming, playing tennis, and jogging, no longer fearing that increasing his HR would lead to a panic attack; indeed, he has not had a panic attack in months, although he admits to experiencing very mild worrying and anxiety. He is still in training to maintain improvements and considers himself to be an optimal performance client now (Figure 8.8).

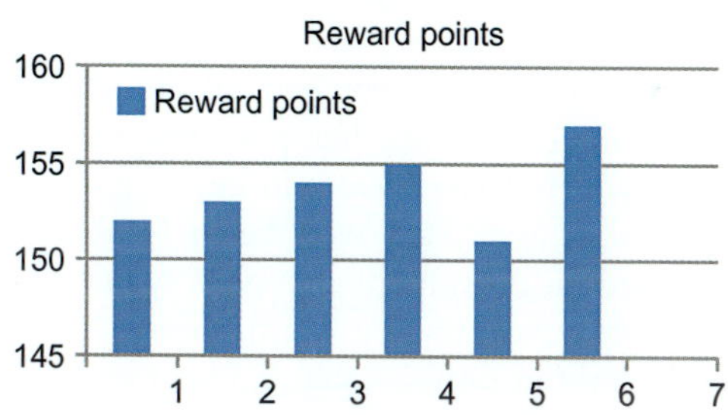

FIGURE 8.8 Within session improvement. 30 min of LNFB were done in this session (six 5-min segments).

During the fifth segment of this session (#5), he was watching an intense part of a movie and scores went down because his anxiety level rose. He was able to rapidly regain calm feeling in segment #6. As previously noted, in the stress assessment discussion, it is not the reaction to stress but the speed and degree of recovery that is important.

CASE 3

A previously athletic, 25-year-old female came for assessment and treatment due to postconcussion symptoms. She had suffered a head injury in a motor vehicle accident 1 year prior to assessment. After her TBI she could no longer function academically, though she had been the top student in her Master's programme prior to injury and so her degree was granted with a few requirements being waived. She had been unable to work for a year, though pre injury she had held a part-time job while also doing her studies. Exercise had been curtailed, too. After 40 sessions of LNFB combined with HRV training, done twice weekly, she no longer required propanolol medication for hypertension, which she had been placed on prior to her injury. She had always worn glasses due to myopia. Post-concussion she had trouble reading and required bifocal glasses. After NFB she no longer had to wear bifocals and her new prescription for distance was not as strong as before her concussion. Her ophthalmologist told her that he had never seen this improvement happen before. With respect to HRV measures, her SDNN improved from 32 up to 74 ms. Total power rose from 454 to 2073 ms^2 and her LF power rose from 149 to 714 ms^2. Regarding ERPs, her P3a response (measured at Cz and reflecting attention and vigilance) indicated faster processing, dropping from 433 to 376 ms. On the continuous performance test reaction, time was about 1/10 s faster, dropping from 544 to 439 ms, and her omission errors dropped from 11.4 to 5.7%. Her scores on the cpt had all moved into the normal range. Concerning EEG measures, her peak frequency had increased from 9.6 to 10 Hz, which is considered an improvement since a higher dominant frequency is associated with being brighter and peak frequency (also termed peak individual alpha) typically drops after a head injury. Another typical finding is a decrease in EEG power post-concussion, particularly in upper alpha and beta ranges (Thayer et al., 2013). These and other QEEG changes can persist, as had been the case with this patient (Korn, Golan, Melamed, Pascual-Marqui, & Friedman, 2005). Her posttreatment EEG demonstrated a global increase in power. The increase in total power correlated with improvement in her symptoms. This may indicate increased neural recruitment and suggests that more neurons are firing synchronously. This positive change may be the result of synaptic changes due to long-term potentiation (LTP).

Note that TBI will usually result in a decrease in blood flow and therefore a deprivation of needed oxygen and nutrients to the neurons in the affected areas. There is also diffuse axonal injury (DAI) that involves stretching and twisting of axons, which can result in a flooding of glutamate into the synaptic junction. This may result in an abnormal increase in sodium and calcium entry into the postsynaptic ending with resulting depression of mitochondrial (Krebs cycle) production of adenosine triphosphate (ATP), which is the energy source for the neurons and, in particular, for active transport across neuronal membranes (Thompson, Thompson, Reid-Chung, and Thompson, 2013). This series of events may be postulated to be part of the reason that there is a decrease in EEG amplitude post injury. Despite all the QEEG findings in cases of mild TBI, it should always be remembered that there is no substitute for reviewing the entire raw EEG. There may be post injury changes that include paroxysmal EEG activity, including brief, but not persistent, high amplitude bursts of any frequency, may not be noticed if you just look at quantitative data because they would produce only a small increase when average amplitude is looked at with the QEEG analysis. The practitioner must therefore look at the whole raw EEG and would be advised to do single point analysis (available using LORETA in the NG program) of any such isolated bursts. If their source correlates with the patient's symptoms then that area can be targeted when doing LNFB, which may be an additional reason for using this approach.

SUMMARY AND CONCLUSION

The networks mentioned above, including affect, executive, salience, and default networks, all have in common involvement of the cingulate gyrus and other CMSs. Dysfunction involving CMSs may be reflected in the surface EEG at, and between, Fz, Cz, and Pz, in addition to other sites. Surface NFB training at midline sites, due in part to having an influence on the cingulate gyrus and its many connections, when combined with the client assuming a functionally appropriate mental state, may encourage changes in the network(s) that are important for efficient and appropriate mental functioning. LNFB can more directly target the central midline and ventral structures involved in these networks; thus LNFB may have the potential to decrease the number of training sessions necessary to achieve clinical improvement. HRV training also has effects on many of the same cortical and subcortical areas and networks that are affected by NFB training and, when combined with surface NFB or LNFB, may reasonably be assumed to enhance the client's self-regulation, especially with respect to emotions and stress management, and further enhance outcomes.

The final key to the most effective interventions may still be the client–trainer connection. The positive expectations and the support of an effective NFB provider both help the client achieve an appropriate mental state that corrects the targeted dysfunction. Being in a positive mental state while doing the LNFB combined with HRV should, theoretically, reinforce this state and assist the client in achieving their training goals.

References

Applehans, B. M., & Lueken, L. J. (2006). Attentional processes, anxiety, and regulation of cortisol reactivity. *Anxiety, Stress & Coping: An International Journal, 19*(1), 81–92.

Baguley, I. J., Heriseanu, R. E., Felmingham, K. L., & Cameron, I. D. (2006). Dysautonomia and heart rate variability following severe traumatic brain injury. *Brain Injury, 20*(4), 437–444.

Beauregard, M., & Levesque, J. (2006). Functional magnetic resonance imaging investigation of the effects of neurofeedback training on the neural bases of selective attention and response inhibition in children with attention-deficit/hyperactivity disorder. *Applied Psychophysiology and Biofeedback, 31*(1), 3–20.

Beniamini, Y., Rubenstein, J. J., Zaichkowsky, L. D., & Crim, M. C. (1997). Effects of high intensity strength training on quality-of-life parameters in cardiac rehabilitation patients. *The American Journal of Cardiology, 80*, 841–846.

Giardino, N. D., Lehrer, P. M., & Edelberg, R. (2002). Comparison of finger plethysmograph to ECG in the measurement of heart rate variability. *Psychophysiology, 39*(2), 246–253.

Grippo, A. J., & Johnson, A. K. (2009). Stress, depression and cardiovascular dysregulation: A review of neurobiological mechanisms and the integration of research from preclinical disease models. *Stress, 12*(1), 1–21.

Hassett, A., Radvanski, D., Vaschillo, E., Vaschillo, B., Sigal, L., Karavidas, M., et al. (2007). A pilot study of the efficacy of heart rate variability (HRV) biofeedback in patients with fibromyalgia. *Applied Psychophysiology and Biofeedback, 32*(1), 1–10.

Karavidas, M., Lehrer, P., Vaschillo, E., Vaschillo, B., Marin, H., Buyske, S., et al. (2007). Preliminary results of an open label study of heart rate variability biofeedback for the treatment of major depression. *Applied Psychophysiology and Biofeedback, 32*(1), 19–30.

Klabunde, R. E. (2013). *Cardiovascular physiology concepts*. <http://www.cvphysiology.com>.

Korn, A., Golan, H., Melamed, I., Pascual-Marqui, R., & Friedman, A. (2005). Focal cortical dysfunction and blood–brain barrier disruption in patients with postconcussion syndrome. *Journal of Clinical Neurophysiology, 22*, 1–9.

Kropotov, J. D. (2009). *Quantitative EEG, event-related potentials and neurotherapy*. San Diego, CA: Academic Press, Elsevier, pp. 292–309.

La Rovere, M. -T., Pinna, D., & Raczak, G. (2008). Baroreflex sensitivity: Measurement and clinical implications. *Annals of Noninvasive Electrocardiology, 13*(2), 191–207.

Lehrer, P. M. (2007a). Biofeedback training to increase heart rate variability. In P. M. Lehrer, R. L. Woolfolk, & W. E. Sime (Eds.), *Principles and Practice of Stress Management* (3rd ed., pp. 148–227). New York: Guilford Press.

Lehrer, P. M. (2013). How does heart rate variability biofeedback work? Resonance, the baroreflex, and other mechanisms. *Biofeedback, 41*, 26–31.

Lehrer, P., & Vaschillo, E. (2008). The future of heart rate variability (HRV) biofeedback. *Biofeedback, 36*, 11–14.

Lehrer, P., Vaschillo, E., Lu, S. -E., Eckberg, D., Vaschillo, B., Scardella, A., et al. (2006). Heart rate variability biofeedback: Effects of age on heart rate variability, baroreflex gain, and asthma. *Chest, 129*, 278–284.

Lehrer, P. M., & Eddie, D. (2013). Dynamic processes regulation and some implications for biofeedback and behavioral interventions. *Applied Psychophysiology and Biofeedback, 38* (2), 143–155.

Lehrer, P. M., Karavidas, M. K., Lu, E. -E., Feldman, J., Kranitz, L., Abraham, S., et al. (2008). Psychological treatment of comorbid asthma and panic disorder: A pilot study. *Journal of the Anxiety Disorders, 22*, 674–683.

Lin, G., Xiang, Q., Fu, X., Wang, S., Wang, S., Chen, S., et al. (2012). Heart rate variability biofeedback decreases blood pressure in prehypertensive subjects by improving autonomic function and baroreflex. *Journal of Alternative and Complementary Medicine, 18*(2), 143–152.

Lloyd, D. (2007). Brownell Professor of Philosophy, Trinity College, 300 Summit Street, Hartford, CT (Personal Communications).

Mikosch, P., Hadrawa, T., Laubreiter, K., Brandl, J., Pilz, J., Stettner, H., et al. (2010). Effectiveness of respiratory-sinus-arrhythmia biofeedback on state-anxiety in patients undergoing coronary angiography. *Journal of Advanced Nursing, 66*(5), 1101–1110.

Monastra, V. J., Lubar, J. F., Linden, M., et al. (1999). Assessing attention deficit hyperactivity disorder via quantitative electroencephalography: An initial validation study. *Neuropsychology, 13*, 424–433.

Nagai, M., Hoshide, S., & Kario, K. (2010). The insular cortex and cardiovascular system: A new insight into the brain–heart axis. *Journal of the American Society of Hypertension, 4* (4), 174–182.

Northoff, G., Heinzel, A., de Greck, M., Bermpohl, F., Dobrowolny, H., & Panksepp, J. (2006). Self-referential processing in our brain—A meta-analysis of imaging studies on the self. *NeuroImage, 31*, 440–457.

Nunez, P. L. (1981). *Electrical fields of the brain*. New York, NY: Oxford University Press.

Nunez, P. L. (1995). *Neocortical dynamics and human EEG rhythm*. New York, NY: Oxford University Press.

Peper, E., Shaffer, F., & Lin, I. -E. (2010). Garbage in; garbage out–identify blood volume pulse (BVP) artifacts before analyzing and interpreting BVP, blood volume pulse amplitude, and heart rate/respiratory sinus arrhythmia data. *Biofeedback, 38*(1), 19–23.

Porges, S. W. (2007). The polyvagal perspective. *Biological Psychiatry, 74*, 116–143.

Prinsloo, G. E., Rauch, H. G., Lambert, M. I., Muench, F., Noakes, T. D., & Derman, W. E. (2011). Effectiveness of respiratory-sinus-arrhythmia biofeedback on state-anxiety in patients undergoing coronary angiography. *Journal of Advanced Nursing, 66* 1101–1110.

Reid, A., Nihon, S., Thompson, L., & Thompson, M. (2013). The effects of heart rate variability training on sensorimotor rhythm: A pilot study. *Journal of Neurotherapy: Investigations in Neuromodulation, Neurofeedback, and Applied Neuroscience, 17*(1), 43–48.

Reiner, R. (2008). Integrating a portable biofeedback device into clinical practice for patients with anxiety disorders: Results of a pilot study. *Applied Psychophysiology and Biofeedback, 33*, 55–61.

Seeley, W., Menon, V., Schatzberg, A., Keller, J., Glover, G., Kenna, H., et al. (2007). Dissociable intrinsic connectivity networks for salience processing and executive control. *The Journal of Neuroscience, 27*(9), 2349–2356.

Shah, S. G., Klumpp, H., Angstadt, M., Nathan, P. J., & Phan, K. L. (2009). Amygdala and insula response to emotional images in patients with generalized anxiety disorder. *Journal of Psychiatry Neuroscience, 34*(4), 296–302.

Supekar, K., Uddin, L. Q., Prater, K., Amin, H., Greicius, M. D., & Menon, V. (2010). Development of functional and structural connectivity within the default mode network in young children. *Journal of Neuroimage, 52*, 290–301.

Sykora, M., Diedler, J., Rupp, A., Turcani, P., & Steiner, T. (2009). Impaired baroreceptor reflex sensitivity in acute stroke is associated with insular involvement, but not with carotid atherosclerosis. *Stroke, 40*, 737–742.

Task Force of The European Society of Cardiology, & The North American Society of Pacing and Electrophysiology (1996). Heart rate variability: Standards of measurement, physiological interpretation, and clinical use. *European Heart Journal, 17*, 354–381.

Thayer, J. F., Åhs, F., Fredrikson, M., Sollers, J. J., III, & Wager, T. D. (2012). A meta-analysis of heart rate variability and neuroimaging studies: Implications for heart rate variability as a marker of stress and health. *Neuroscience and Behavioral Reviews, 36*, 747–756.

Thatcher, R. W. (2012). Handbook of quantitative electroencephalography and EEG biofeedback: Scientific Foundations and Practical Applications. <www.appliedneuroscience.com>.

Thompson, J., & Hagedorn, D. (2012). Multimodal analysis: New approaches to the concussion conundrum. *Journal of Clinical Sport Psychology, 6*, 22–46.

Thompson, M., Thompson, J., & Wenqing, W. (2008). *Brodmann areas, 10–20 sites, primary functions booklet.* San Rafael, CA: ISNR Publications.

Thompson, M., & Thompson, L. (2001). "Setting-Up-For-Clinical-Success" Suite. Biofeedback Federation of Europe: Amsterdam.

Thompson, M., & Thompson, L. (2003). *The neurofeedback book: An introduction to basic concepts in applied psychophysiology.* Wheat Ridge, CO: Association for Applied Psychophysiology. Polish translation 2012.

Thompson, M., & Thompson, L. (2007). Neurofeedback for stress management. In P. M. Lehrer, R. L. Woolfolk, & W. E. Sime (Eds.), *Principles and practice of stress management* (3rd ed., pp. 249–287). New York, NY: Guilford Publications.

Thompson, M., & Thompson, L. (2010). Functional neuroanatomy and the rationale for using EEG biofeedback for clients with asperger's syndrome. *Journal of Applied Psychophysiology and Biofeedback, 35*(1), 39–61.

Thompson, M., Thompson, L., & Reid, A. (2010). Functional neuroanatomy and the rationale for using EEG biofeedback for clients with Asperger's syndrome. *Journal of Applied Psychophysiology and Biofeedback, 35*(1), 39–61.

Thompson, M., Thompson, L., Reid-Chung, A., & Thompson, J. (2013). Managing TBI: Appropriate assessment and a rationale for using neurofeedback and biofeedback to enhance recovery in postconcussion syndrome. *Biofeedback, 41*(4), 158–173.

Thompson, M., Thompson, L., Thompson, J., & Hagedorn, D. (2011). Networks: A compelling rationale for combining neurofeedback, biofeedback and strategies. *NeuroConnections*, 8–17. Summer 2011.

Thompson, M., Thompson, L., Thompson, J., Reid, A., & Hagedorn, D. (2013). Heart–brain connections underlie effective neurofeedback plus biofeedback interventions: Complex case with depression. *NeuroConnections*, 11–26. Winter 2013.

Zoeller, R. F. (2007). Physical activity: Depression, anxiety, physical activity, and cardiovascular disease: What is the connection? *American Journal Lifestyle Medicine, 1*, 175–180.

Zöllei, E., Paprika, D., & Rudas, L. (2003). Measures of cardiovascular autonomic regulation derived from spontaneous methods and the Valsalva manoeuver. *Autonomic Neuroscience, 103*(1–2), 100–105.

CHAPTER

9

Treating Anxiety Disorders Using Z-Scored EEG Neurofeedback

William A. Lambos, PhD
and Rebecca A. Williams, BSc
ABF Behavioral Health, Tampa, FL, USA

To grapple with and understand anxiety is, in some sense, to grapple with and understand the human condition…The syndromes described by Hippocrates are recognizably the same clinical phenomena described in the latest issues of the Archives of General Psychiatry *and* Bulletin of the Menninger Clinic…*Their similarities bridge the yawning gap of millennia and circumstances that separate them, providing a sense of how, for all the differences in culture and setting, the physiologically anxious aspects of human experience may be universal.*

— From: Scott Stossel, "My Age of Anxiety," iBooks, https://itun.es/us/KOtkQ.1

INTRODUCTION

There is no behavioral or mental health problem that affects more individuals than the group of conditions classified as anxiety disorders. The incidence rate in American and European cultures is estimated at having a lifetime prevalence of greater than 25%. And given the stigma that continues to be associated with mental health conditions in many areas, especially in the USA (where there persists a cultural ethos of rugged individualism—the so-called Marlboro Man persona), we suspect that the actual rate at which anxiety disorders are experienced is considerably higher than the reported incidence figures.

Z Score Neurofeedback.
DOI: http://dx.doi.org/10.1016/B978-0-12-801291-8.00009-1

Nor does anxiety typically come "in the door" alone. In at least 50% of cases, the patient with anxiety also presents as comorbid with depression, rumination, or other issues. Considering what has been learned in the last 5–10 years about brain networks based on nodal concentrations of specific neural activity sharing broad interconnections with other nodes (Hagmann et al., 2008), this is not surprising. Momentary and situation-appropriate anxiety serves a useful purpose, and as we shall see, involves a complex interplay among affective, limbic, executive, arousal-related, and thalamic synchronization areas of both cortical and subcortical areas of the brain. It is therefore not unexpected that when one or more aspects of such complex networks become dysregulated, other interrelated networks also fall into dysregulation and result in comorbidity.

Thus, no one practicing the treatment of behavioral health issues is likely to avoid confronting the patient who suffers from anxiety disorders—and their comorbidities and complications—for very long. And, as is very likely well known to readers of this volume, the standard existing treatments for anxiety disorders are hardly satisfactory. The two main approaches, while by no means the only avenues available to therapists, can be categorized as (a) pharmacotherapy and (b) cognitive–behavioral therapy. The former relies largely on two groups of medications, those intended for affective regulation (typically antidepressants and mood stabilizers), and drugs that inhibit the release of the inhibitory neurotransmitter gamma-aminobutyric acid (GABA). The most common of latter group of substances are the benzodiazepines, which include Xanax and Valium, and are among the most abused substances in industrialized nations.

The latter group of therapies—those based on cognitive–behavioral or other forms of counseling—have similarly fallen short (Hollander & Simeon, 2003).

For all the prescriptions written for Wellbutrin, Ativan, and Lexipro, and for the thousands of talk therapy sessions aimed to treat anxiety that take place every day, anxiety disorder has not decreased in prevalence. Rather, its incidence appears to be increasing (Stossel, 2013). An alternative treatment to this most widespread of mental health disorders would surely be of no small value to patients and therapists alike, and to our society as a whole.

We have been treating clients for anxiety disorders using Z-scored electroencephalogram (EEG) biofeedback since 2006. Beginning with four-channel protocols for reducing excess normative high beta over C–Z or other sites (based on quantitative electroencephalogram (qEEG) mapping), we have had increasing success in helping clients overcome chronic and even disabling anxiety. Long-term recovery of normative daily functioning has been the outcome in the majority of these cases, and the trend appears to be one of increasing efficacy in a decreasing number of training sessions. In addition, the majority of our clients have been able to cease the regular use of anxiolytic medications following treatment. At our clinic today, we continue to offer several modalities of treatment for anxiety disorders, but the great majority of patients receive low-resolution EEG tomographic analysis (LORETA) 19-channel symptom-guided EEG biofeedback combined with ongoing cognitive–behavioral support. Some, with a history of traumatic experience, also receive eye movement desensitization and reprocessing (EMDR) therapy (Silverman, 2011) in between EEG biofeedback sessions. For such patients, the combination of therapies has proved quite synergistic.

Overall, our practice with 19-channel Z-scored EEG biofeedback has demonstrated that the outcomes for patients presenting with anxiety disorders continue to improve, and we consider anxiety disorders among the most readily treatable of behavioral health issues. The data we present in this chapter are intended to support this assertion.

THE INITIAL ASSESSMENT OF ANXIETY DISORDER PATIENTS

Every patient at our clinic begins his or her experience with a lengthy diagnostic interview lasting 60–90 min. The first 25–40 min or so normally consists of a free-form exploratory discussion in which we ask the patient (and family members if present) to explain why they have come, stated as attempting to answer the question "What are we trying to achieve via treatment?" At times, the goal must be restated more or less operationally depending on the circumstance and sophistication level of the client. It is very important to observe the behavior of the patient during this interview, as his or her nonverbal cues reveal a great deal about their level of distress and coping mechanisms. The second half of the interview consists of a dozen or so structured questions that address medical and neurological issues (i.e., the patient's health history, evidence of past brain injury and of infectious diseases of the brain, epileptic symptoms, cerebral edema, etc.) as well as a biopsychosocial summary, educational, vocational, substance use, and related background questions.

Following this interview, if the patient is deemed an appropriate candidate for further assessment and agrees to pursue it, he or she will be scheduled for a 19-channel qEEG mapping as well as a number of other assessments appropriate to his or her age and presenting condition. For the patient with any of the anxiety disorders, he or she is requested to take the Beck Anxiety Inventory and/or the Clarke–Beck OCD Inventory, as well as the Personality Assessment Inventory (Adult or Adolescent version, as appropriate), if over the age of 12 years. If they are under 12 years old, then behavior scales for two parents or home caregivers and two teachers are requested instead. We have used the Conners Behavioral

Rating Scales (CBRS), the Conners Early Childhood Scales (CECS), the Multidimensional Anxiety Scale for Children (MASC), the Pediatric Behavior Rating Scale (PBRS), or others as deemed appropriate.

What is important from the practitioner's perspective is to collect multiple sources of independent data one hopes will be convergent. In addition, some of the tests can be given posttreatment to reassess the client to help collect normative data on the degree and magnitude of change that has taken place over the course of treatment.

Following the scoring of the assessments and analysis and interpretation of the qEEG maps, a written report is compiled and shared with the client. This report summarizes the patient's presenting symptoms and history, outlines the consistency of the assessment metrics, the markers of anxiety disorder found in the qEEG maps, and suggests a treatment plan if treatment is deemed likely to be beneficial for the particular patient.

THE BRAIN'S ANXIETY NETWORK

Thatcher (2012) has summarized the components of the areas and interconnections that are considered the core components of the brain's anxiety network. His diagram summarizing the interconnections is shown in Figure 9.1.

The figure is interesting not in the least, because the majority of the components of the anxiety network lie outside the cortex. Although both the hippocampus and the amygdala contain apical dendrites and therefore generate EEG that can be seen with LORETA imaging, the fact is most of this network is not amenable to neuromodulation with EEG biofeedback.

This begs the question: Why does 19-channel Z-scored symptom-driven EEG biofeedback as a treatment for the anxiety disorders appear to be so effective if the majority of the central nervous system structures that mediate the fear response are insensitive to EEG-based neuromodulation techniques?

The case studies and other data from our client population we present in the following pages are an attempt to answer this question. We do not claim to offer a definitive answer. However, our experience of many years in working with these patients does suggest a hypothesis, which can be more or less succinctly summarized as the following assertion:

> *Anxiety disorders are characterized by chronic activation of subcortical fear- and arousal-related structures that are no longer under the inhibitory control of the cortical structures that generally suppress their activity in nonclinical individuals. Therefore, effective treatment of anxiety disorders involves restoring such inhibitory cortical control to cortical areas over these subcortical regions.*

Thus, in the absence of a fear-inducing stimulus appropriate to a given situation (i.e., the sound of an intruder in one's home late at night), the

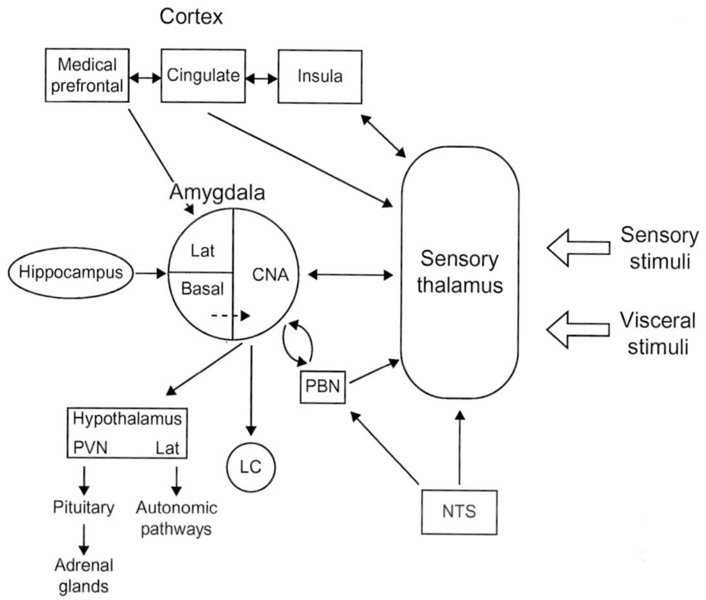

FIGURE 9.1 The brain's anxiety network. Note the large number of subcortical and brain stem structures relative to cortical areas that play a prominent role in mediating anxiety. *From Thatcher (2012) reprinted with permission.*

amygdala, hypothalamus, locus ceruleus, and/or other subcortical structures remain inappropriately activated over long periods of time, resulting in persistent hypervigilance and exhaustive stress that characterizes chronic anxiety (Kim et al., 2011). Moreover, the cortical structures normally responsible for inhibiting this activation appear to have lost their ability to do so (Etkin, Prater, Schatzberg, Menon, & Greicius, 2009).

We do not expect the reader to receive this hypothesis as novel or innovative. What is surprising, however, is the apparent efficacy with which LORETA Z-score-guided EEG biofeedback is able to achieve restoration of cortical control and, therefore, afford lasting relief from the suffering associated with various manifestations of chronic anxiety.

qEEG MARKERS OF ANXIETY DISORDERS

Given the former discussion, we would expect to see certain markers in qEEG brain maps among anxiety patients, and indeed, this is often the case. Three markers appear regularly in these patients' qEEG maps:

1. Excess Z-scored power activity in the cingulate gyrus and/or the insula. These are most typically in the central cingulate, but we often

see them in the anterior cingulate and, more rarely, the posterior cingulate gyrus as well. They are always excesses in power, never deficits.

2. Aberrant Z-scored power activity in the areas that can be imaged on LORETA near the amygdala, which include the parahippocampal gyrus and the hippocampus. Depending on the exact area of this region of the brain, these discrepancies from the norm may be either excess or deficient in Z-scored power. For example, the more distal with respect to the temporal lobes the locus of dysregulation, the more likely the aberration is power appears to be below the norm rather than in excess of it. This suggests that loci in these areas exert an inhibitory influence on the limbic arousal structures such as the amygdala. When these areas do not generate sufficient power to inhibit their targets, anxiety may result.
3. Aberrant Z-scored connectivity metrics between the dorsolateral prefrontal cortex (DLPFC) and the areas near the amygdala (again, the parahippocampal gyrus and the hippocampus). There is also, in some cases, wider dysregulation in connectivity measures among other cortical areas, including between the DLPFC, the insula, and parietal lobe regions.

These three mechanisms are in agreement both with the current neuroscience literature on arousal, anxiety, and fear (Kent, Sullivan, & Rauch, 2002), and with pre- and posttreatment qEEG maps we have seen in our own clinic over the years. We have treated over 100 patients for one or another type of anxiety disorder, 30 of them using 19-channel Z-scored symptom-driven LORETA EEG biofeedback. We will address our overall outcome measures in the conclusion of the chapter. For the present, we turn to the case studies to support our working hypothesis—anxiety disorders as a group share a failure of inhibitory control of lower-level (reptilian brain) structures by higher-level (executive control) structures. Therefore, successfully treating anxiety must involve restoring this higher-level control to the patient. The following three case studies hope to present a cogent argument and consistent data with respect to this assertion.

ANXIETY DISORDER CASE STUDIES

Case 1, male client of age 58 years, presented with ongoing generalized anxiety for the last 40 years. In the more recent 5 years, he was prescribed benzodiazepines. Case 1 received 20 sessions of 19-channel LORETA Z-scored symptom-driven neurofeedback. He reported after the sessions that his anxiety had been relieved significantly, and he no longer had trouble falling asleep at night. He also reported waking without feelings of anxiety and having better coping skills in his high-stress work environment.

The absolute power maps, in Figure 9.2, show the excess surface power at sites above the limbic system structures such as the cingulate gyrus, a well-known marker associated with anxiety. The dysregulation shows improvement to normative measures after training with symptom-driven LORETA neurofeedback. Similar reductions in aberrant LORETA current source density power are seen in Figure 9.3. As noted, and consistent with known markers, excess current source density measures are seen in the insula region at more than four standard deviations from the reference population. A noteworthy reduction in aberrant power to within neurotypical range is observed.

What is notable about this case is that prior to the availability of symptom-driven protocols including LORETA connectivity measures, the usual standard of care for neurotherapy would have been to down-train the excess Z-scored power emanating from the insula. But looking at connectivity metrics associated with the anxiety network revealed broad yet focal additional dysregulation in connectivity between the DLPFC and the limbic Brodmann areas. Adding these to the treatment protocol (as was suggested by the symptom checklist match in neuroguide neurofeedback) appears to have been an important component of this patient's outcome.

This is demonstrated by comparing pre- and posttreatment LORETA coherence graphs in Figure 9.4. After the 20 sessions of LORETA neurofeedback, there are highly significant improvements in LORETA coherence measures observed between Brodmann areas 8, 9, 10, and 46 and the amygdala and hippocampus. This case shows how LORETA neurofeedback is effective in frontal-limbic associated dysregulations that are markers for anxiety disorders even where focal excess power of limbic or cortical structures is revealed in qEEG maps.

Case 2 involves a male client of age 15 years who presented with severe social anxiety. His symptoms negatively impacted his life to the point he was unable to participate in class, avoided social interactions, and was hesitant to learn how to drive. He reported his symptoms had been ongoing for approximately 2 years and had seen it worsening with age. Case 2 received 20 sessions of 19-channel LORETA Z-scored symptom-driven neurofeedback. He reported after the sessions his social interactions had greatly improved in both group settings and with new people. He reported becoming more talkative and readily made eye contact with people as a rule, whereas before, this was nearly impossible for him.

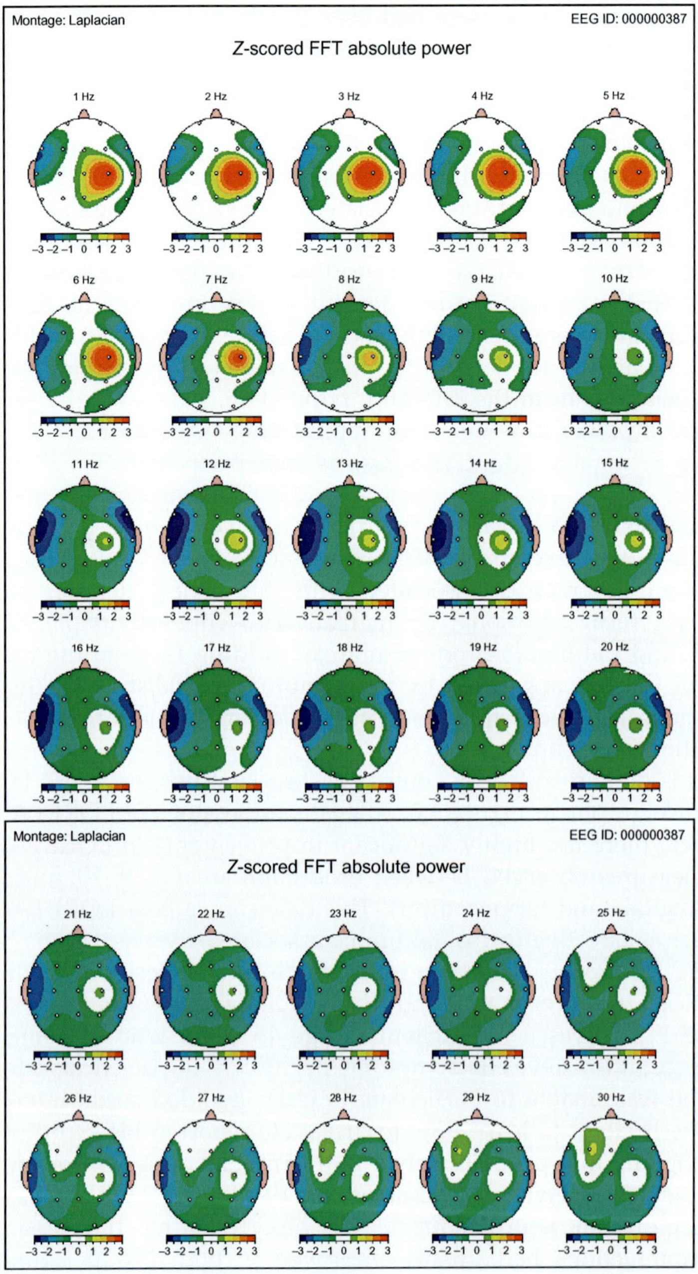

FIGURE 9.2 Pretreatment (left) and post-20 sessions (right) of LORETA neurofeedback Z-scored Fast Fourier Transform (FFT) absolute power maps in the Laplacian montage for Case 1 in the eyes closed condition.

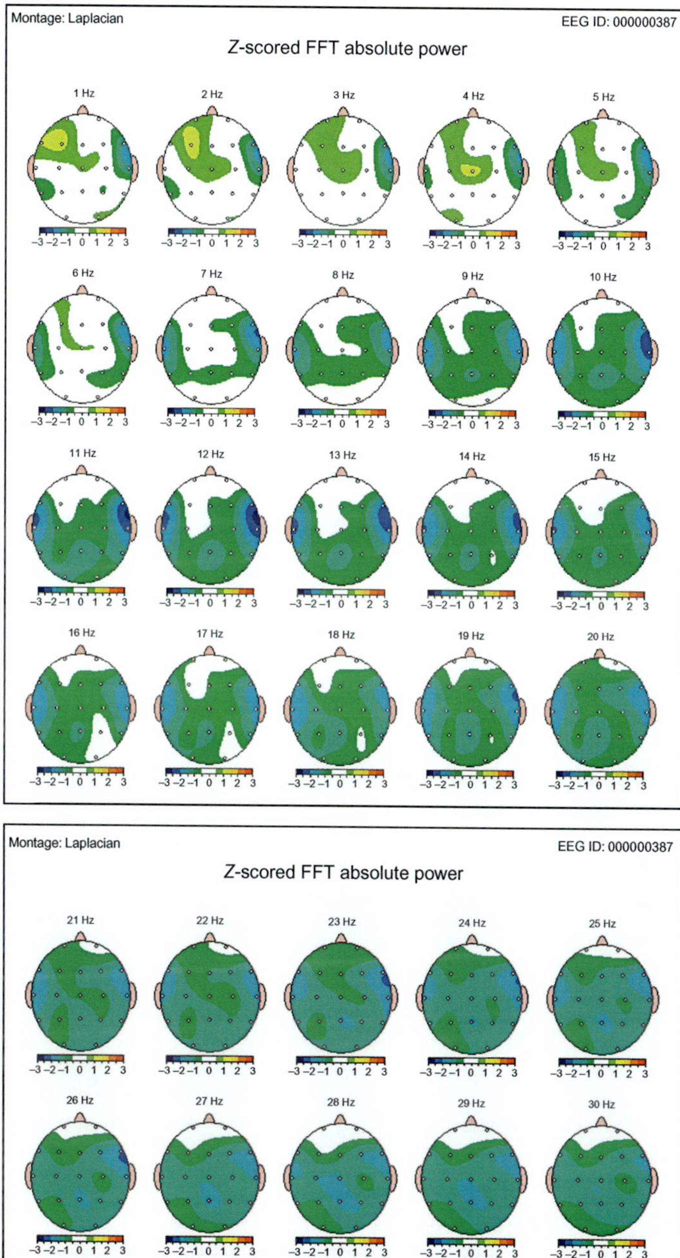

FIGURE 9.2 (Continued)

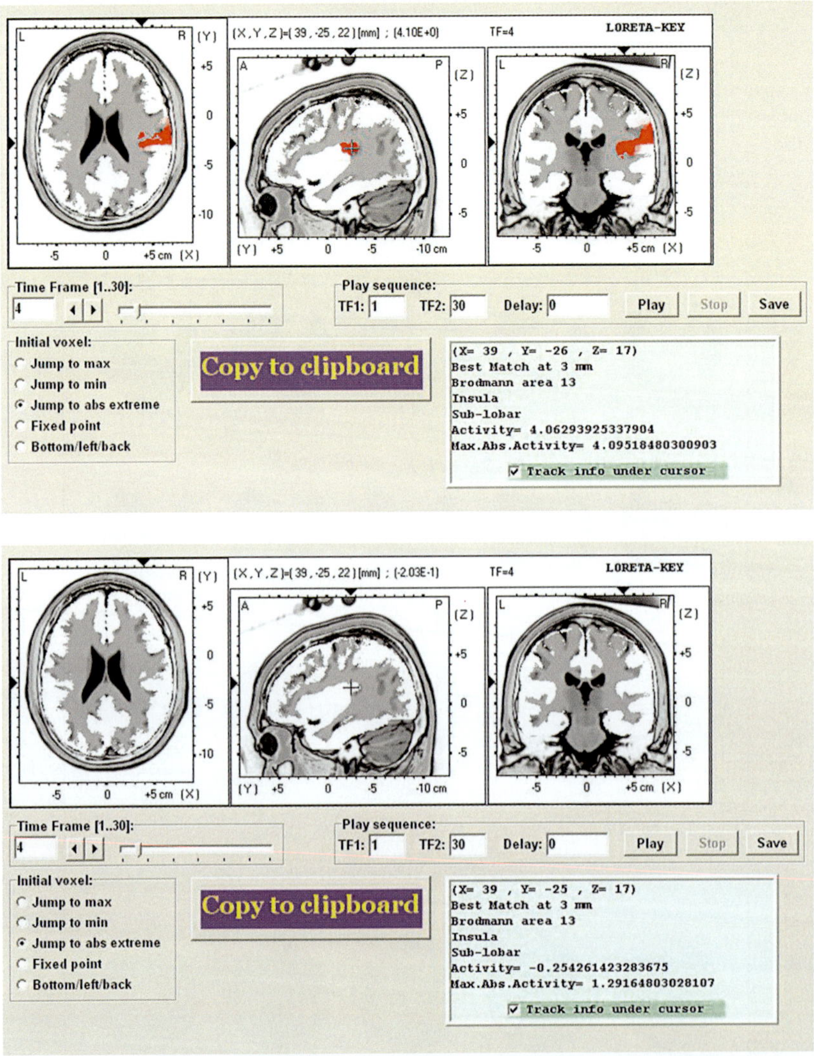

FIGURE 9.3 Pretreatment (top) and post-20 sessions (bottom) of LORETA neurofeedback Z-scored LORETA current source density maps for Case 1 in the eyes closed condition. Dysregulation is seen in the insula.

Figure 9.5 shows the excess surface power in the maps of Case 2 (again, Laplacian montage) to be in frontal lobe areas in delta, theta, and alpha frequencies and excess parietal power in alpha frequencies. These surface findings are cortical–cortical in nature. Following the 20 sessions of LORETA neurofeedback, the dysregulation in surface power normalized at these frequencies. With respect to surface power, all measures are well within the normative boundaries.

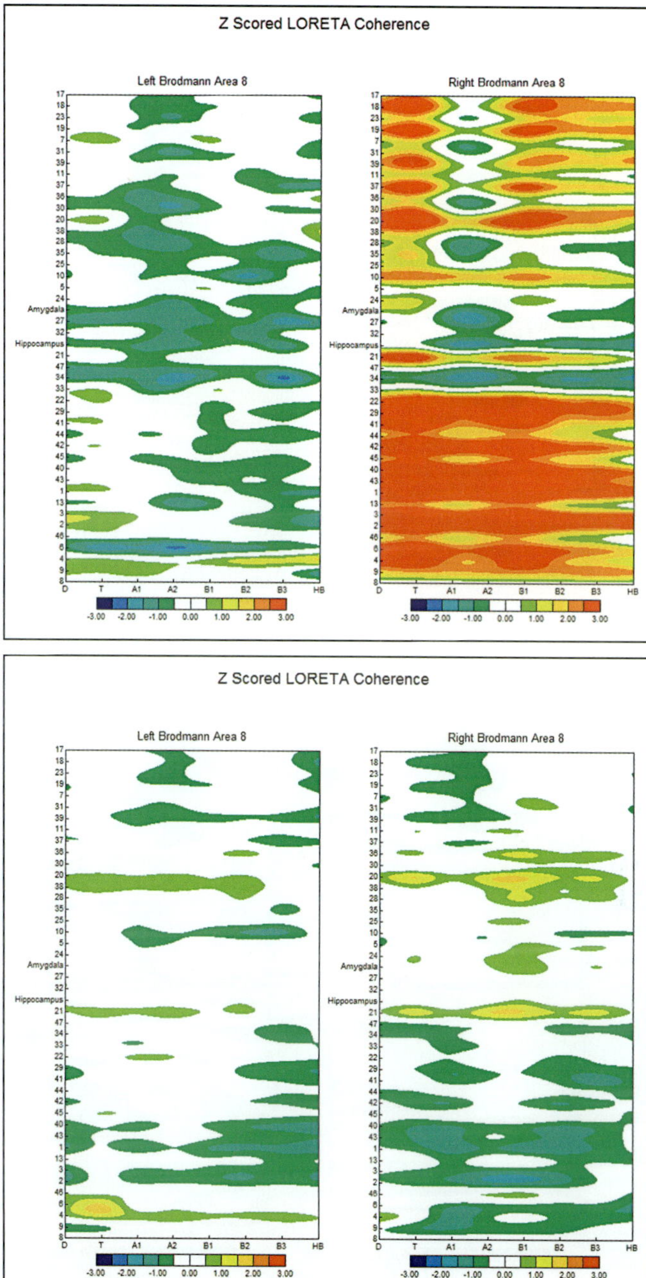

FIGURE 9.4 Case 1 LORETA coherence maps pretreatment (top) and following 20 sessions of LORETA 19-channel *Z*-score-based neurofeedback (bottom). The aberrant coherence shows normalization after treatment.

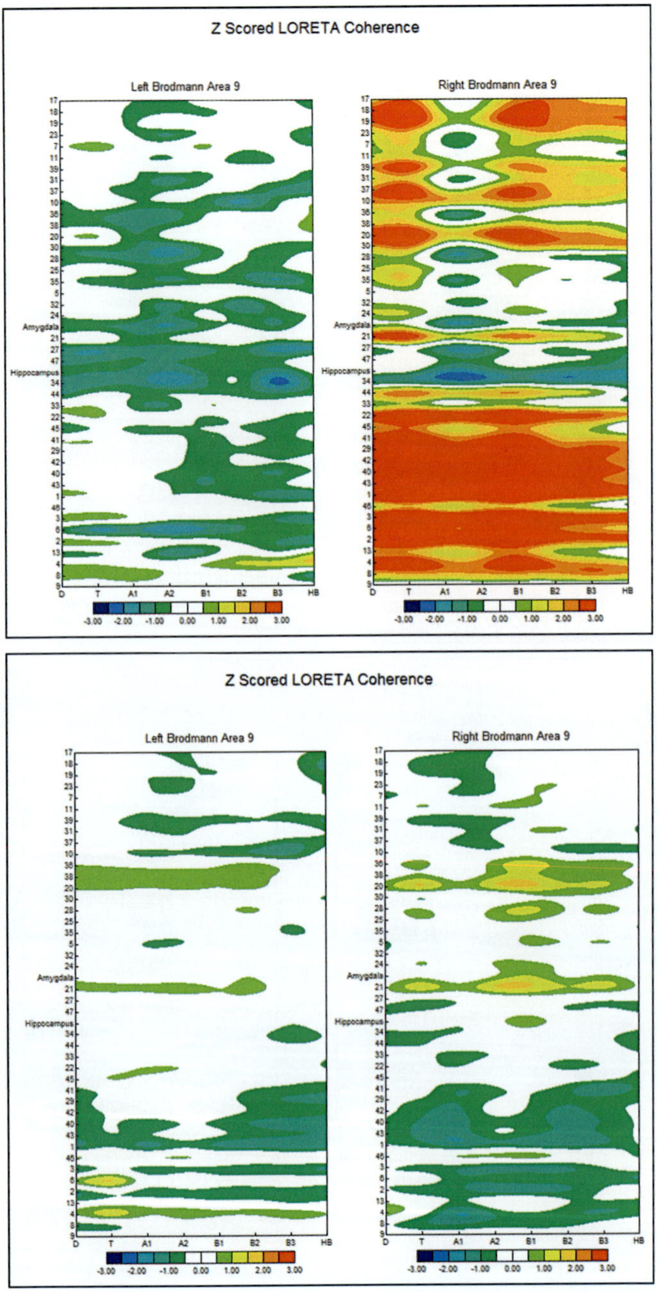

FIGURE 9.4 (Continued)

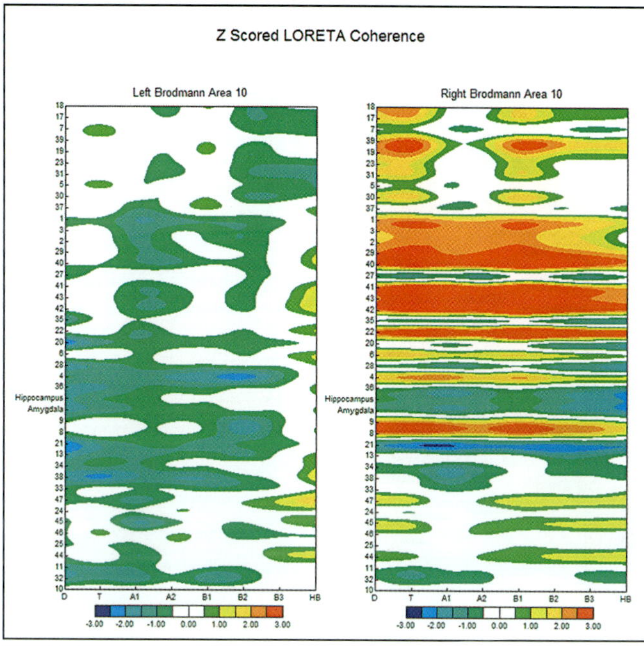

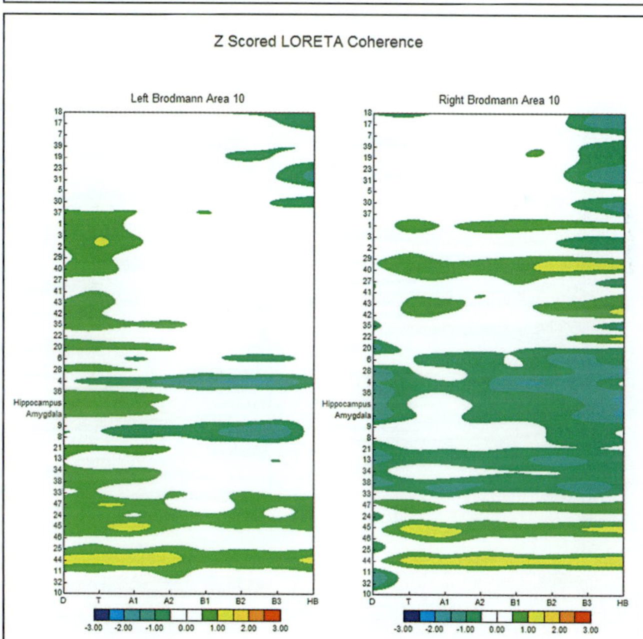

FIGURE 9.4 (Continued)

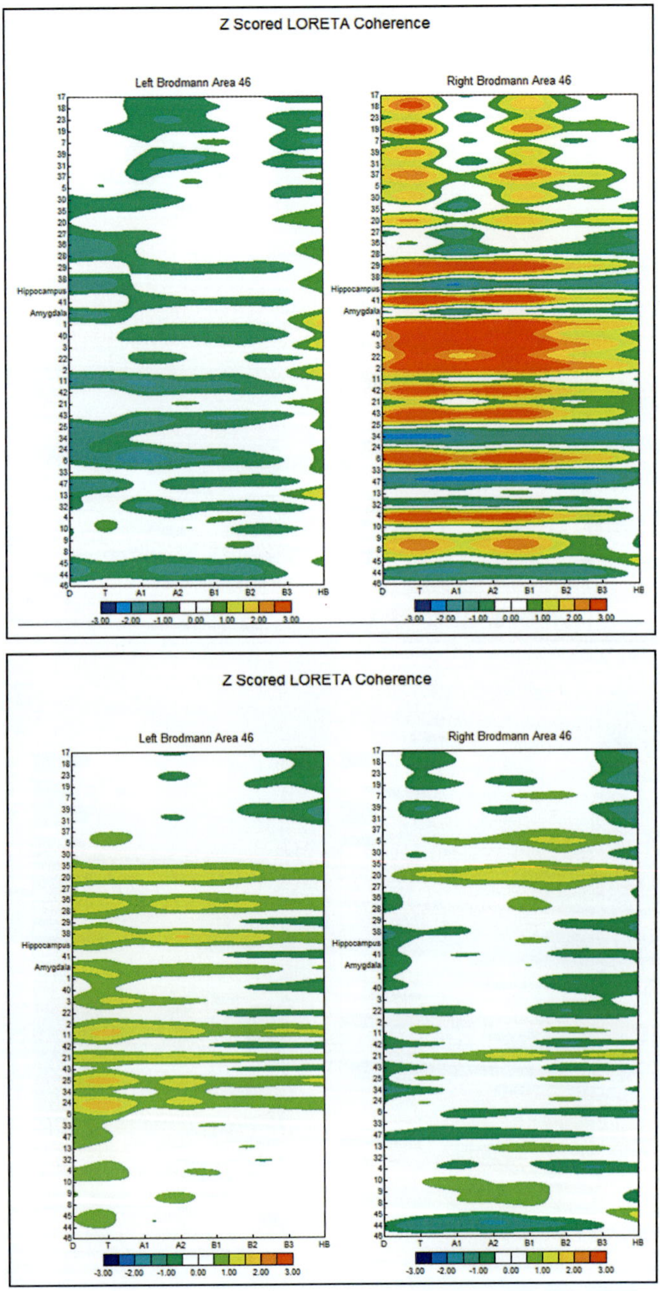

FIGURE 9.4 (Continued)

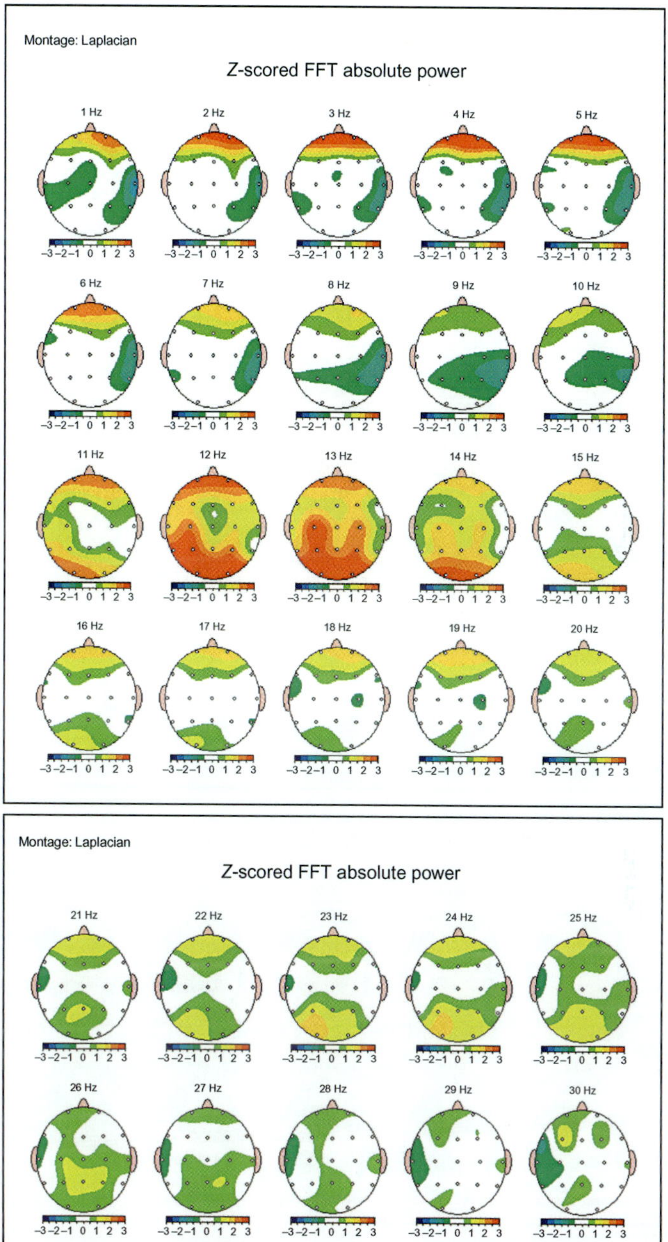

FIGURE 9.5 Pretreatment (left) and post-20 sessions (right) of LORETA neurofeedback *Z*-scored FFT absolute power maps in the Laplacian montage for Case 2 in the eyes closed condition.

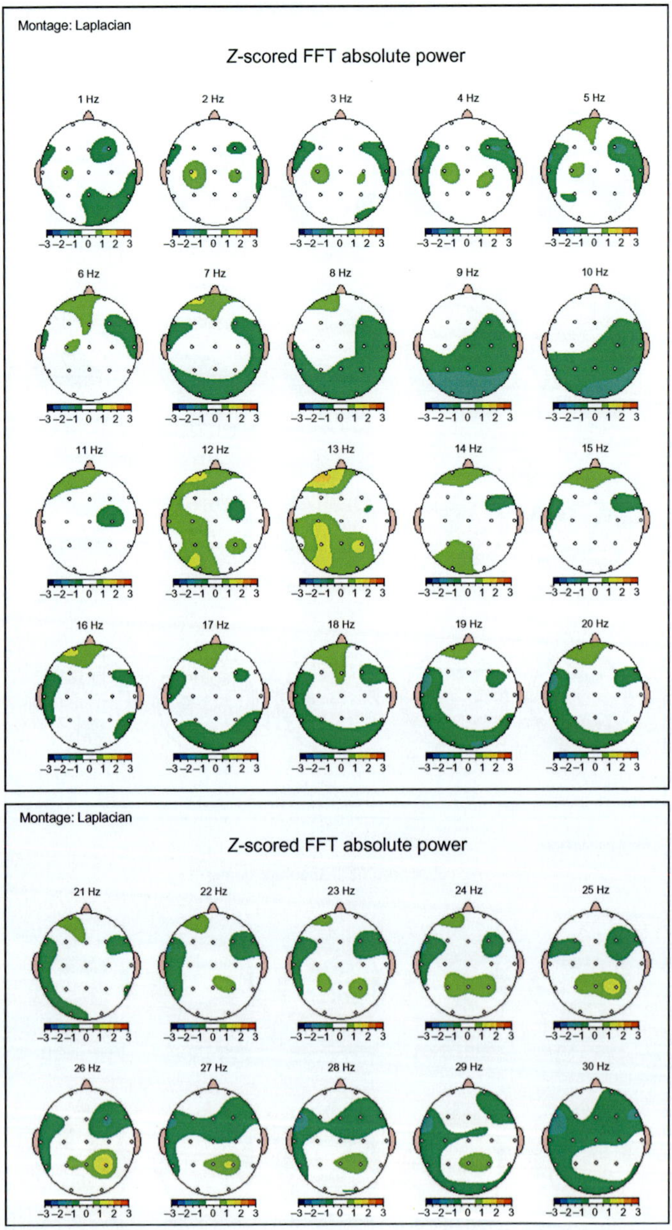

FIGURE 9.5 (Continued)

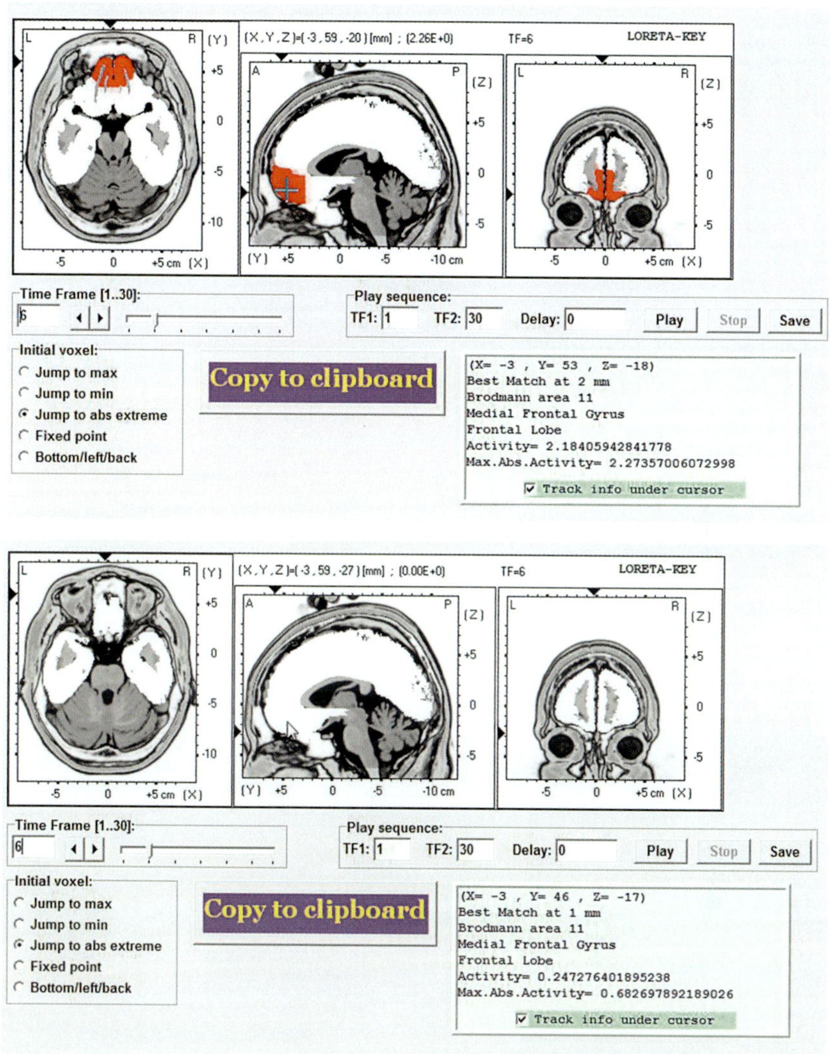

FIGURE 9.6 Pretreatment (top) and post-20 sessions (bottom) of LORETA neurofeedback Z-scored LORETA current source density maps for Case 2 in the eyes closed condition. Dysregulation is seen in the medial frontal gyrus and anterior cingulate.

Figures 9.6 and 9.7 show excess current source density measures in the medial frontal gyrus and in the parahippocampal gyrus, respectively. This relationship is more centered between the limbic cortical areas (including the medial temporal lobes) than the pattern seen in Case 1, but the pretreatment dysregulations in the anxiety network are obvious nonetheless. LORETA neurofeedback, including rewarding the

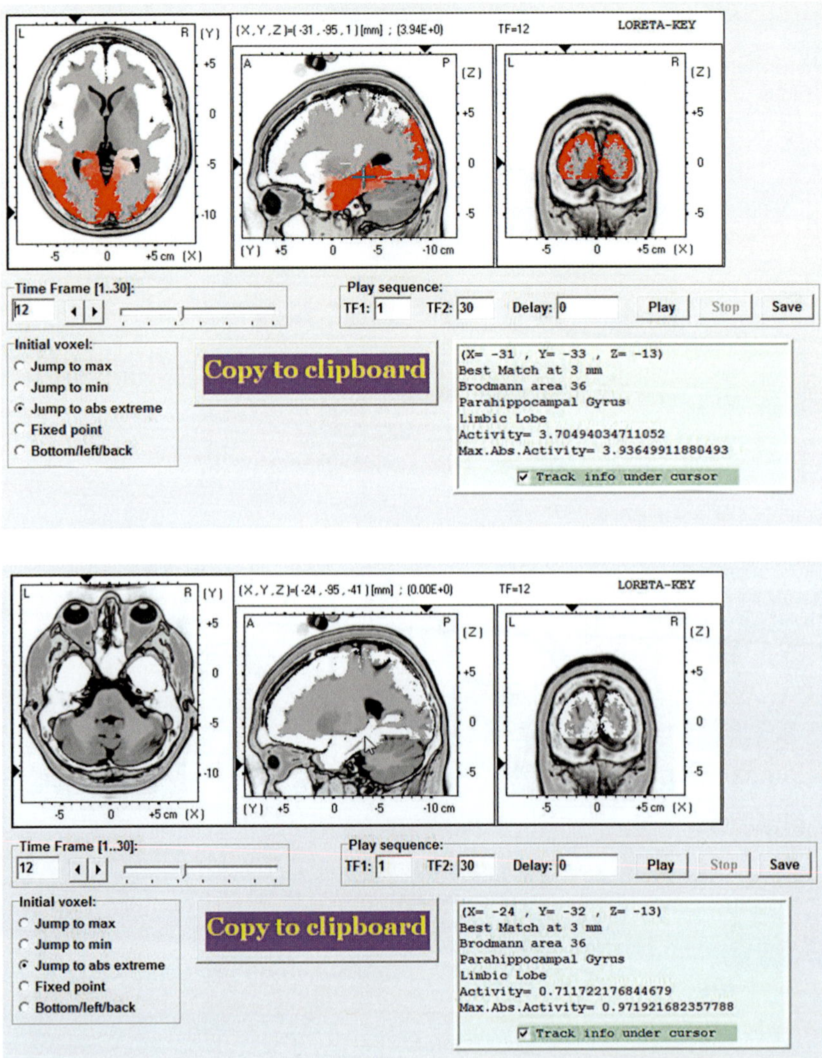

FIGURE 9.7 Pretreatment (top) and post-20 sessions (bottom) of LORETA neurofeedback Z-scored LORETA current source density maps for Case 2 in the eyes closed condition. Dysregulation is seen in the parahippocampal gyrus.

patient for normalizing LORETA coherence among these areas, again showed to be effective in normalizing dysregulation in the measures of current source density after 20 sessions. The improvement change is by nearly two standard deviations in this comparison. When normalized, improved connectivity between these regions also resulted.

Figure 9.8 shows the connectivity measures between the amygdala, hippocampus, and Brodmann area 46. Significant hypercoherence is of note between these limbic areas, contributing to symptoms of anxiety. This parietal-limbic anxiety dysregulation responds positively to LORETA neurofeedback training, in this case, correlated with Case 2's greatly improved ability to function in social settings and, as he reported, to "just act normal again."

Case 3 is a 62-year-old female who presents with anxiety and agoraphobia. Her symptoms began after menopause and seemed to have worsened after she was hospitalized for a myocardial atrial fibrillation and associated complications 2 years prior to visiting our clinic. She was a self-appointed caregiver to her sister, who she described as paranoid and mentally unstable.

Case 3 received 10 sessions of 19-channel LORETA *Z*-scored symptom-driven neurofeedback. After the sessions, she reported an increase in socialization, improved sleep, and reduced anxiety while driving. She also reported being able to return to the gym and attend weekly social gatherings with friends.

Figure 9.9 shows, in her pretreatment maps, excess surface power at frontal and left parietal locations in delta and theta frequencies. Parietal excess surface power is seen in high-beta frequencies. These findings are also consistent with hypothesized markers for anxiety disorders. After the 10 sessions of training, aberrant surface power in the delta and theta frequencies show complete normalization. Beta frequency dysregulation shows reductions in excess surface power by at least one standard deviation.

Case 3 also showed notable excess current source density measures in the parahippocampal gyrus and right temporal gyri. Aberrant current source density measures in the parahippocampal gyrus, pretreatment, were over four standard deviations from the reference population. After 10 sessions, LORETA power decreased by three standard deviations to within the normative range, see Figure 9.10. Figure 9.11 shows a reduction in excess current source density measures from over two standard deviations to nearly 1.5 standard deviations. This reduction in aberrant power is within the reference range after 10 LORETA neurofeedback sessions.

Figure 9.12 shows the coherence maps pretreatment and after 10 sessions of LORETA neurofeedback. Hypercoherence is significant between Brodmann areas 42 and 43 and the amygdala and parahippocampal gyrus. These findings are seen in nearly every frequency band and are strongly consistent with the anxiety markers as described earlier. Notable improvements in connectivity are seen following 10 sessions, and coherence measures are largely normalized in all bandwidths at

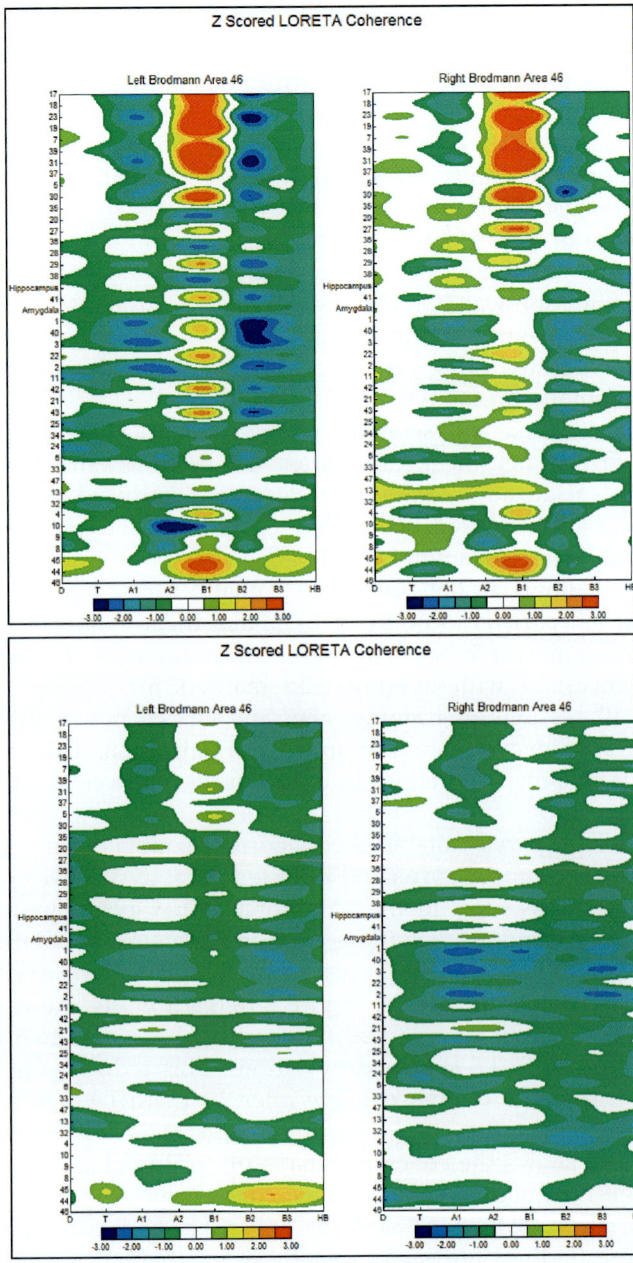

FIGURE 9.8 Case 2 LORETA coherence maps pretreatment (top) and following 20 sessions of LORETA 19-channel Z-score-based neurofeedback (bottom). The aberrant coherence shows normalization after treatment.

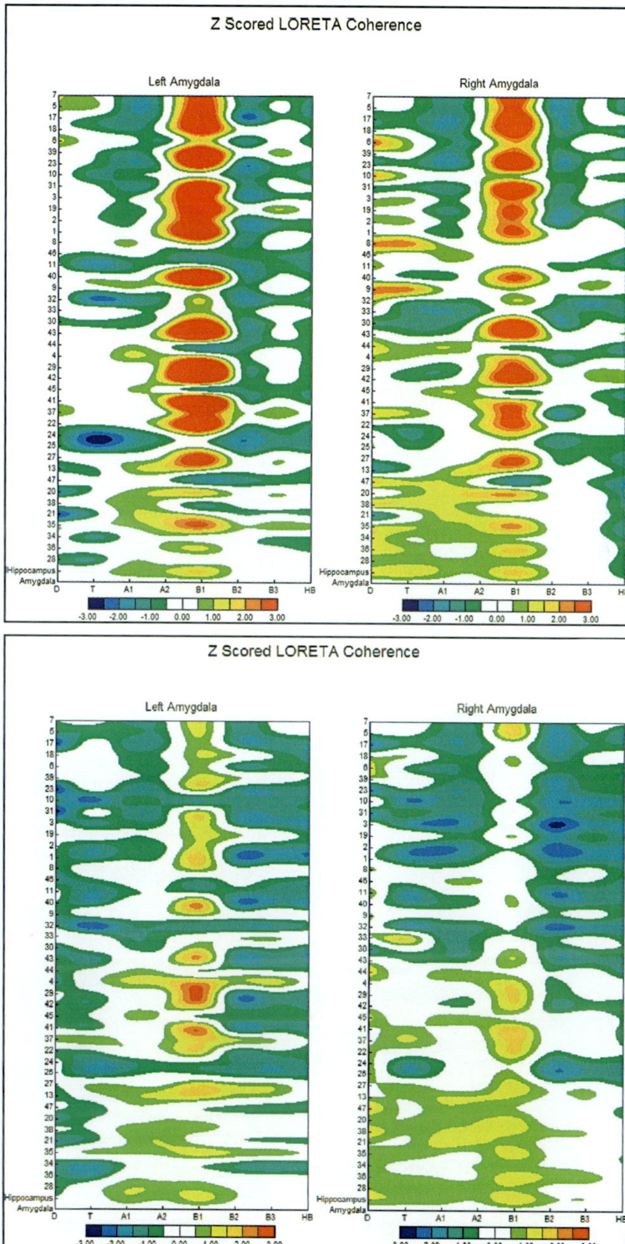

FIGURE 9.8 (Continued)

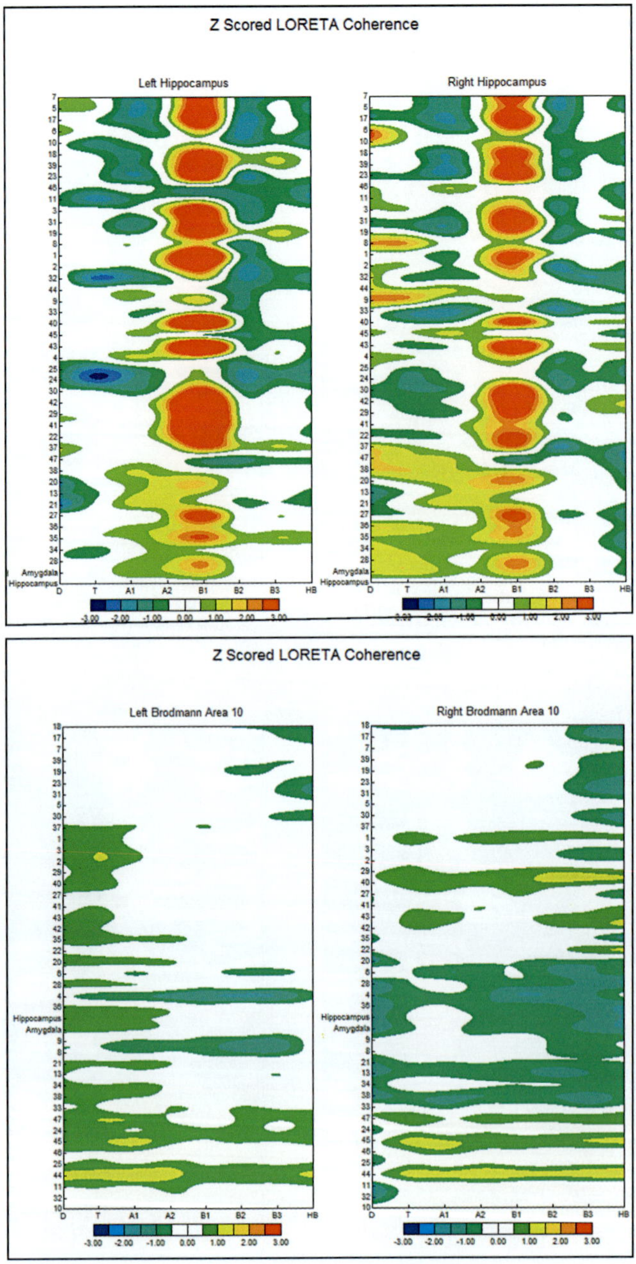

FIGURE 9.8 (Continued)

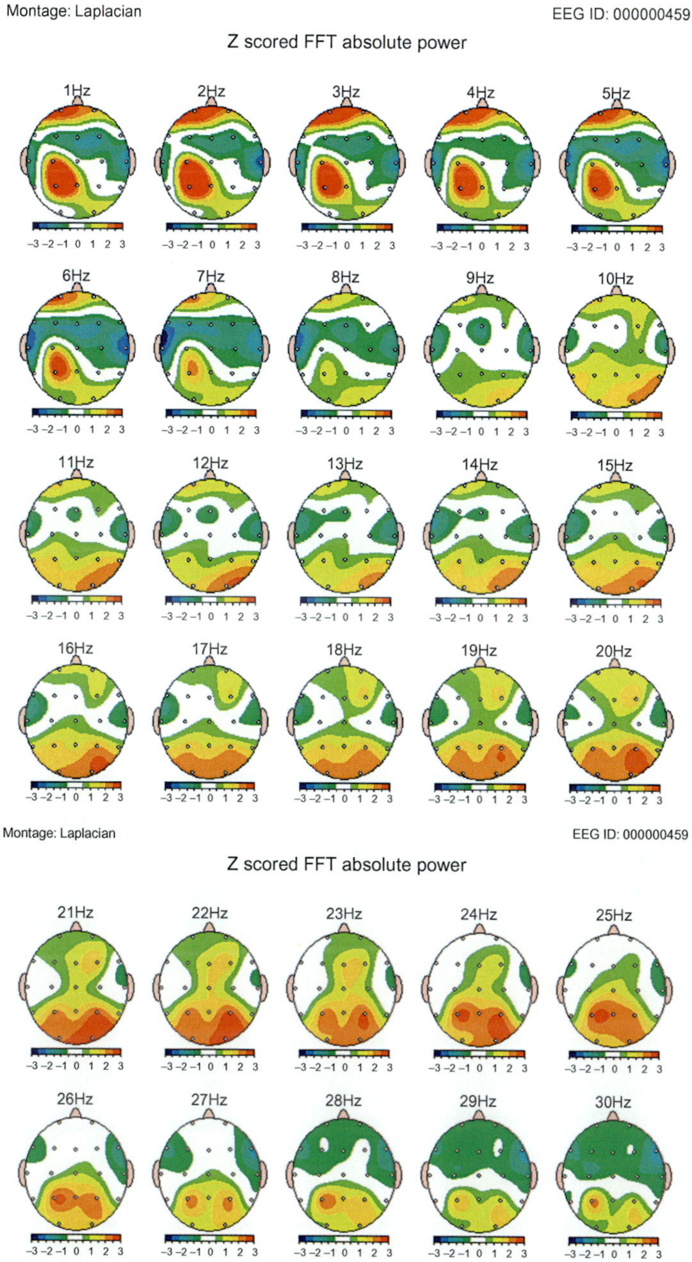

FIGURE 9.9 Pretreatment (left) and post-10 sessions (right) of LORETA neurofeedback Z-scored FFT absolute power maps in the Laplacian montage for Case 3 in the eyes closed condition.

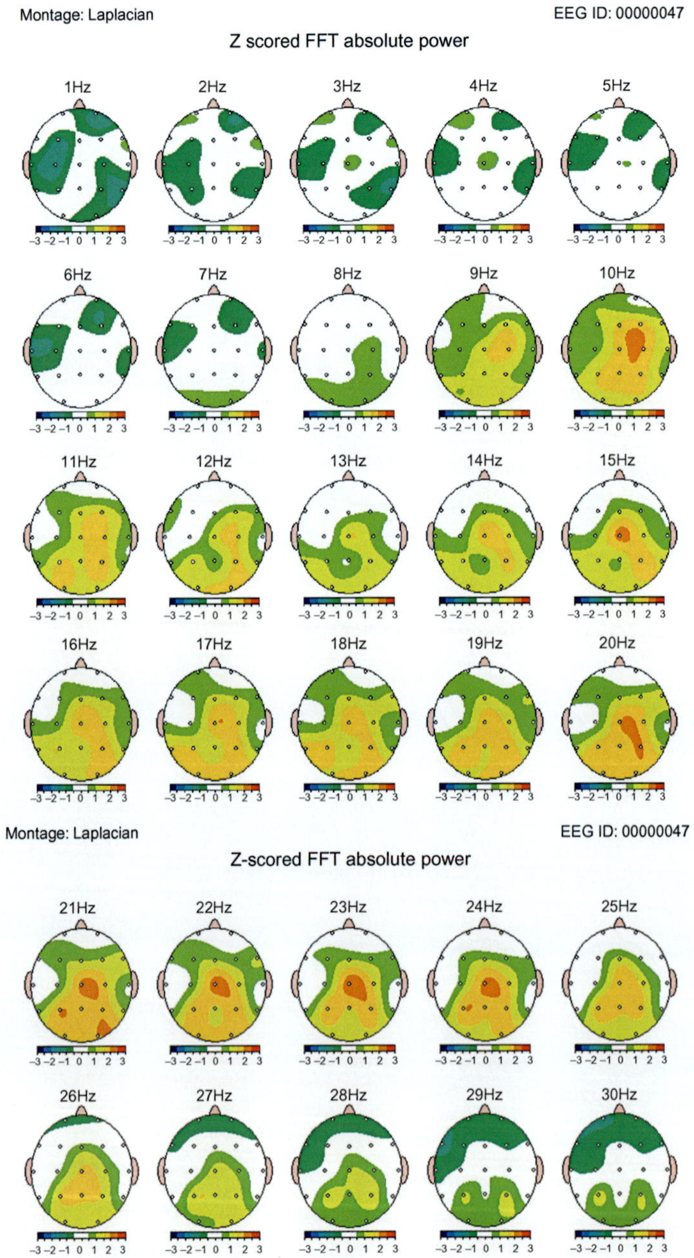

FIGURE 9.9 (Continued)

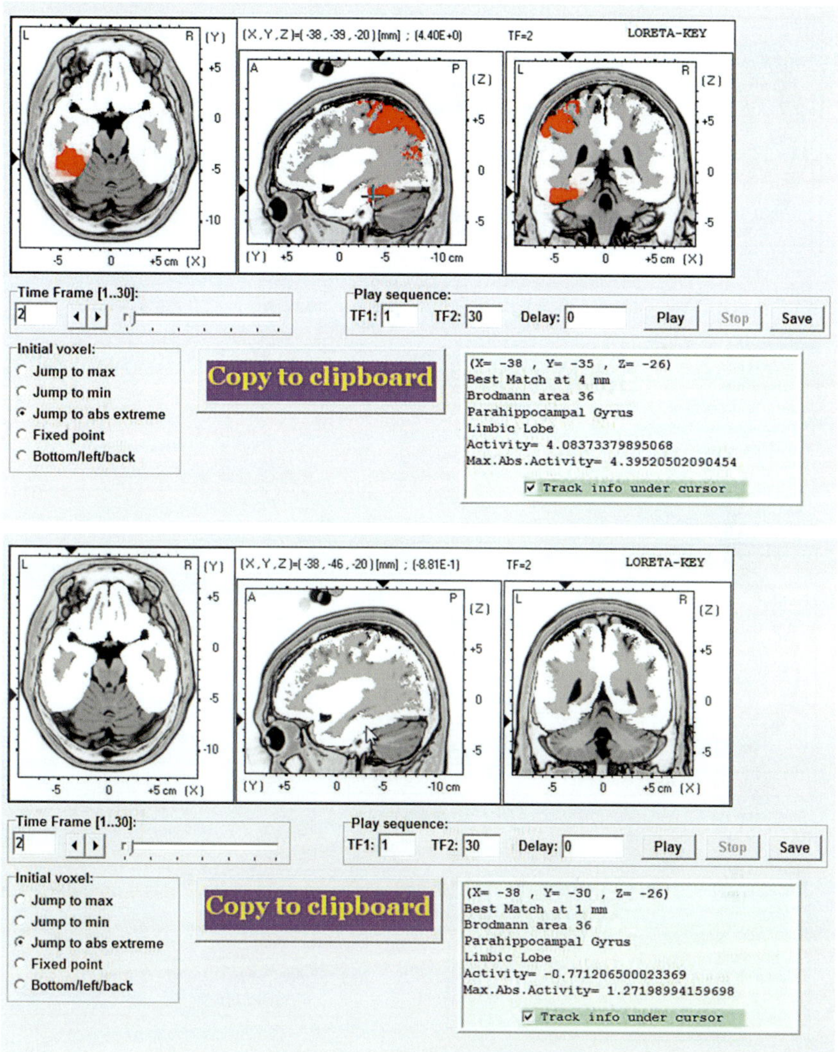

FIGURE 9.10 Pretreatment (top) and post-10 sessions (bottom) of LORETA neurofeedback Z-scored LORETA current source density maps for Case 3 in the eyes closed condition. Dysregulation is seen in the parahippocampal gyrus.

these Brodmann areas. This case exemplifies a frontotemporal-limbic anxiety case, and how symptom-driven LORETA 19-channel neurofeedback is effective, particularly when connectivity dysregulations between frontal lobe and limbic areas are corrected.

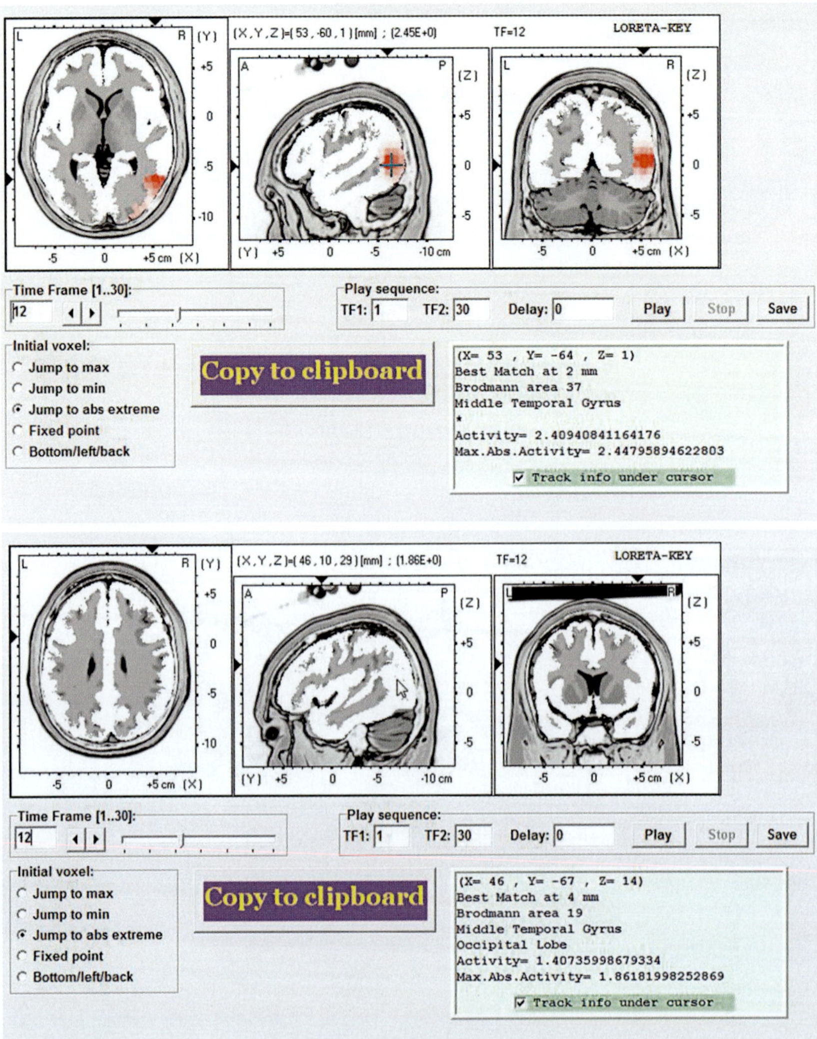

FIGURE 9.11 Pretreatment (top) and post-10 sessions (bottom) of LORETA neurofeedback Z-scored LORETA current source density maps for Case 3 in the eyes closed condition. Dysregulation is seen in the right temporal gyri.

CONCLUSION

The three case studies reviewed in this chapter were chosen because (a) each is prototypical of one of three dysregulatory mechanisms we observe and treat in anxiety patients on a regular basis and (b) all three cases demonstrate, albeit from different perspectives, our hypothesis

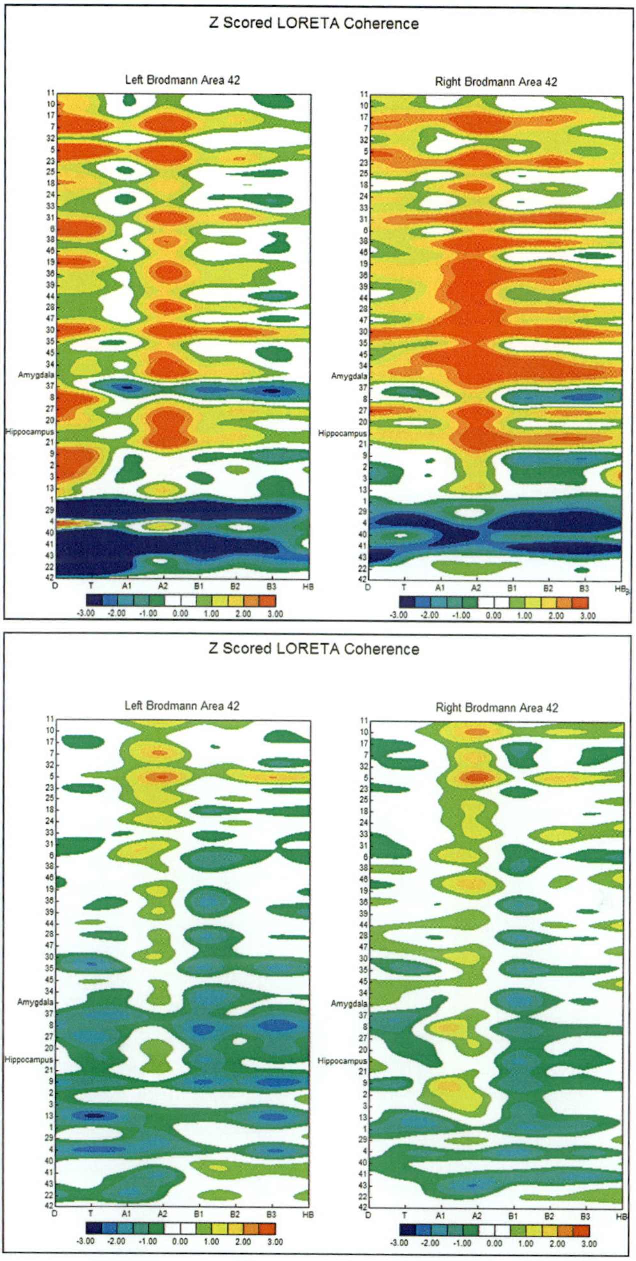

FIGURE 9.12 Case 3 LORETA coherence maps pretreatment (top) and following 10 sessions of LORETA 19-channel *Z*-score-based neurofeedback (bottom). The aberrant coherence shows normalization after 10 sessions.

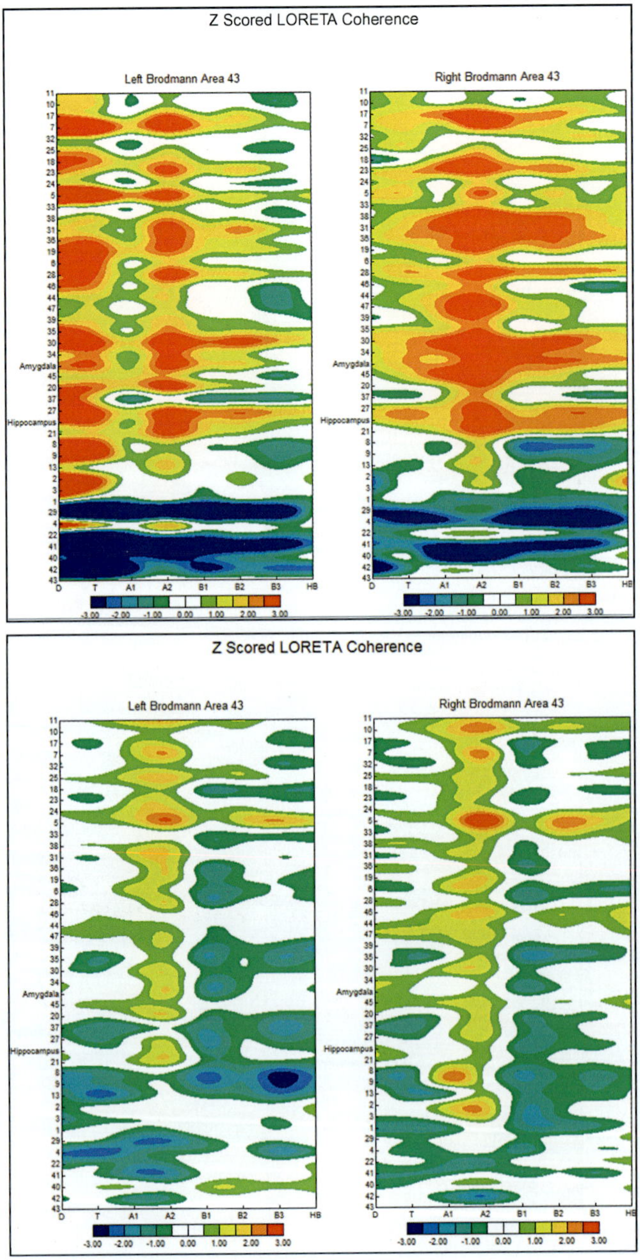

FIGURE 9.12 (Continued)

with respect to that which is common to the anxiety orders as a class: loss of inhibitory control by higher-level frontal lobe structures over lower-level limbic structures. The exact mechanisms of the loss of regulatory control vary among different patients, but in every case, where there is aberrant power, there is also aberrant connectivity, as demonstrated by LORETA coherence (and/or phase) metrics.

From the time 19-channel Z-scored symptom-driven LORETA neurofeedback has been available, we have treated 30 anxiety patients using the approach. Our long-term success rates, based on a combination of subjective patient reports (including follow-up contacts with patients) and posttreatment mapping data such as that presented in this chapter, have allowed us to estimate a success rate of 70–90% improvement per average patient (defined as "a significant improvement in both biometric and subjective data, as well as a reduction in their need for anxiolytic medications").

We do not offer these studies as the equivalent of clinical trial data. We are a treatment center, not a study site. We do not run controlled studies, nor do we randomly assign subjects to treatment conditions. However, we believe the data presented herein make a good case for funding such studies, and we also believe we may have elucidated some subtle interventions (i.e., assess and correct connectivity dysregulations first) that may well proven to be a cornerstone of an accepted standard of care in the future. These shortcomings notwithstanding, we hope the reader is now in a better position to share our enthusiasm for the potential power of using Z-scored LORETA feedback for the treatment of anxiety.

References

Etkin, A., Prater, K. E., Schatzberg, A. F., Menon, V., & Greicius, M. D. (2009). Disrupted amygdalar subregion functional connectivity and evidence of a compensatory network in generalized anxiety disorder. *Archives of General Psychiatry*, *66*(12), 1361–1372.

Hagmann, P., Cammoun, L., Gigandet, X., Meuli, R., Honey, C. J., Wedeen, V. J., et al. (2008). Mapping the structural core of human cerebral cortex. *PLoS Biology*, *6*, e159.

Hollander, E., & Simeon, D. (2003). *Concise guide to anxiety disorders*. Washington, D.C.: American Psychiatric Publishing.

Kent, J. M., Sullivan, G. M., & Rauch, S. L. (2002). Neural circuitry and signaling in anxiety. In G. B. Kaplan, & R. P. Hammer (Eds.), *Brain circuitry and signaling in psychiatry: Basic science and clinical implications*. Washington, DC: American Psychiatric Publishing.

Kim, M. J., Loucks, R. A., Palmer, A. L., Brown, A. C., Solomon, K. M., Marchante, A. N., et al. (2011). The structural and functional connectivity of the amygdala: From normal emotion to pathological anxiety. *Behavioural Brain Research*, *223*(2), 403–410.

Silverman, S. J. (2011). Effecting peak athletic performance with neurofeedback, interactive metronome, and EMDR: A case study. *Biofeedback*, *39*(1), 40–42.

Stossel, S. (2013). *My age of anxiety: Fear, hope dread and the search for peace of mind*. New York, NY: Alfred A Knopf.

Thatcher, R. W. (2012). *Handbook of quantitative electroencephalography and EEG biofeedback*. St. Petersburg, FL: ANI Publishing Co.

CHAPTER

10

Therapy of Seizures and Epilepsy with Z-Score LORETA Neurofeedback

J. Lucas Koberda, MD, PhD[1]

Tallahassee NeuroBalance Center, Tallahassee, FL, USA

INTRODUCTION

Seizures are abnormal discharges from the cortex which frequently manifest as jerking movements of the extremities. Seizures may be caused by metabolic problems or by structural dysfunction of the cortex. Epilepsy is diagnosed as reoccurring seizures frequently caused by cortical injury. Seizures may affect only a small, localized portion of the cortical area without spreading electrical discharge to the whole cortex. This is sometimes associated with symptoms of short lasting confusion. In such cases, the patient is diagnosed with a partial complex seizure. When the electrical discharge becomes generalized (thus affecting the whole cortex) after focal initiation then the patient is diagnosed with secondary generalized seizures.

Depending on the location of the initial neuronal discharge initiating the seizure, a different type of aura (prodromal symptoms) may be experienced by the patient. Temporal lobe epilepsy is frequently associated with aura described as a "déjà vu" sensation. Seizures originating in the primary sensory area may produce a strange sensation before seizure onset. Primary generalized epilepsy produces generalized epileptic discharges in cortical neurons with frequently thalamic and frontal origin of the seizure (Moeller et al., 2011; Wang et al., 2012). In secondary generalized epilepsy, the tonic–clonic seizure is frequently preceded by focal onset discharges which in many cases can be detected by conventional electroencephalography (EEG).

[1]www.TallahasseeNeuroBalanceCenter.com

Z Score Neurofeedback.
DOI: http://dx.doi.org/10.1016/B978-0-12-801291-8.00010-8

THE ETIOLOGY OF EPILEPSY

The prevalence of epilepsy is estimated at 1 in 200 persons. An epileptic seizure is a result of the dysfunction of the brain resulting in abnormal electrical discharge of cortical neurons. The dysregulation between cortical and thalamic connections may be a contributing factor in epileptic seizure formation. Thalamocortical cells have excitatory (predominantly glutamatergic) projections to the cortex. Cortical neurons, in turn, are reciprocally connected by excitatory connections with the thalamus. Inhibitory neurons whose neurotransmitter is γ-aminobutyric acid (GABA) are located throughout the cortex as well as the thalamus, but a layer of almost pure GABAergic neurons is located in the lateral parts of the thalamus. This is the thalamic reticular nucleus (nRT), a special portion of the thalamus that receives collaterals of the thalamocortical and corticothalamic axons. These collaterals excite the cells of the nRT. The GABAergic cells in the nRT project back to the thalamus and also connect with other nRT cells via inhibitory synapses (Blumenfeld, 2003). Enhanced burst firing in corticothalamic neurons may increase $GABA_B$ receptor activation in the thalamus, leading to the slower, more synchronous oscillations seen in spike-and-wave seizures (Blumenfeld, 2003). In addition, other subcortical structures may contribute to epileptic seizures control. For instance, the GABAergic projections from substantia nigra pars reticulata (SNR) to thalamocortical neurons of the ventral medial (VM) thalamic nucleus were reported to provide a potent network for the control of seizures by basal ganglia (Paz et al., 2007). The hippocampus is particularly susceptible to epileptogenic activity and is frequently the source of epileptic seizures. Seizures activate N-methyl-d-aspartate (NMDA-) receptors and strengthen connections between the exited neurons. Long-term potentiation (LTP) may contribute to promotion of ongoing epileptic activity and could explain why seizure activity at particular site often spreads to involve other synaptically connected cortical regions. The repetitive cortical activation potentiates excitatory transmission and depresses inhibitory transmission, creating self-perpetuating excitatory circuit and facilitating excitation of neighboring neurons. The abnormal electrical activity generated by seizure spreads throughout the brain to other regions utilizing various connector structures including corpus callosum.

Brain damage can also produce seizure activity. A head injury frequently produces neuronal damage with scar tissue formation and subsequent abnormal electrical discharge generation. Most seizures initiate within 1 year since head injury, however, remote seizures occurring many years after a brain trauma were also reported. A vascular malformation which may be prone to blood extravasation and cortical irritation maybe also responsible for epileptic seizures. Venous angiomas or arteriovenous malformations are inborn abnormalities which may produce seizures. Neuronal damage caused by ischemic or hemorrhagic stroke may also generate seizures.

Cortical developmental abnormalities or hereditary disorders like tuberous sclerosis frequently contribute to epilepsy (Jones, 2012). Brain tumors either primary or metastatic also may produce recurrent seizures due to vasogenic edema and neuronal damage. Brain infections including encephalitis may produce mesial temporal sclerosis which often presents as temporal lobe epilepsy.

THE CLINICAL PICTURE OF EPILEPSY

Depending on location of the seizure onset, the beginning of the seizure may manifest as tingling or other type of somatosensory phenomena. Visual or auditory aura maybe experienced by the patient. Focal motor tonic–clonic extremity movements, facial grimacing or autonomic symptoms like epigastric sensation may be also present (Rowland and Pedley, 2010). In partial complex seizures, by definition alteration of consciousness needs to be present. Psychomotor phenomena like chewing movements or automatisms such as picking at clothing are frequently experienced by the patient. In primary generalized epilepsy and secondary generalized epilepsy, the development of tonic and clonic muscle contraction is typical with postictal confusion.

Unless there is major structural lesion in the brain, a neurological examination between seizures is frequently unremarkable.

Absence seizures, previously called Petit Mal seizures, are mostly seen in the pediatric population. It presents in children becoming inattentive and confused for a short period of time. Eye fluttering is often noted during these episodes. EEG provides definitive diagnostic confirmation and typically demonstrates brief generalized bilaterally synchronous 3 Hz spike-and-wave discharges. Hyperventilation may precipitate absence seizures. Juvenile myoclonic epilepsy is a primary generalized epilepsy that usually begins during the teenage years and is associated with morning myoclonic jerks soon after awakening. Many of the patients have intermittent generalized seizures. EEG frequently shows bilaterally synchronous spike-and-wave or polyspike discharges at variable frequency.

DIAGNOSTIC CONSIDERATIONS

Multiple other neurological conditions may mimic epileptogenic seizures. The most common neurologic condition that may be confused with seizure is syncope. Postictal confusion, tongue biting, and generalized tonic–clonic movements are suggestive of seizure or epilepsy. Another condition which is frequently difficult to distinguish from epilepsy is psychogenic seizure. Many patients with this condition are having combined epileptic and nonepileptic seizures. In the case of normal interictal EEG, ambulatory 24 h EEG or video EEG telemetry is needed in many cases to provide the final diagnosis. In cases of nonepileptogenic seizures, video EEG telemetry shows no epileptogenic abnormalities despite typical clinical manifestation of the symptoms. Sometimes sleep disorders such as parasomnia including night terrors may produce seizure-like activity. Less frequently, migrainous events may be mistaken for seizures, especially when associated with lethargy and loss of consciousness. These types of symptoms may be associated with basilar type of migraine. A similar situation may be noticed during transient ischemic attack, when a patient may present with altered consciousness or focal weakness leading to a fall which may be mistaken for epilepsy. Psychiatric manifestations like anxiety with panic attacks and hyperventilation may also be mistaken for seizure. Initial evaluation would include standard EEG or ambulatory EEG. Brain imaging including magnetic resonance imaging (MRI) (in order to rule out focal abnormalities) is usually recommended. Supplementary testing if needed may include video EEG telemetry where the patient is observed for 24 h or even longer with continuous EEG and video monitoring. Nuclear and functional imaging with position emission tomography (PET) and single photon emission tomography (SPECT), functional magnetic resonance imaging (fMRI) may be of benefit in more complex cases. Another condition which is frequently difficult to distinguish from epilepsy is psychogenic nonepileptogenic seizure. Many patients with this condition are having combined epileptic and nonepileptic seizures. In case of normal interictal EEG, ambulatory 24 h EEG or video EEG telemetry is needed in many cases to provide the final diagnosis. In cases of nonepileptogenic seizures, a video EEG telemetry shows no epileptogenic abnormalities despite typical clinical manifestation of the symptoms. Sometimes sleep disorders show abnormalities in blood oxygenation in different areas of the brain. PET shows abnormalities in glucose metabolism in the areas affected by neuronal damage responsible for the seizure. Ictal SPECT shows increased blood flow in the epileptic region of the brain.

TREATMENT OF EPILEPSY

Despite major progress in the treatment of epilepsy, unfortunately approximately 30% of patients are still refractory to medical treatment. Surgical treatment may be an option for some of those patients, however, many patients may not be interested or eligible for surgical therapy. Therefore, there is a need to develop alternative treatments which would be able to offer a substantial seizure reduction. Currently, a mainstay of therapy in epilepsy is pharmacotherapy. Multiple medications are available on the market for different types of epilepsy. Some of them are broad-spectrum medications which cover both primary generalized and secondary generalized epilepsy. Other relatively narrow spectrum medications are effective mostly in certain type of seizures. Phenobarbital which is one of the oldest antiseizure medications binds with the $GABA_A$ receptor and potentiates its neuronal inhibitory activity. Several anticonvulsants, including phenytoin, fosphenytoin (a phenytoin prodrug), carbamazepine, oxcarbamazepine (an active metabolite of carbamazepine), lamotrigine and valproate, produce block of voltage-gated sodium channels in the brain and inhibit the development of seizure foci as well as the spread of epileptiform activity in the brain while leaving normal neuronal activity relatively intact. Valproic acid in addition to inhibition of sodium ion influx through voltage-gated sodium channels has a number of actions including inhibition of GABA transaminase and inhibition of calcium ion influx through T-type calcium channels. The succinamides including ethosuximide act primarily via inhibition of T channels. The mechanism of action of topiramate is not clear but seem to involve inhibition of voltage-gated sodium channels, enhancement GABA-mediated synaptic inhibition, and antagonism of amino-methyl proprionic acid/kainate (AMPA/KA) sensitive receptors and inhibition of carbonic anhydrase.

Unfortunately, approximately 30% of patients with epilepsy do not respond to pharmacological treatment. These patients are classified as medically refractory and other forms of treatment need to be applied in order to reduce frequency of seizures. In the pediatric population, the ketogenic diet has been found effective in reducing seizure numbers in selected patients. Surgical options include minor surgery like vagus nerve stimulator implantation, or major surgery including lesion resection or even lobectomy. Neurofeedback (NFB) has been found to be an effective treatment modality in patients who do not respond to pharmacological treatment (Sterman, 2010).

Dr. Sterman from UCLA initiated NFB experiments which have proven the effectiveness of sensory motor rhythm (SMR) entrainment in epilepsy treatment (Sterman, 2010; Sterman & Egner, 2006). His protocols were based on the one or two electrode type of NFB, which resulted in significant seizure reduction in drug refractory patients. Approximately 60% seizure frequency reduction was noted in clinical studies with SMR entrainment (Sterman, 2010). Currently, newer NFB protocols are being tested for effectiveness in the treatment of epilepsy including Z-score NFB.

Z-score surface and low-resolution electrode-magnetic tomography analysis (LORETA) 19-electrode (cap system) was recently introduced to the market (Applied Neurosciences, Inc.). This system has the potential for faster results based on the larger number of electrodes applied to treatment. LORETA-based therapy also enables targeting activity in cortex deeper than that monitored by standard EEG-based NFB. In addition, relatively inexpensive computer software and EEG hardware make this procedure potentially cost effective. Preliminary data coming from my office indicate successful primary and secondary generalized seizure response to this type of therapy.

Table 10.1 presents a summary of 10 patients who were treated with LORETA and/or surface Z-score NFB in my office.

Since we have not had so far any seizure patients who have not (at least partially) responded to this type of NFB, we can, so far, report 100% effectiveness of this therapy. The response to NFB therapy is defined as reduction of seizure frequency. In the following pages, I will give some more information on the patients.

TABLE 10.1 Summary of Patients Suffering from Seizures

Z-score NFB of epilepsy patients:

1. 18 F with intractable epilepsy with secondary generalization.
2. 17 F with intractable primary idiopathic epilepsy with generalization.
3. 44 M with frontal epilepsy with generalization—S/P tumor resection.
4. 46 F with focal epilepsy and intermittent generalization and cognitive dysfunction—S/P tumor resection.
5. 16 F with intractable absence epilepsy with cognitive problems.
6. 59 M with intractable generalized epilepsy and cognitive problems (ETOH).
7. 18 M with autistic spectrum and intractable partial complex epilepsy.
8. 23 M with autism and frequent generalized seizures.
9. 28 F pharmacist with frequent intractable generalized seizures.
10. 19 M with well-controlled generalized epilepsy on valproate desiring discontinuation of medication.

CASE 1

Eighteen-year-old female high school senior who's seizures started at age 11, sometimes proceeded by eye blinking episodes. Her current medications included Keppra XR 1500 mg daily and Lamictal 150 mg daily. Prior MRI of the brain was reported to be normal. EEG showed multiple sharps in several locations including P3, P4 T5, T6, O1, O2.

Cognitive testing showed low information processing speed and memory (Figure 10.1). Despite extensive neurological evaluations at UCLA and multiple medications, no seizure reduction was observed. Her mother even reported an increase in seizure numbers with use of antiepileptic mediations. Dr. Barry Sterman was also consulted and SMR NFB was initiated with some seizure reduction noted. However, despite 90–100 sessions of NFB completion seizures were still occurring, but with lower frequency. This patient presented to my office for 1 week of intensive therapy with Z-score LORETA NFB (twice a day). LORETA imaging showed multiple areas of cortical electrical dysregulations (Figure 10.2). After completion of eight NFB sessions, longer remission (previously seizures were occurring more frequently) was achieved (approximately 4 months seizure free). Further NFB therapy was continued at another location but with much lower frequency. Since the initiation of Z-score LORETA NFB therapy (approximately 11 months), only two seizures were noted. In addition, marked improvement of cognitive status was found with resultant admission to college and very good grades during the freshman year (mostly A's).

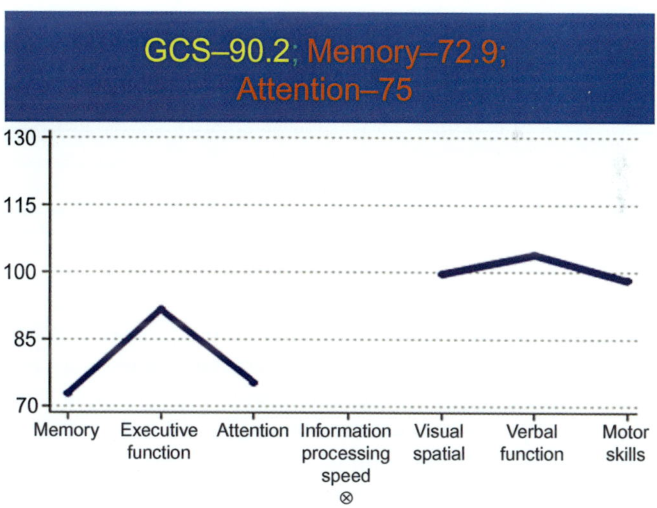

FIGURE 10.1 Lower than expected cognitive score especially memory and attention as well as information processing speed (too low to be scored). Expected score (100) with standard deviation (SD) (15). GCS, Global Cognitive Score.

continued

CASE 1 *(cont'd)*

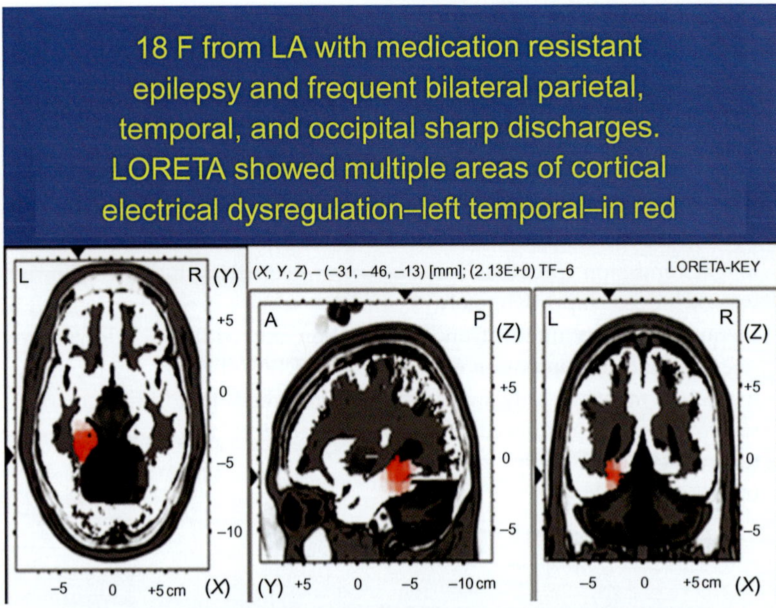

FIGURE 10.2 LORETA imaging before NFB initiation—only one of many areas of cortical dysregulations is shown.

CASE 2

Seventeen-year-old female well known to my practice for the last 3 years was diagnosed with primary generalized epilepsy resistant to pharmacological therapy. Her seizures consisted of multiple short lasting confusion episodes with intermittent generalization. Patient was previously on multiple medications including valproic acid, lamotrigine, clonazepam, zonisamide, levetiracetam, topiramate frequently in combination. Unfortunately her medications were also producing side effects including memory problems and drowsiness. Despite multiple adjustments of medications (lately included lamotrigine and zonisamide), patient still had intermittent breakthrough seizures. Patient also

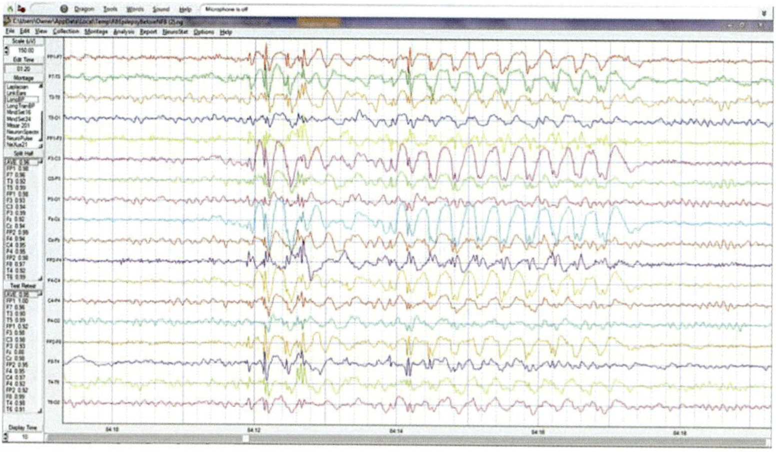

FIGURE 10.3 EEG of 17-year-old female with primary generalized epilepsy and frequent electrographic seizures—see generalized spike-and-wave episode which lasted 6 s followed by normal EEG background.

reported worsening of her school performance due to seizures and medications side effects.

Patient workup included normal MRI of the brain. EEG showed multiple generalized electrographic seizures of few seconds duration (Figure 10.3) in practically every EEG recording (multiple EEG in the past).

Subsequent video EEG telemetry completed at University of Florida epilepsy section confirmed diagnosis of primary generalized epilepsy. Patient's computerized neuropsychological testing (Figure 10.4) showed global cognitive score of 85 (expected score 100) with deficiency in memory, information processing speed as well as other domains (Figure 10.4).

Due to her resistance to medications, the patient volunteered to try Z-score NFB focusing on normalization of grossly abnormal electroencephalogram with multiple spike-and-wave generalized discharges throughout the recording. Z-score LORETA NFB is one of the newest forms of NFB where usually 19-electrode simultaneous therapy is conducted in order to normalize aberrant EEG with a goal of reaching a Z-score close to 0 (Koberda et al., 2012; Thatcher, 2010; Thatcher, 2013). Only 8 out of 10 planned sessions were completed due to the fact that the patient decided to withdraw from NFB therapy. Subsequent follow-up visits revealed no more clinical seizures. Two follow-up

continued

CASE 2 *(cont'd)*

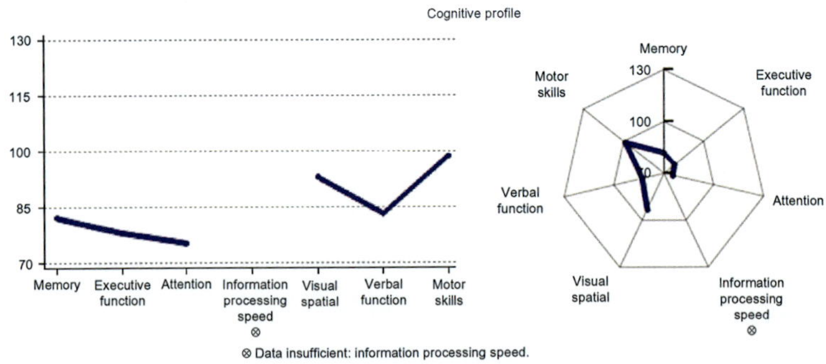

Global Cognitive Score: 85
Memory: 82.1
Executive function: 78
Attention: 75.2
Visual spatial: 92.9
Verbal function: 83.2
Motor skills: 98.8

FIGURE 10.4 Seventeen-year-old patient with epilepsy and cognitive problems—NeuroTrax is a computerized neuropsychological testing which compared this patient to age and education matched controls with mean (100) and standard deviation (SD) (15). In most of the domains tested, these patients scored below expected mean value. Information processing was the weakest with poor performance preventing from being scored.

electroencephalograms were completed which showed complete normalization of EEG with no more evidence of electrographic seizures. In addition, quantitative EEG (QEEG) analysis also showed marked improvement (Figure 10.5A and B) of previously abnormal spectral pattern. This patient remains seizure free for more than a year since NFB initiation and continues being on lamotrigine and zonisamide. The patient also reported improvement in her cognitive function and school performance.

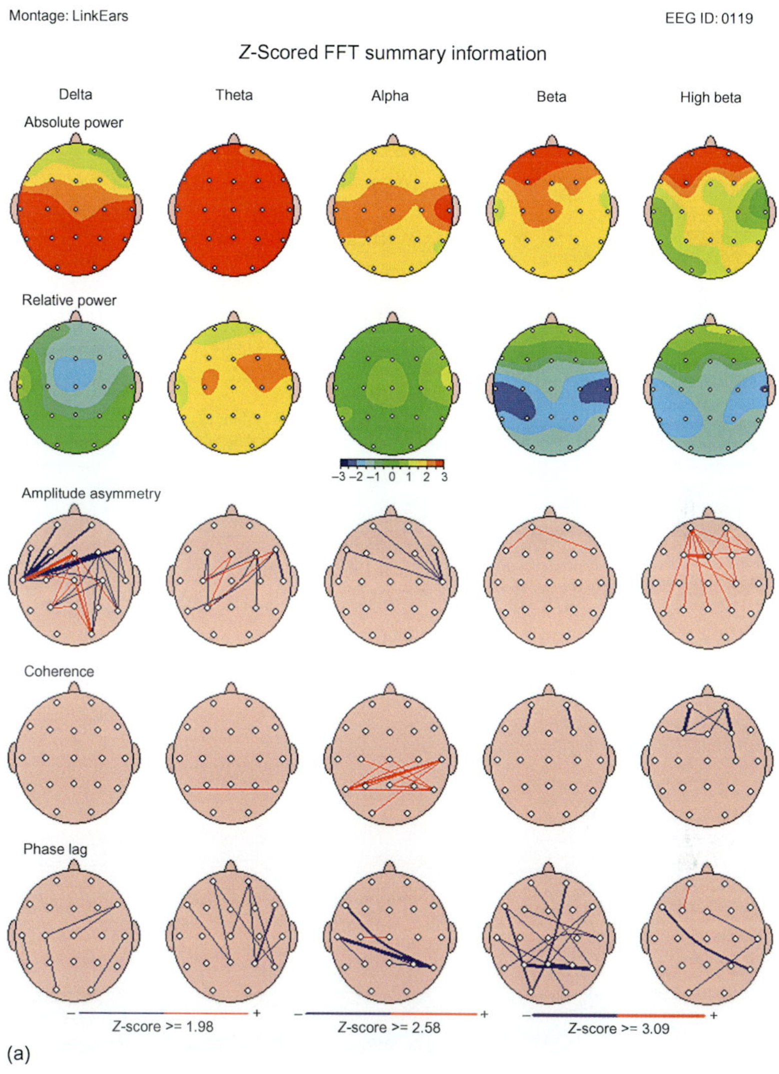

FIGURE 10.5 (A) QEEG maps which are color coded (before NFB). Patient's EEG was compared to normal controls. Areas in green are between 0 and 1 standard deviation (SD); area in yellow between 1 and 2 SD; and in red between 2 and 3 SD from the norm. Marked increase in Delta, Theta, and frontal Beta power was recorded.

continued

CASE 2 (*cont'd*)

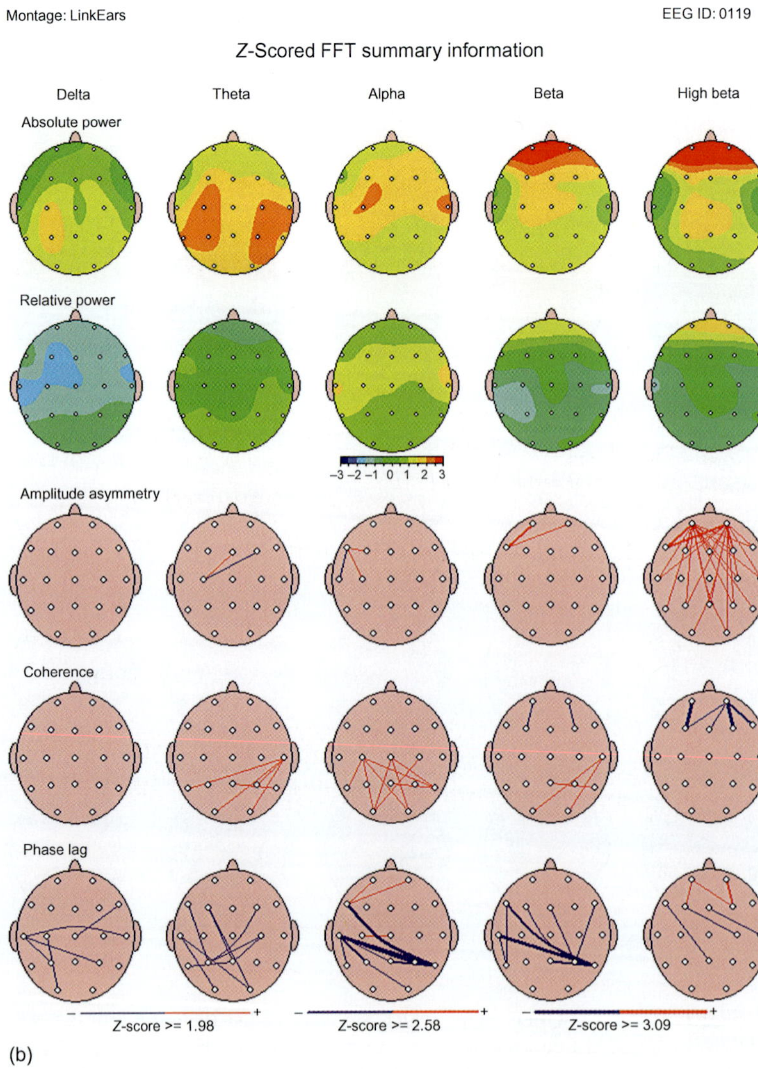

FIGURE 10.5 (B) Marked improvement of Delta and Theta power overexpression. There is still elevation of frontal Beta power most likely related to frontal muscle artifact.

CASE 3

A 40-year-old man noticed his first seizure after experiencing several episodes of the left upper extremity numbness associated with a headache. Generalized seizure was preceded by jerking movements of the left upper extremity. Several more seizures with an identical pattern were subsequently noted by the patient. The patient reported that, on a few occasions, he developed incontinence and tongue biting during a generalized seizure. The patient never experienced similar episodes in the past. The patient reported no other significant medical problems. The patient denied excessive alcohol consumption or smoking. MRI revealed a right frontal central contrast enhancing lesion-likely meningioma. EEG showed right frontal sharp waves and was diagnosed with secondary generalized seizures.

The patient was started on antiseizure medication levetiracetam (Keppra) for seizure prevention. Neurosurgical consultation was requested at Johns Hopkins University and indicated high likelihood of meningioma. Subsequent surgery included frontal craniotomy and tumor resection, which confirmed a diagnosis of meningioma. Unfortunately, despite being on levetiracetam, the patient still

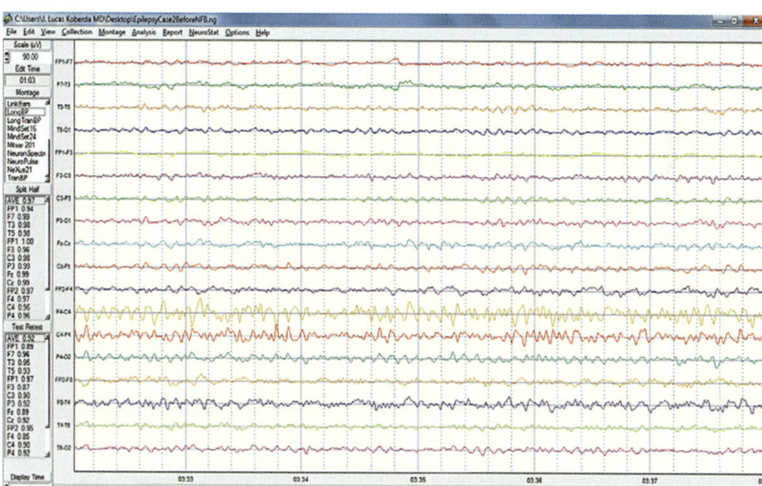

FIGURE 10.6 Forty-year-old male patient with partial complex epilepsy with frequent generalization—EEG shows a breach rhythm with epileptiform activity including sharp contoured waves with frequent phase reversals at C4.

continued

CASE 3 *(cont'd)*

experienced breakthrough seizures most likely due to one scar tissue formation after the surgery. Subsequent EEG showed left frontal central breach rhythm with possible sharp contoured activity (Figure 10.6).

Subsequent Z-score NFB (10 sessions) resulted in clinical remission with no further clinical seizures. This patient comes periodically for "refresher" NFB sessions (he worries about return of seizures) and the dose of Keppra has been gradually reduced from initial 1000 mg twice a day to 750 mg and subsequently 500 mg twice a day. Medication reduction was also associated with subjective improvement (feeling less drowsy) and he has continued to be free of seizures for more than 2 years.

CASE 4

Fifty-year-old female was seen in follow up of hospitalization for seizures due to frontal meningioma—status post tumor resection. Patient complained of cognitive problems and occasional seizures despite being on Keppra 1000 mg twice a day. Her cognitive computerized testing before NFB showed global cognitive score 81.7 with memory score of 45.4 and information processing speed 66.7. 10 sessions of LORETA Z-score NFB resulted in complete seizure elimination and marked cognitive enhancement with global cognitive score 87, memory increased to 54.9 and higher information processing speed 88.5. This patient has been seizure free for more than 2 years.

CASE 5

Sixteen-year-old female presented for neurological evaluation due to absence seizures, and cognitive and visual integration problems. Due to "bullying" in school, her parents decided to convert her to a home schooling program. Initial computerized cognitive testing showed

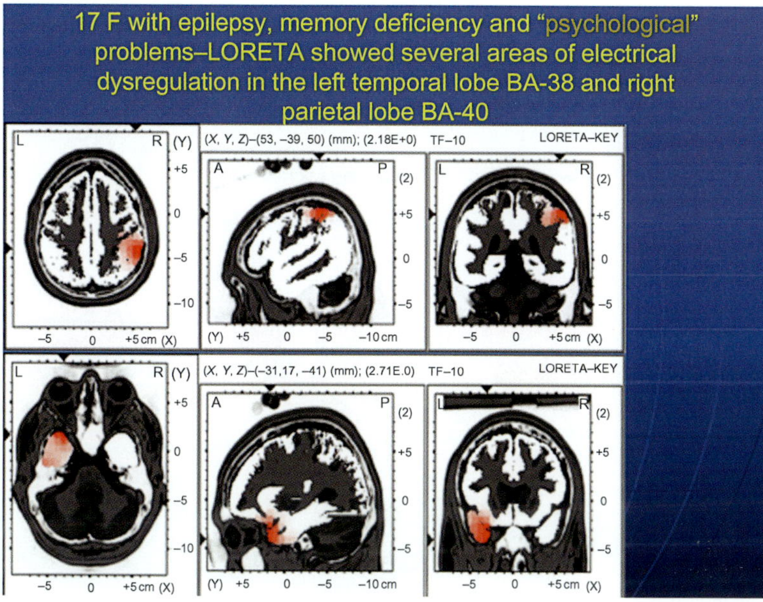

FIGURE 10.7 LORETA before NFB showed several areas of electrical dysregulation including BA-38 and 40 (in red).

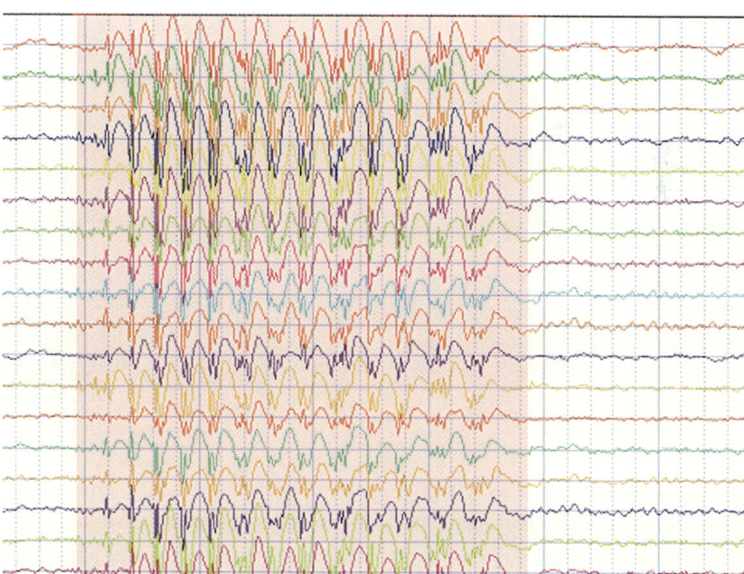

FIGURE 10.8 EEG of 16-year-old female (before NFB) showing generalized spike-and-wave discharges typical of absence seizure (several seconds duration).

continued

CASE 5 (*cont'd*)

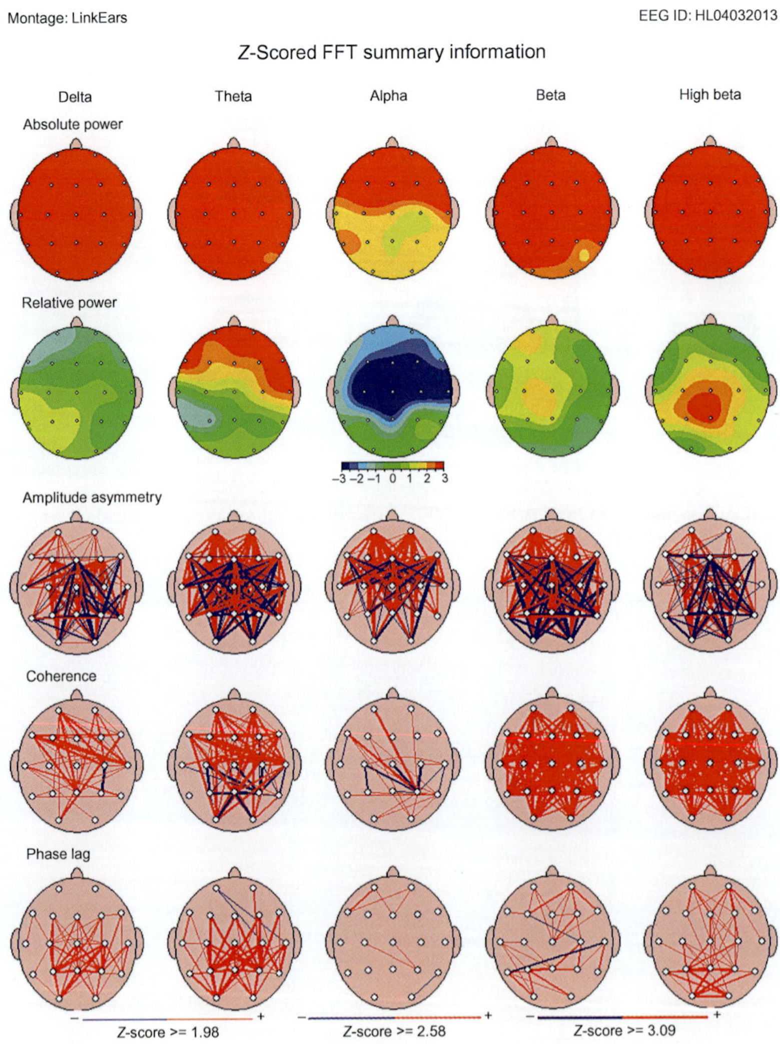

FIGURE 10.9 QEEG of selected seizure fragments—before NFB—shows marked increase of coherence and amplitudes of most of frequency bands.

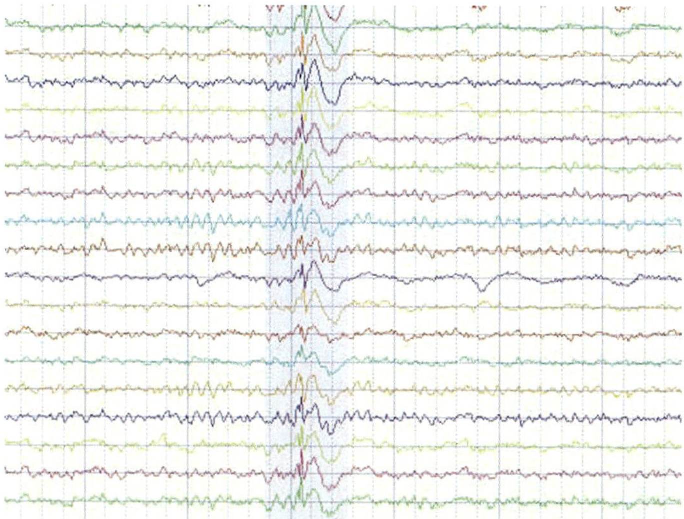

FIGURE 10.10 Sixteen-year-old female with epilepsy—Just a few NFB sessions caused marked reduction of frequency and duration of electrographic absence seizures (only 1 s of generalized spike-and-wave discharge was noted).

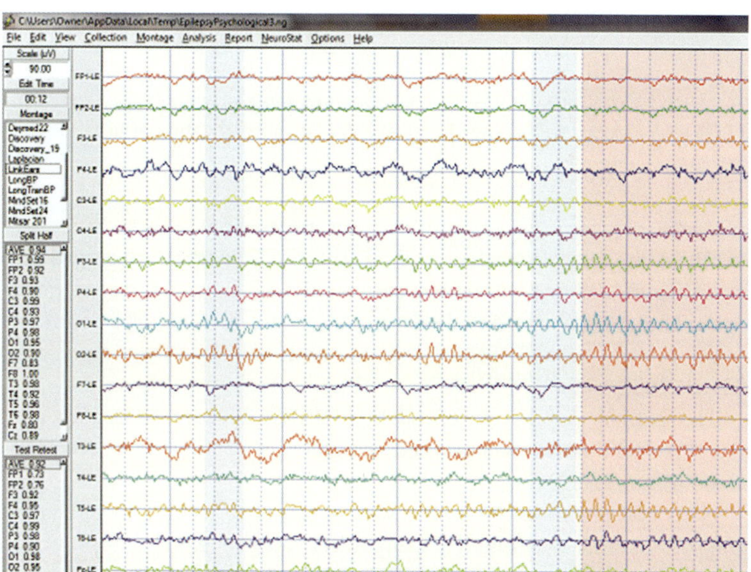

FIGURE 10.11 Sixteen-year-old female—EEG after 10 sessions of NFB-total resolution of epileptic discharges.

continued

CASE 5 *(cont'd)*

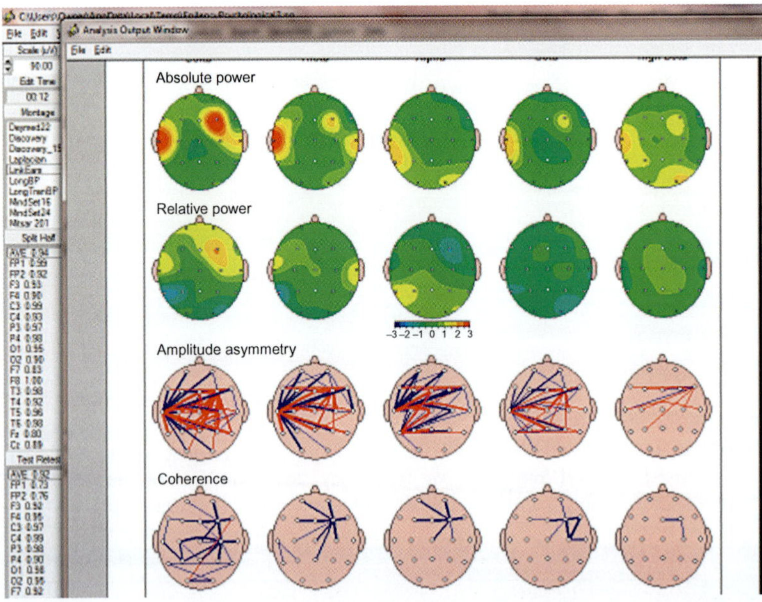

FIGURE 10.12 Sixteen-year-old female with epilepsy—QEEG after 10 sessions of LORETA Z-score NFB showed almost complete normalization of her QEEG.

evidence of memory and information processing speed difficulties. LORETA imaging revealed several areas of electrical dysregulation including BA-38 and 40, which correlated with her cognitive deficiencies. (These areas are involved in regulation of memory, cognition, emotion, and visual processing in addition to other functions.) (Figure 10.7–10.9).

The patient decided to enroll in LORETA Z-score NFB, and after just three NFB sessions a marked reduction of seizures frequency was noted (Figure 10.10).

After completion of 10 NFB sessions, complete resolution of electrographic seizures was noted (Figure 10.11) and repeated computerized cognitive testing showed marked improvement of her memory.

Repeated QEEG also showed marked improvement of previously identified abnormalities including power and coherence (Figure 10.12).

CASE 6

Fifty-nine-year-old male with longstanding history of alcohol abuse was diagnosed with multiple recurrent generalized seizures. In addition, cognitive problems and peripheral neuropathy were also identified, likely also related to his long history of alcohol abuse. The patient was placed on medications including Keppra, clonazepam, and gabapentin, however, he still had intermittent breakthrough seizures on a monthly basis. His interictal EEG was normal. After completion of a course of Z-score NFB (total of 23 sessions) his seizures subsided and he has been seizure free for approximately 1 year. In addition, his wife also reported an improvement of his cognitive status.

CASE 7

Eighteen-year-old male who was diagnosed with high functioning autistic spectrum disorder and frequent partial complex seizures. EEG was read as normal on multiple occasions. Z-score NFB therapy caused seizure frequency reduction and improvement in his cognition, however, seizures were not completely eradicated.

CASE 8

Twenty-three-year-old male diagnosed with low functioning autistic spectrum disorder characterized as major cognitive dysfunction with aphasia and social interaction problems. In addition, frequent generalized seizures were reported despite valproic acid administration. EEG was read as normal. QEEG showed increase in frontal delta and theta power (Figure 10.13). After a course of LORETA Z-score NFB seizures completely subsided (for more than 22 months), and an improvement in social functioning was noted. Repeated QEEG also showed an improvement of previously overexpressed beta power (Figure 10.14).

continued

CASE 8 *(cont'd)*

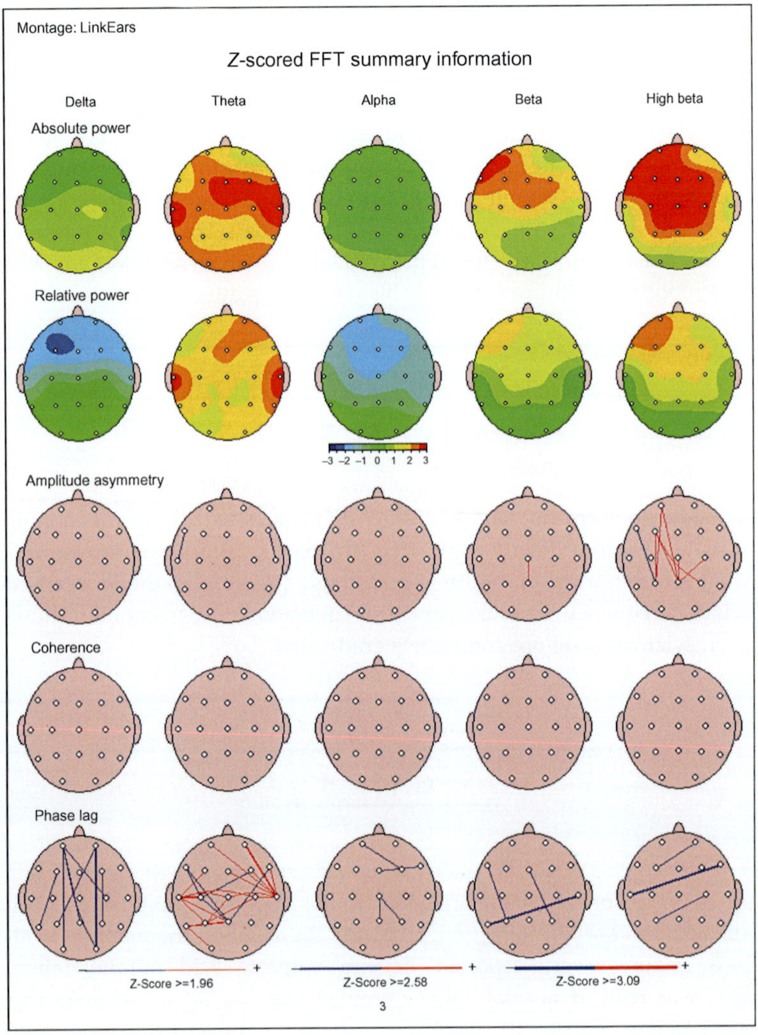

FIGURE 10.13 QEEG of 23-year-old autistic male—before completion of NFB. Markedly increased frontal beta power was recorded as well as frontal and temporal theta power.

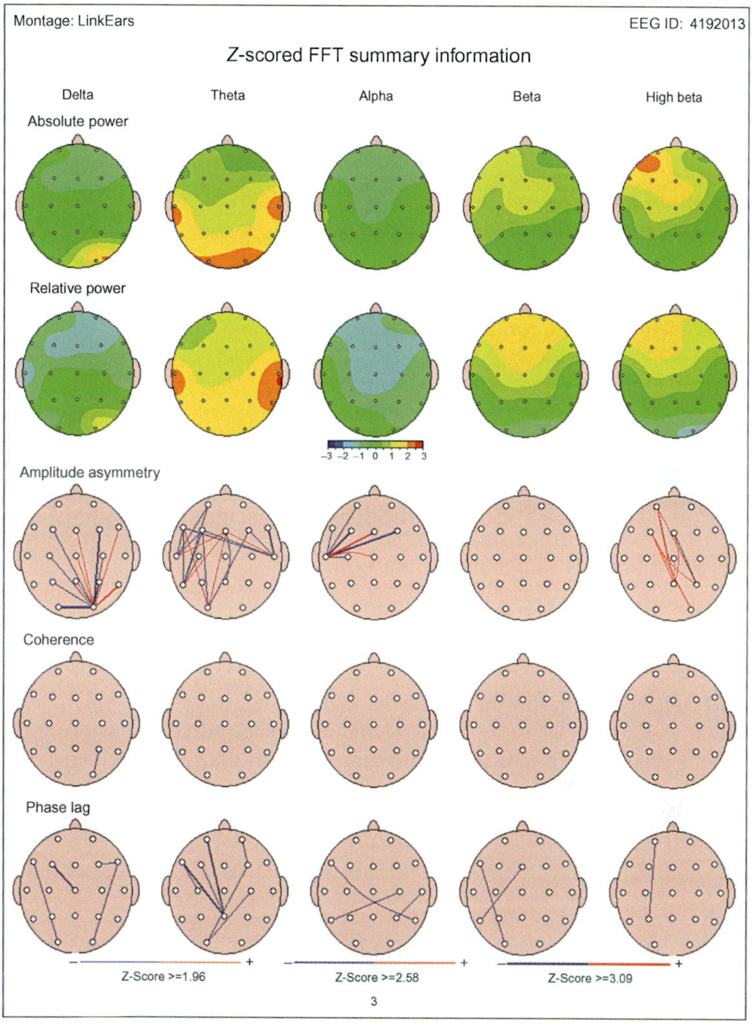

FIGURE 10.14 QEEG after completion of the course of NFB-marked reduction of previously overexpressed beta and theta power is noted.

CASE 9

A 25-year-old pharmacist was complaining of frequent generalized seizures especially in the morning on awakening. Multiple EEGs were normal as well as EEG telemetry completed at University of Florida. Her MRI was also normal. Seizures continued despite use of multiple anticonvulsant medications, including Keppra 1000 mg twice a day, Topamax 200 mg twice a day, and subsequently Vimpat 150 twice a day.

After a course of Z-score LORETA NFB (total of 18 sessions), the seizures subsided and all seizure medications were gradually discontinued. This patient continues to be seizure-free (21 months).

CASE 10

A 19-year-old male was diagnosed with probable juvenile myoclonic epilepsy with frequent generalization, which was well controlled on Depakote. His interictal EEG was normal. Patient was interested in discontinuation of medication with help of NFB therapy. During the course of Z-score LORETA NFB, Depakote was gradually discontinued. Patient was seizure free for approximately 6 months after which intermittent myoclonic jerks started reoccurring. Patient elected to be back on his antiepileptic medication due to fear of losing driving privileges.

SUMMARY

These 10 epilepsy patients from our clinic subjected to surface/LOTERA Z-score NFB showed marked clinical improvement in all examples (and in some cases also showed electrographic improvement), including long-lasting clinical remissions or seizure frequency reduction regardless of type of epilepsy.

Many patients reported marked improvement after only two to five sessions of LORETA NFB.

Most of the patients reported some cognitive improvement, which could have been related to NFB in addition to seizure reduction.

The minimum frequency of NFB was once per week, however, more frequent NFB sessions seem to give more benefits.

The above cases illustrate the great potential of LORETA Z-score NFB as a therapy for a variety of seizure types including primary generalized and secondary generalized epilepsy. There is also the possibility that this type of therapy may prove to be effective for nonepileptogenic seizures.

Acknowledgment

I would like to give a special thanks to Dr. Eric Harris who contributed in editing of this chapter.

References

Blumenfeld, B. H. (2003). From molecules to networks: Cortical/subcortical interactions in the pathophysiology of idiopathic generalized epilepsy. *Epilepsia*, *44*(Suppl. 2), 7–15.

Jones, H. R. (2012). *Netter's neurology*. Philadelphia, PA: Elsevier.

Koberda, J. L. (2012). Comparison of the effectiveness of Z-score surface/LORETA 19-electrode neurofeedback to standard 1-electrode neurofeedback. *Journal of Neurotherapy*, *7*, 302.

Koberda, J. L., et al. (2012). Cognitive enhancement using 19-electrode Z-score neurofeedback. *Journal of Neurotherapy*, *3*, 224–230.

Moeller, F., Maneshi, M., Pittau, F., Gholipour, T., Bellec, P., Dubeau, F., et al. (2011). Functional connectivity in patients with idiopathic generalized epilepsy. *Epilepsia*, *52* (3), 515–522.

Paz, A. -J. T., et al. (2007). Activity of ventral medial thalamic neurons during absence seizures and modulation of cortical paroxysms by the nigrothalamic pathway. *Journal of Neuroscience*, *27*, 929–941.

Rowland, L. P., & Pedley, T. A. (2010). *Merritt's neurology*. Philadelphia, PA: Lippincott.

Sterman, M. B. (2010). Biofeedback in the treatment of epilepsy. *Cleveland Clinic Journal of Medicine*, *77*(Suppl. 3), S60–S67 (Review).

Sterman, M. B., & Egner, T. (2006). Foundation and practice of neurofeedback for the treatment of epilepsy. *Applied Psychophysiology and Biofeedback*, *31*(1), 21–35 (Review).

Thatcher, R. W. (2010). LORETA Z score biofeedback. *Neuroconnections*9–13.

Thatcher, R. W. (2013). Latest developments in live Z-score training: Symptom check list, phase reset, and Loreta Z-score biofeedback. *Journal of Neurotherapy*, *17*, 69–87.

Wang, Z., Zhang, Z., Jiao, Q., Liao, W., Chen, G., Sun, K., et al. (2012). Impairments of thalamic nuclei in idiopathic generalized epilepsy revealed by a study combining morphological and functional connectivity MRI. *PLoS One*, *7*(7), e39701.

CHAPTER

11

LORETA Neurofeedback in Alcohol Use Disorders: A Case Study

Wesley D. Center

Liberty University, Lynchburg, VA, USA; Focus for Living, PLLC, Burleson, TX, USA

INTRODUCTION

Alcohol use disorders (AUDs) affect an estimated 17 million Americans (Grant et al., 2004). In 2012, an estimated 87.6% of people over the age of 18 reported drinking alcohol at some point in their life, 71% reported drinking alcohol in the past year, and 56.3% reported drinking in the past month (SAMHSA, 2013). While the image in the popular culture of those with AUDs is a person from a low socioeconomic status, the reality is that most of the people affected by AUDs are, by all appearances, successful and productive (Aldhous, 2010).

Importantly, of those affected by AUDs, only an estimated 15% ever seek treatment (Grant et al., 2004; Huebner & Kantor, 2011). For the vast majority of those who do seek traditional allopathic models of treatment or 12-step recovery programs, treatment failure is the norm (Dodes & Dodes, 2014). AUDs rarely occur in isolation from other psychiatric disorders. Mood disorders, sleep disorders, anxiety disorders, posttraumatic stress disorder, mild traumatic brain injury (mTBI), attention deficit/hyperactivity disorder, and schizophrenia are common comorbid psychiatric conditions encountered in AUD treatment (CSAT, 2005; Fergusson, Boden, & Horwood, 2009; Grant et al., 2004; Hasen & Grant, 2002; Petrakis, Gonzalez, Rosenheck, & Krystal, 2002; Schuckit, 2005, 2006, 2008; Smith, Molina, & Pelham, 2002). Suicide is also much more common among those with AUDs than in the general population

Z Score Neurofeedback.
DOI: http://dx.doi.org/10.1016/B978-0-12-801291-8.00011-X

(Chachamovich, Ding, & Turecki, 2012; Conner et al., 2006; Frierson, Melikian, & Wadman, 2002). It is important then to assess the patient who is presenting with an AUD not only for alcohol use patterns but also for comorbid psychiatric conditions and their overall impact on biopsychosocial functioning (Glasner-Edwards & Rawson, 2010).

ETHANOL'S EFFECTS ON BRAIN FUNCTION

Ethyl alcohol (ethanol or ETOH), the form of alcohol most commonly ingested in alcoholic beverages, has specific pharmacological effects in the brain. What is not well understood is which of these effects result in intoxication. The ETOH molecule is relatively small and is both water and lipid soluble (Jones, 1996), making its transport across the blood–brain barrier relatively rapid following ingestion (Kranzler & Ciraulo, 2005). Ethanol does not appear to prefer specific receptor sites, but affects the actions of several different neurotransmitters (NTs) and interferes with the actions of messenger molecules within the neuron (Gilpin & Koob, 2008; Knapp, Ciraulo, & Kranzler, 2008; Lovinger, 2008). Among the many NT systems affected by ETOH are dopamine (DA), γ-aminobutyric acid_A (GABA_A), glutamate (especially *N*-methyl-D-aspartate, NMDA), endocannabinoids, nicotinic, norepinephrine, and voltage-gated calcium ion channels (Cruz, Bajo, Schweitzer, & Roberto, 2008; Feltenstein & See, 2008; Knapp et al., 2008; Koob & Valkow, 2010). Ethanol has excitatory effects on release of DA and taurine in the ventral tegmental area (VTA) and nucleus accumbens (NAc) (Brodie, Pesold, & Appel, 1999; Ikemoto, 2007; Lammel, et al., 2008; Ericson et al., 2011; Yorgason, Ferris, Steffensen, & Jones, 2014). Ethanol has psychoactive effects on the GABA_A (agonist) and NMDA (antagonist) receptors in the VTA, where there is the greatest concentration of DA neurons in the brain.

The NT most associated with goal-directed behavior and reward—and by implication the addiction–reward network—is DA, and the connections between the mesoaccumbens pathway and reward have been well established in the literature for decades. There is also evidence that DA is involved in reward prediction between the NAc and the VTA, a factor in associative learning, not merely Pavlovian reward learning (Day & Carelli, 2007; Schultz, Dayan, & Montague, 1997; Yin, Ostlund, & Balleine, 2008). The overactivation of VTA neurons and the general reward circuit as a consequence of ETOH addiction results in increased levels of glutamate and decreased GABA, thereby dysregulating the neurochemistry of the addiction–reward network (Brodie et al., 1999). "From the brain's perspective, DA does not appear to be directly involved in the emergence of pleasure *per se*; rather, the firing rate of dopaminergic neurons in pleasure centers is likely to encode the saliency of a stimulus as a function of current expectations, and to facilitate the consolidation of memory traces connected to such a stimulus" (Volkow & Baler, 2007). It is this complex interaction of salience, outcome expectation, and memory that present such significant challenges in treating addiction.

Importantly, the learning processes associated with ETOH addiction involve not only episodic and procedural memories but also emotional components associated with the initial pleasure from ETOH consumption (Kropotov, 2009; Linden, 2011). As the addiction deepens, the pleasure of consumption diminishes and the compulsion to drink, *wanting*, increases (Berridge & Robinson, 1995; Linden, 2011; Robinson & Berridge, 2003). Associative learning is critical in using neurofeedback (NFB) to treat addicts because addictive behaviors are gained through reward-guided learning and sustained by drug-paired cues (Day & Carelli, 2007; Hogarth, Balleine, Corbit, & Killcross, 2013). Components of those very same learning networks (dorsal lateral prefrontal, orbitofrontal, anterior cingulate, and motor/premotor cortices) are important for goal-directed learning (including operant conditioning) and targeted for NFB training of patients presenting with AUDs. Repeated and extended training should affect the networks associated with instrumental learning.

Alcohol, like other drugs, also affects the electrophysiology of the brain. Little and McAvoy (1952) reported that the EEG of alcoholics was typified by elevated slow and fast activity and deficient alpha. Other early studies of ETOH effects on the EEG looked at abnormal brain activity associated with acute withdrawal and long-term abstinence (Begleiter & Platz, 1972; van Sweden, 1983). Most early studies concluded that ETOH has the effect of long-term pathologic changes in the EEG of chronic users (persistent arrhythmia, dysrhythmia, spiking, increased low-voltage slow waves) and short-term effects (proneness to seizure) in the case of acute alcohol withdrawal. Electroencephalographic mapping (tEEG) has also been used to accurately predict relapse in alcohol-dependent patients, with high frequency beta being the predictor of relapse (Bauer, 1994 & 2001; Winterer et al., 1998). Other studies have sought to use EEG as a marker of vulnerability to developing alcoholism (Elhers & Schuckit, 1990; Enoch et al., 1999; Gabrielli et al., 1982; Spehr & Stemmler, 1985; Winterer et al., 1998). Most EEG studies of alcoholics from the 1950s through the late 1990s have found increase in beta (>12 Hz), and less commonly, increases in alpha (8–12 Hz) in the chronic alcohol-using population (Costa & Bauer, 1997).

A number of tEEG studies of alcoholics, relative to normal controls, have found decreased delta/theta and alpha absolute power in frontal regions of the brain, and significantly increased beta absolute and relative power in wide distributions (Kiloh, McComas, Osselton, & Upton, 1981;

Niedermeyer & Lopes da Silva, 1982). Saletu-Zyhlarz et al. (2004) hypothesize that "the low-voltage fast desynchronized patterns may be interpreted as hyperarousal of the CNS" (p. 233) but also caution, as have others (Bauer, 2001; Coutin-Churchman, Anez, & Vergara, 2006; Winterer et al., 1998), that frontal dysregulation in alcoholics may be a premorbid condition that contributes to the development of alcohol dependence. Other changes in the EEG, such as decreased alpha (Propping, 1983), increased beta (Gabrielli et al., 1982), or increased coherence (Winterer et al., 2003), may also reflect premorbid and predisposing factors in the development of alcoholism.

Coutin-Churchman and Moreno (2004) suggest that deficits in delta absolute power are common in alcoholics and alcoholics with comorbid depression, though the current source deficits differ. Their analysis via low-resolution electromagnetic tomographic analysis (LORETA) indicated that the depressed alcoholics had significantly reduced current sources in delta bilaterally in the parahippocampal gyrus relative to normal healthy controls. The nondepressed alcoholics had deficient current sources in delta in the left parahippocampal gyrus and medial areas, as well as bilaterally in the posterior cingulate relative to the controls. Coutin-Churchman et al. (2006) suggest that the decreased power in delta/theta in alcoholic patients may be indicative of alcohol-related brain atrophy or damage, while the increase in the beta frequency may be related to a number of endogenous and exogenous variables effecting cortical excitability.

In contrast to those studies finding decreased slow wave absolute power among alcoholics, a number of other studies find that prolonged use of ETOH increases delta and theta amplitude in chronic alcoholics. Some have theorized that slow wave excesses in chronic alcoholics' EEGs may be indicative of permanent brain changes due prolonged exposure to ETOH (Johannesson, Berglund, & Ingvar, 1982; Spehr & Stemmler, 1985). In comparing recovered alcoholics (>5 years in recovery) to nonalcoholic controls, Pollock, Schneider, Zemansky, Gleason, and Pawluczyk (1992) found significantly elevated bilateral anterior and posterior theta amplitude in the recovered alcoholics. Rangaswamy et al. (2003) found that theta absolute power was elevated in all surface sites in their alcohol-dependent subjects, hypothesizing that the increase in theta might be reflective of an information processing deficit in alcoholics.

While slow wave amplitude has been implicated in most of the tEEG studies in AUDs, there is not a single or definitive EEG marker for AUDs. Importantly, the topographical/spatial resolution of EEG is limited, and tEEG remains subject to a number of physiological and mathematical confounds that make it vulnerable to artifact and distortion (John et al., 1994; John, Prichep, Fridman, & Easton, 1988; Kahn et al., 1988). Prior to LORETA and its successors (sLORETA and eLORETA), our knowledge of how the deeper cortical generators contribute to the topographical representations of EEG data taken from scalp locations was also limited (Pascual-Marqui & Biscay-Lirio, 1993; Pascual-Marqui & Lehmann, 1993; Günther et al., 1997; Pascual-Marqui, 1999, 2002; Pascual-Marqui, Michel, & Lehmann, 1994; Thatcher, North, & Biver, 2005, 2012). Since the origin of slow wave activity lies in the subcortical projections of the thalamus and in the anterior medial frontal cortex of the waking brain (Knyazev, 2012; Michel, Henggeler, & Brandeis, 1993; Michel, Lehmann, & Henggeler, 1992), and the direct effects of ETOH on the brain are largely in the mesocorticolimbic pathway, LORETA would appear to be uniquely suited among other EEG neuroimaging techniques for assessing and addressing AUDs (Saletu, Anderer, & Saletu-Zyhlarz, 2006).

NFB and Substance Abuse Treatments

The treatment of substance use disorders (SUDs) using alpha/theta NFB was pioneered by Elmer and Alyce Green in the Voluntary Controls Program at the Menninger Foundation as an augment to psychotherapy (Green, Green, & Walters, 1974; Trudeau, 2005). Eugene Peniston's work with veterans using alpha/theta NFB in combination with temperature and electromyographic biofeedback training and psychotherapy is widely regarded as the first use of NFB to treat SUDs (Peniston & Kulkosky, 1989, 1990; Trudeau, 2005; Sokhadze, Trudeau, & Cannon, 2014; Peper & Shaffer, 2010). The Peniston Protocol (which included deep, relaxed state training via skin temperature biofeedback and scripted autogenic phrases, and alpha/theta NFB) is an example of an approach to NFB using predetermined electrode placement(s) and reward/inhibit thresholds under the assumption that the protocol addresses the patient's symptoms. Other protocols to address SUDs, such as the Scott–Kaiser modification of the Peniston Protocol, have demonstrated effectiveness in improving treatment outcomes, yet NFB as a standard approach to treating SUDs has not been widely adopted (deBeus, 2007; Kelly, 1997; Khalily, Clarke, & Jahangir, 2009; Scott & Kaiser, 1998; Scott, Kaiser, Othmer, & Sideroff, 2005; Trudeau, 2005).

NFB for the treatment of SUDs is not a stand-alone approach (Dehghani-Arani, Rostami, & Nadali, 2013; Myers & Young, 2012; Sokhadze et al., 2014; Trudeau, Sokhadze, & Cannon, 2009). While NFB is not an evidence-based treatment for SUDs, it may be incorporated with evidence-based treatments such as pharmacotherapies, cognitive behavioral psychotherapies, community reinforcement approaches, and motivational enhancement therapy. As discussed below, quantitative electroencephalogram (qEEG)-guided LNFB permits the clinician to match the patient's symptoms to dysregulated networks and modules associated with the patient's symptoms. Matching dysregulated brain networks and modules to symptoms ensures that the selected protocol(s) address(es) the network of the patient's brain that is dysregulated/weak while ensuring that compensatory/helper networks are not targeted for training (Thatcher, 2012; Trudeau, 2005). The qEEG-guided LNFB approach has great promise to improve treatment outcome as well as reduce the number of training sessions due to its specificity in matching symptoms to the patient's dysregulated brain networks and modules.

Understanding the neurocircuitry of addiction helps to guide the NFB clinician's assessment of weak/dysregulated systems to be trained using LORETA Z-scored NFB, and compensatory systems that will not be the clinical focus in training. Explanatory models of addiction from a neurobehavioral perspective help the clinician to conceptualize assessment and treatment of SUDs. For example, Koob, Lloyd, and Mason (2009) propose a three-stage cycle of addiction, consisting of (i) binge/intoxication, (ii) withdrawal/negative effect, and (iii) preoccupation, involving allostatic changes in the brain's reward and stress systems. Different networks of the brain mediate each of the three stages. The mesocorticolimbic DA system mediates the positive reinforcing effects of ETOH in the first stage, where pleasure accompanies consumption (Kauer & Malenka, 2007; Hikosaka et al., 2008; Alcaro, Huber, & Panksepp, 2007). The third stage (preoccupation and anticipation, craving, or *wanting*) involves the circuitry of the glutamatergic projections of the amygdala and NAc from the prefrontal cortex (orbital, medial, and cingulate nuclei) and from the basolateral amygdala (conditioned cues). The withdrawal stage not only involves the neural circuitry of the positive reinforcing effects of drugs but also involvement of the brain's stress response systems (Koob, 2008; Koob, Boutrel, & Valdez, 2013). These distinctions are important in hypothesis formation as well as clinical decision making regarding the approach to LNFB training. For example, a clinician treating a patient who continues to receive pleasure from ETOH consumption may hypothesize that the pleasure network may be dysregulated, and if confirmed, may begin LNFB training on that network. Another patient deeper in the cycle of addiction may no longer have the pleasure associated with consuming ETOH but feels the compulsive *wanting* associated with the above model of addiction. In the event that the clinician's hypothesis of a dysregulated addiction–reward network is confirmed, that network should be targeted for LNFB training.

For our purposes in LORETA NFB training using *NeuroGuide Deluxe 2.8* (Thatcher, 2014), we consider the addiction network to be synonymous with the reward network. The addiction–reward network is involved in valuing the intrinsic attractiveness (positive valence) of environmental stimuli as diverse as objects, goals, persons, outcomes, etc., and internal representations that create "pleasure" (Brody et al., 2002; Hammer, 2002; Linden, 2011; Sutherland, McHugh, Pariyadath, &

Stein, 2012). Though there are overlaps (bolded), the addiction–reward network (BAs 13, **24**, 25, **32**, **34**, **44**, **45**, **46**, and **47**) differs from the pleasure network (BAs 8, 9, 10, **24**, 30, **32**, 33, **44**, **45**, **46**, **47**, the amygdala, and hippocampus) in terms of brain "real estate" (Thatcher, 2012, 2014). Additionally, any of the patient's symptoms that are comorbid with the AUD but determined by the clinician to be distinct from the etiology and/or pathology of the AUD will be included in the hypothesis formation tested using the qEEG, linking the patient's symptoms to functional networks and modules of the brain (Thatcher, 2012).

CASE PRESENTATION

Presenting Problems

Jack (pseudonym) is a 55-year-old male who self-describes as a "functioning alcoholic." His primary care physician referred him to NFB treatment after unsuccessful attempts to stop drinking using traditional allopathic models of treatment and 12-step recovery programs. Jack describes his drinking pattern as moderate daily consumption accompanied by episodic binge drinking, and he has consumed alcohol in this pattern for most of his adult life. Alcoholism and substance abuse is a family pattern among first and second degree maternal and paternal relatives. Jack also has a history of sports-related head trauma extending back into adolescence, with his most recent "ding" resulting from a motor vehicle accident 6 months prior to entering treatment. Upon entering treatment, Jack was hypertensive and that was not well controlled by antihypertensive medications.

Jack presented with self-reported depressed mood and effect, mood instability, sleep disturbances (insomnia and hyposomnia), angry outbursts, negative internal dialog, inefficient self-quieting/self-soothing, chronic pain, intermediate and short-term memory deficits, distractibility, and transient cognitive cloudiness (which he described as "brain fog") persisting for more than 36 months without relent. Although retired, Jack remains physically active, engaging in a moderate level of exercise three to five times per week. He was diagnosed with arthritis in his dominant hand and aggravated a mechanical low back injury during the course of treatment while exercising.

Assessment Procedures, Results, and Diagnosis

Following the patient's acknowledging the limitations of confidentiality, informed consent (including a description of the procedure, intended use of qEEG and NFB, risks, benefits, and alternatives to NFB training, and the potential that training might lead to a distaste for alcohol or a negative reaction to alcohol), the assessment of the patient began. A clinical interview was administered at intake, as well as administration of several screening instruments, including: Amen Clinics' self and other report screens (Adult General Symptom Checklist, Brain System Checklist, Anxiety and Depression Type Questionnaire, which indicated prefrontal cortex and anterior cingulate dysregulation) (Amen, 2004a), the Depression, Anxiety and Stress Scale-42 Item version (DASS-42), which indicated severely depressed mood (Brown, Chorpita, Korotitsch, & Barlow, 1997; Parkitny & McAuley, 2010), the Alcohol Use Disorders Identification Test (AUDIT) (Babor, La Fuente, Saunders, & Grant, 1992; Reinert & Allen, 2007), and Michigan Alcohol Screening Test (MAST) (Selzer, 1971), which indicated the presence of an AUD. The initial and subsequent risk assessments indicated that Jack was not a risk to harm self or others. We also inquired about diet, exercise, and sleep habits and asked the patient to inform the clinician if there were any changes to these patterns during the course of training.

Jack was also administered the MicroCog™ assessment of cognitive functioning and the QIK™ visual continuous performance task (CPT) test. The results of the pretreatment MicroCog™ assessment (Table 11.1) suggested reduced cognitive competence due to inaccurate cognitive processes and memory impairment relative to age- and education-matched peers. The QIK™ CPT (Table 11.2) did not reveal any deficits in attention or mental control and was consistent with the MicroCog™ in terms of information processing speed.

The pretreatment QIK™ CPT results are given in Table 11.2.

The results of the assessment support the diagnosis of an AUD with comorbid mood disorder. Jack's self-reported symptoms and functional impairments were confirmed by the testing and assessment, and by qEEG hypothesis testing. The initial hypotheses were that there would be reduced delta/theta and alpha absolute power over frontal regions, increased beta absolute power in a wide distribution, and dysregulation in the functional networks associated with addiction–reward, pleasure, mood, executive functions, and memory.

The initial EEG recordings were obtained in the Eyes Open and Eyes Closed conditions. The 19-channel recordings were made with a Discovery 24 amplifier using an Electro Cap with tin electrodes and a linked ears referenced montage and were acquired via NeuroGuide Deluxe. For all recordings and LORETA NFB training, impedances at the reference and ground were at or below 2 kΩ and at or below 5 kΩ at all other sites.

The raw EEG in the Eyes Closed condition revealed some well-developed posterior dominant 8 Hz activity spreading forward into the frontal regions with diffuse low-voltage fast activity at 15–25 Hz.

TABLE 11.1 Pretreatment MicroCog™ Results

Age and education corrected norms (age: 55–64, education: >high school)					
	Sum	**Scaled score**	**Percentile**	**95% confidence interval**	**Qualitative description**
Level 3—Indexes					
General cognitive functioning (GCF)	175	85	16	79–91	Average
General cognitive proficiency (GCP)	75	82	12	76–88	**Low average**
Level 2—Indexes					
Information processing speed (IPS)	92	93	32	86–100	Average
Information processing accuracy (IPA)	95	82	12	75–89	**Low average**
Level 1—Indexes					
Attention/mental control (Attn)	70	100	50	90–110	Average
Reasoning/calculation (Reas)	55	91	27	79–103	Average
Memory (Mem)	44	80	9	70–90	**Low average**
Spatial processing (Spat)	33	88	21	78–98	Average
Reaction time (RT)	63	103	58	96–110	Average

TABLE 11.2 Pretreatment QIK™ CPT Results

Pretreatment results	**Data**	**Norm ± SD**	**#SDs**	**Standard score**	**Percentile**
Sustained attention	**0.0%**	0.2 ± 0.3%	−0.7	110	99
Impulse control	**1.6%**	2.2 ± 1.2%	−0.5	107	67
Speed of response	**319.3 ms**	435.9 ± 46.9 ms	−2.5	**137**	99
Consistency of response	**62.4 ms**	71.4 ± 11.6 ms	−0.8	112	78

The raw EEG in the Eyes Open condition revealed diffuse low-voltage fast activity at 15–25 Hz with some alpha activity mixed in throughout the various 10–20 sites. Because there was a history of head injury reported by the patient, a TBI discriminant analysis was performed and the score (−2.19) was not significant.

The computerized power spectral analyses (Figure 11.1) using Thatcher's NeuroGuide linked ears Z-scored FFT Eyes Open database were deviant from normal with deficient absolute power in theta, alpha, and total beta. EEG asymmetry (in beta) and phase (all frequencies) were abnormal, especially in the right temporal region and both parietal regions. Unlike Winterer et al. (2003) findings of increased coherence in depressed alcoholics, our patient's coherence was normal across all frequencies. Inspection of the single herz bins (Figures 11.2 and 11.3) revealed deficient absolute power in 5 Hz in the right central region, 6 Hz in the right occipital region, and in 11–16 Hz especially frontally but also in the occipital region at 14 Hz. There were also decreases in 20 Hz absolute power in the left frontocentral region and in 30 Hz in the right parietal region.

Analysis of the LORETA 3-dimensional sources using NeuroGuide's LORETA Z-scored database was consistent with the surface EEG maps with deficient current sources in the left superior, middle, and medial frontal gyri with a maximum at 4, 5, 6, and 11 Hz (left Brodmann areas 10, 11, and 47). The deficient current sources were maximal at 6 Hz (−4.57 SDs; $X = -38$, $Y = 59$, $Z = -6$; 1st Best Match ($d = 3$ mm); Brodmann area 10, Middle Frontal Gyrus, Frontal Lobe) (Figures 11.4 and 11.5) but widely distributed.

The pattern of dysregulation observed in the surface maps and LORETA analyses was consistent with the patient's self-reported symptoms and the results of testing. The pattern of reduced absolute power in delta/theta and alpha observed in this patient is consistent with the findings of Saletu-Zyhlarz et al. (2004) and Coutin-Churchman and Moreno (2004), in comparing ETOH-dependent patients to normal controls, and depressed ETOH-dependent patients relative to controls, confirming our related hypotheses. Our hypothesis concerning the expectation that there would be a wide distribution of increased absolute power in beta was not confirmed by spectral and LORETA analyses.

The clinical conclusion was that LORETA NFB with biofeedback training could play a role in reducing Jack's symptoms and improving overall functioning because his reported symptoms correlated to dysregulated areas of the brain determined by LORETA normative comparisons in NeuroGuide's surface and LORETA Z-scored databases. Specifically, we expected that training the addiction–reward, default mode, pleasure, working memory, and mood networks would result in a decrease in reported frequency, duration, and severity of symptoms and an overall

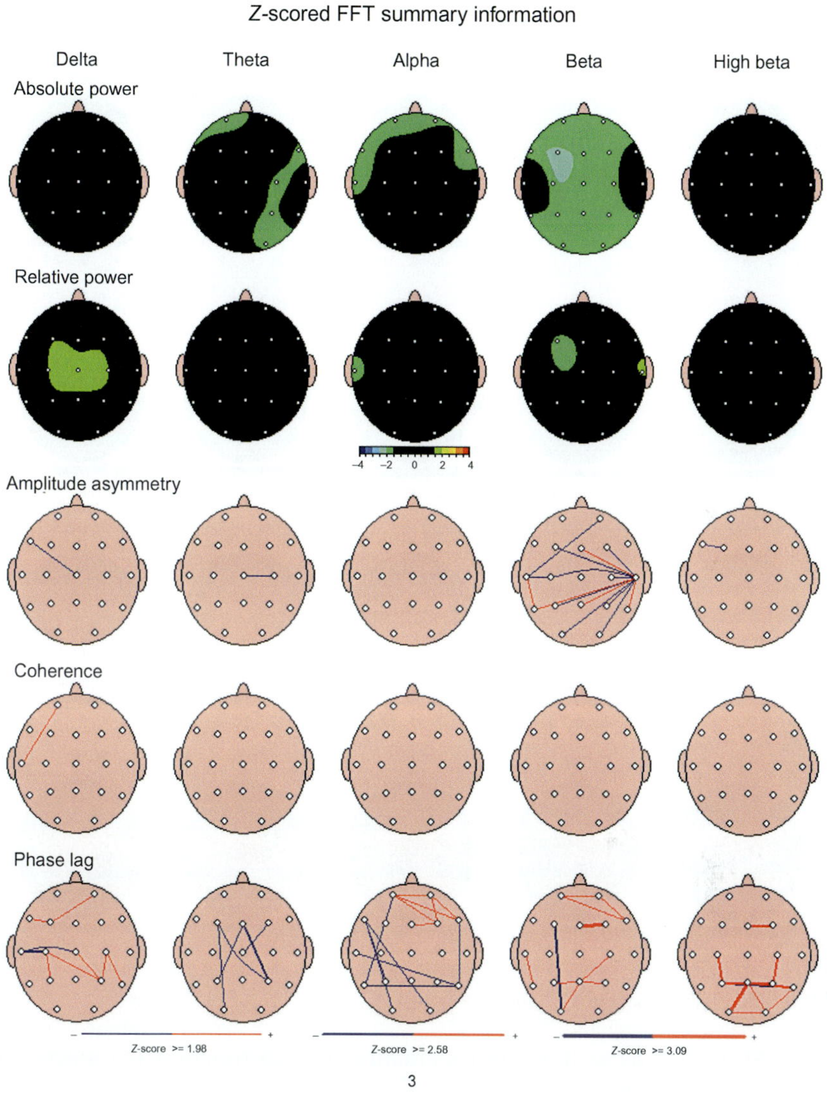

FIGURE 11.1 Eyes open Z-scored FFT summary.

improvement in functioning. With movement of trained *Z* scores toward $Z=0$, we expected reduction, and over time elimination, of Jack's problem drinking, overall improvement in mood and mood stability, improvement in sleep onset, duration, and quality, and improvements in short-term memory. Additionally, we expected posttreatment scores to demonstrate improvement over pretreatment scores on the MicroCog™

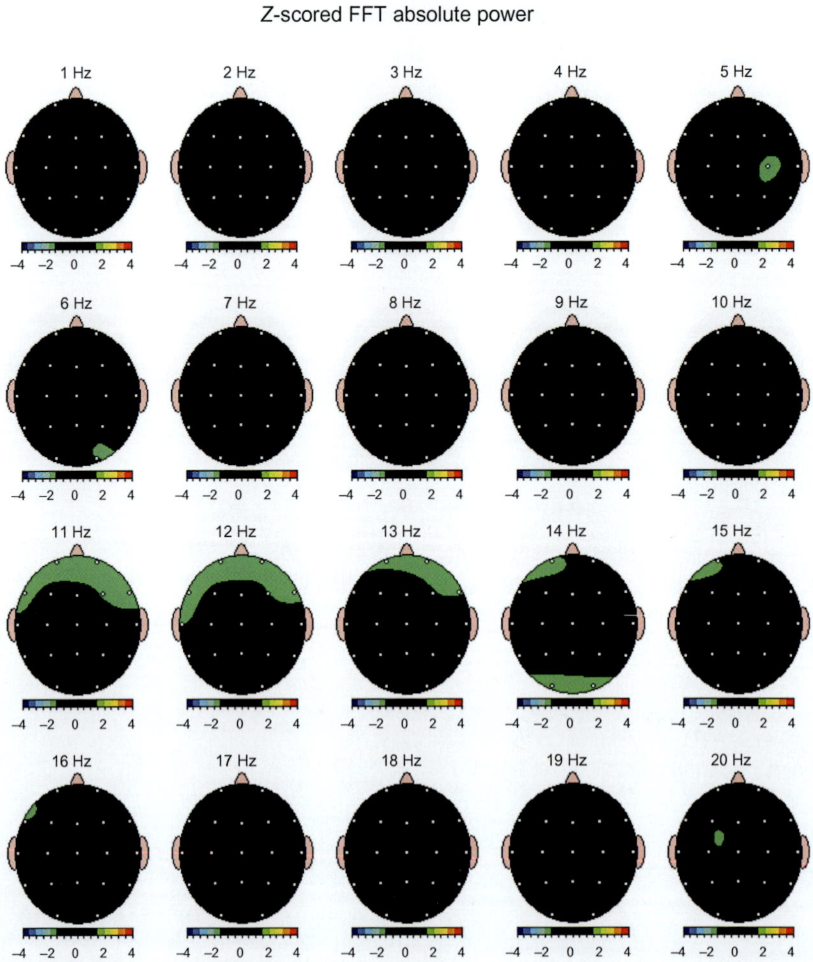

FIGURE 11.2 Z-scored FFT absolute power A.

and QIK CPT™, as well as improvements in brain function as reflected in posttreatment LORETA analyses. Our conclusions and plan for addressing the dysregulated areas of the brain that were correlated with Jack's symptoms were explained to Jack prior to the initiation of training. Jack also agreed to follow up at 6, 9, and 12 months after the end of training for additional EEG recordings and testing.

Training Methods and Procedures

Remembering that NFB is not a stand-alone approach to treating AUDs, Jack was encouraged to explore his thought life for patterns of

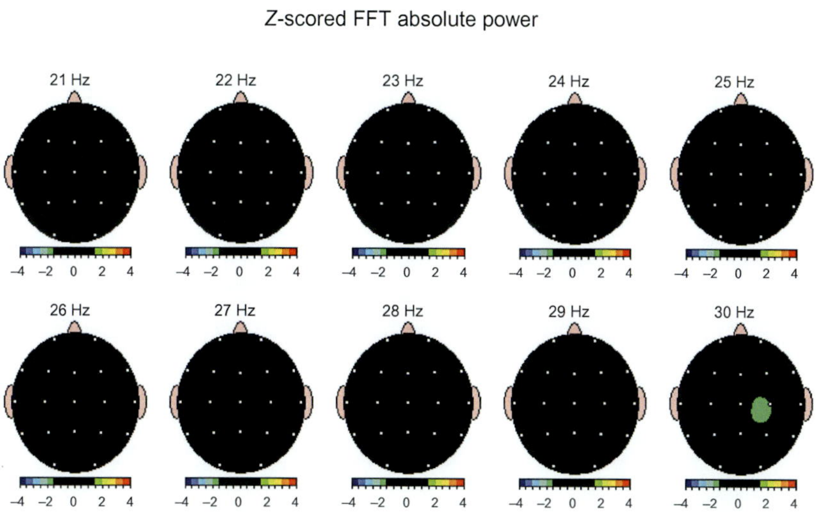

FIGURE 11.3 Z-scored FFT absolute power B.

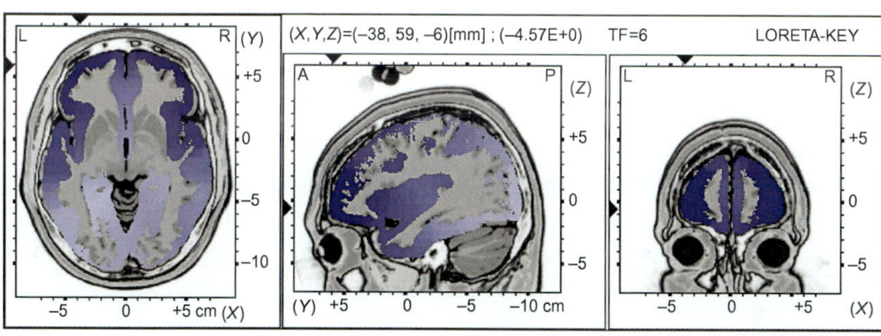

FIGURE 11.4 LORETA current source analysis at 6 Hz.

negative thinking that support and undergird his struggles with alcohol and depression. In the initial training session, Jack was given Amen's (1998, 2004b) *ANT Therapy: How to Develop Your Own Internal Anteater to Eradicate Automatic Negative Thoughts (ANTs)* workbook, and a very brief explanation of how to use the workbook to identify, stop, and replace/edit negative thought patterns. Cognitive behavioral and cognitive restructuring strategies are evidence-based treatments for both AUDs and mood disorders (CSAT, 2005; Drake, Merrens, & Lynde, 2005; Flynn & Brown, 2008). In the initial five sessions, the therapist reviewed Jack's progress in using the ANT identification, stopping, and replacement strategies in the Amen workbook. Each session thereafter, the therapist briefly (5–10 min) inquired as to Jack's progress with

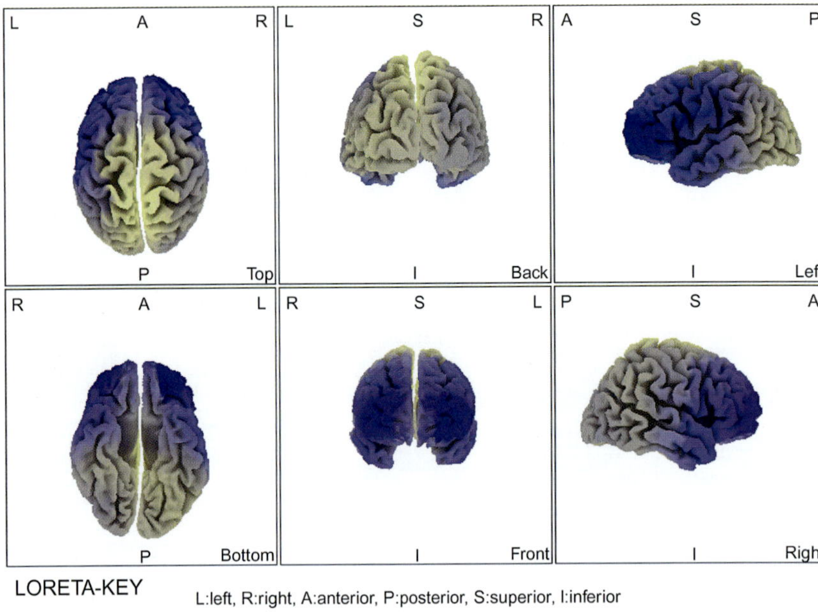

FIGURE 11.5 LORETA current source analysis at 6 Hz orthogonal view.

managing his thought life, normally during the preparation time for the LORETA NFB session.

Prior to each LORETA NFB session, a 10-min heart rate variability (HRV) biofeedback session was conducted. The purpose of HRV training is to achieve synchrony of breathing and the interbeat interval of the heart and thereby reduce anxiety and stress (Antelmi et al., 2004; Zohar, Cloninger, & McCraty, 2013). We have found that using HRV immediately prior to NFB training tends to relax the patient and facilitates a state of relaxed attention for the session's duration.

LNFB uses a brain–computer interface that facilitates learning through auditory and visual feedback to regulate EEG activity. Training was accomplished with a 19-channel array, referenced to linked ears, with band pass filtering (low pass at 40 Hz, high pass at 1 Hz). No additional filtering was employed. All training was done in the Eyes Open condition. Training data was acquired with a BrainMaster Discovery 24 amplifier via NeuroGuide. Training protocols were established using a combination of the patient's self-reported symptoms and a LORETA NFB symptom checklist match generated by NeuroGuide. New symptom checklist matches were created periodically during treatment.

The method employed for all training was Z Tunes. The Z Tunes method employs real-time Z scores to help guide the EEG resonant frequencies and network functioning by reinforcing the movement of trained Z scores toward $Z = 0$ with respect to age-matched peers in the LORETA normative database (Thatcher, Biver, & North, 2002; Thatcher et al., 2005). It is important to note that LORETA Z-scored NFB, as with all Z-scored NFB, does not reward artifact, as by definition, artifact produces Z scores that are moving away from $Z = 0$ and are therefore not reinforced. The LORETA NFB module in NeuroGuide permits training of absolute power, coherence, and phase in as many as 24 Brodmann areas simultaneously, providing those metrics fall outside of the database norms and are linked to the patient's symptoms. Each LORETA NFB session included absolute power, coherence, and phase metrics. The initial session training duration was 15 min (3 rounds of 5 min) for each network/symptom trained working up to 25 min (5 rounds of 5 min) total training duration. Between-round breaks of 60–90 s in duration were provided for coaching in each session.

Audio/video feedback for all training sessions was provided by NeuroGuide's DVD player. The video played normally when the patient's Z scores met the training criteria, and shrank in size and dropped in volume when the Z scores exceeded the training threshold values; this was explained to the patient. Reward points accrued during each round and were displayed to the patient in a separate window on top of the DVD window. In every session, the therapist manipulated the Z-score threshold and Z-score window (Figure 11.6) during the course of training so that the patient received no less than an average of 20 points per minute per round, and no more than an average of 30 points per minute per round, with a single exception noted below.

The only instructions given to the patient were to "Be relaxed and interested in the video. Do not try to change the size of the picture or volume of the feedback consciously. You will accumulate points during each round. Tell yourself that you want to get more points from one round to the next." In between rounds, these instructions were repeated. At the conclusion of the last round of every session, the session was reviewed by displaying the round by round scores to the patient and reviewing his training behaviors (on task behaviors, artifact producing behaviors, and insight into goal-directed performance). The patient was also asked to describe any side effects or changes in cognitive or emotional state since the beginning of the session.

Prior to the first session, the patient completed a symptom checklist (Thatcher, 2012, pp. 556–558) identifying symptoms that he was most concerned with addressing in training. The patient's chief complaints on the initial day of training were sleep and negative thinking, followed by addiction and depressed mood. The symptom checklist was reviewed with the patient prior to each session and he completed a new symptom checklist every 4–7 sessions for the duration of 27 training sessions that took place over the course of 4 months (late September 2012 to the

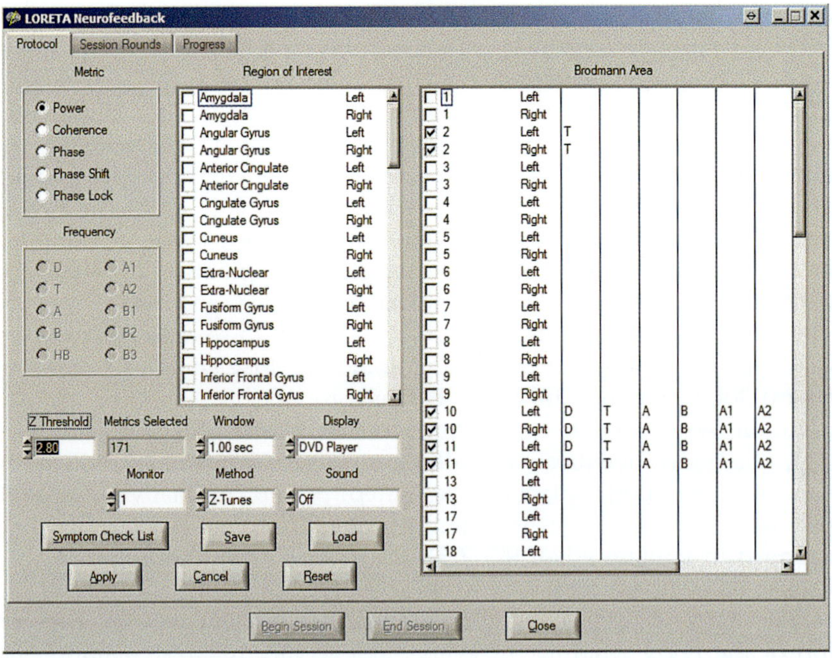

FIGURE 11.6 LORETA NFB setup panel.

end of January 2013). There were three 1-week breaks during training (the weeks of Thanksgiving, Christmas, and New Year).

Because the patient's chief complaints via the symptom checklist at the initiation of training were sleep and negative thinking, which are self-related processes, the initial training protocol focused on the default mode network (DMN) (Buckner & Carroll, 2007; Gusnard, Akbudak, Shulman, & Raichle, 2001; Raichle & Snyder, 2007; Uddin, Clare-Kelly, Biswal, Castellanos, & Milham, 2009; Wicker, Ruby, Royet, & Fonlupt, 2003). This decision was based on our clinical experience that dysregulation in the DMN often manifests in sleep disturbances related to negative thought processes, and that sleep disturbances interfere significantly with NFB training. The upper and lower Z-score thresholds for identifying training metrics were established at ±2.80 *Z*, yielding 171 metrics (absolute power, coherence, and phase) selected for training (refer Figure 11.6). Bilateral Brodmann areas trained were 2, 10, 11, 19, 29, 30, 35, and 40. The DMN locations were trained for five sessions. The initial training session was three rounds of 5 min, after which the patient reported being mentally fatigued. The beginning session *Z* threshold was 2.80 *Z* and the ending session *Z* threshold was 2.00 *Z*. The patient achieved 339 points during the session, averaging 28.3 points per minute.

By the fifth DMN training session, the patient's ending Z threshold was 0.90 Z, with an average of 28.3 points per minute, for the session. The patient averaged 28.3, 27.7, 28, 30.4, and 28.3 points per minute per round in the five sessions, respectively. During the course of the five sessions, the patient reported overall improvement in sleep quality and duration and a reduction of negative thinking, particularly at bedtime. He also reported experiencing fewer cravings for alcohol during the 2-week period of the initial five sessions.

The second network trained was the addiction network. With the symptom checklist match Z-score threshold set to ±3.00 Z, there were 224 metrics (absolute power, coherence, and phase) identified for training in bilateral Brodmann areas 13, 24, 25, 32, 34, 44, 45, 46, and 47. The addiction network was trained for seven consecutive sessions. The initial session settings for training the addiction network was at a Z threshold of 2.60 Z and Z window of 1.00 s and the ending Z threshold at the seventh session was 0.80 and a Z window of 1.00 s. The patient averaged 29.2, 24.5, 24.5, 25.4, 24.8, 23.6 and 28.3 points per minute per round in the seven sessions, respectively. During the course of training the addiction network, the patient reported a continuing decrease in the *wanting* of alcohol.

The third symptom trained was working memory and it was trained for five sessions. With the symptom checklist match Z-score threshold set to ±3.40 Z, there were 246 metrics (absolute power, coherence, and phase) identified for training in bilateral Brodmann areas 8, 9, 24, 32, in right Brodmann area 40, and the right hippocampus. The initial session settings for training working memory were at a Z threshold of 3.00 Z and Z window of 1.00 s and the ending Z threshold at the fifth session was 0.80 and a Z window of 1.00 s. The patient averaged 27.1, 26.3, 27, 23.3, and 24 points per minute per round in the five sessions, respectively.

The pleasure network was the fourth area addressed in training. With the symptom checklist match Z-score threshold set to ±3.60 Z, there were 116 metrics (absolute power, coherence, and phase) identified for training in bilateral Brodmann areas 9, 10, 24, 32, 45, and 47, in right Brodmann areas 8 and 44. The initial session settings for training the pleasure network was at a Z threshold of 2.50 Z and Z window of 1.00 s and the ending Z threshold at the fifth session was 0.80 and a Z window of 1.00 s. The patient averaged 28.5, 27.8, 20.9, 26.25, and 22.9 points per minute per round in the five sessions, respectively.

We returned to the addiction network for a single session at the patient's request. The patient initially indicated that he desired reassurance that "training is working." Using a new LORETA symptom checklist match, and a Z-score threshold set to ±3.70, there were 74 metrics (absolute power, coherence, and phase) selected for training in the addiction network. The beginning Z threshold was set at 3.30 Z and the ending Z threshold was set at 0.90 Z. The patient averaged 24.3 points per round in the session. The patient disclosed at the end of the session that he drank a partial glass of wine two nights prior to the session, had found the taste of the wine to be unpleasant, and did not finish the glass. This reaction to alcohol following a course of NFB training, particularly during alpha/theta training, has been referred to as the "Peniston Flu" (Robins, 2008, p. 169) or "Peniston effect" (Demos, 2005, p. 247).

The mood network was trained last. With the symptom checklist match Z-score threshold set to ±3.50 Z, there were 107 metrics (absolute power, coherence, and phase) identified for training in bilateral Brodmann areas 10, 11, 24, 32, 44, 45, and 47, and in left Brodmann area 13. The initial session settings for training the pleasure network was at a Z threshold of 3.50 Z and Z window of 1.00 s and the ending Z threshold at the fourth session was 0.70 and a Z window of 1.00 s. The patient averaged 23.7, 23.2, 19.6, and 15.8 points per minute per round in the four sessions, respectively. The last session's average score was negatively affected by moving the Z threshold too rapidly in the third and fourth rounds. At the end of the last training session, the patient complained of being very fatigued mentally, reminiscent of earlier in training. We believe that this side effect is a direct result of attempting to move too rapidly in training.

Posttreatment Analyses

Training terminated by mutual consent when the patient's goals for training were met. At the conclusion of training during the review of goals for therapy, the patient reported a significant decrease in ETOH consumption (<1–2 standard drinks per month since the beginning of training), an overall improvement in mood and mood stability, increase in sleep onset, quality, and duration, and a significant improvement in short-term memory. He also reported being less irritable, more resilient to stress, and no further instances of "brain fog." His posttreatment DASS-42 scores were within normal limits (<1.0 Z) for depression, anxiety, and stress. The first of three posttreatment EEG recordings was obtained in the Eyes Open condition the week following the last training session. Subsequent recordings were made at 6, 9, and 14 months posttraining with no significant differences in the recordings.

Jack was administered the MicroCog™ assessment of cognitive functioning and the QIK™ visual CPT test 14 months after his last training session. The results of the posttreatment MicroCog™ assessment (Table 11.3) suggested improved cognitive competence due to improved cognitive processes and no memory impairment relative to age- and

TABLE 11.3 Posttreatment MicroCog™ Results

Age and education corrected norms (age: 55–64, education: >high school)					
	Sum	Scaled score	Percentile	95% Confidence interval	Qualitative description
Level 3—Indexes					
General cognitive functioning (GCF)	210	106	66	100–112	Average
General cognitive proficiency (GCP)	98	99	47	93–105	Average
Level 2—Indexes					
Information processing speed (IPS)	111	110	75	103–117	Average
Information processing accuracy (IPA)	120	100	50	93–107	Average
Level 1—Indexes					
Attention/mental control (Attn)	71	101	53	91–111	Average
Reasoning/calculation (Reas)	73	122	93	110–134	**Above average**
Memory (Mem)	63	104	61	94–114	Average
Spatial processing (Spat)	43	105	63	95–115	Average
Reaction time (RT)	71	112	79	105–119	Average

education-matched peers. Jack's pretraining scores in the areas of general cognitive proficiency (pre = 82, 12‰, post = 99, 47‰), information processing accuracy (pre = 82, 12‰, post = 100, 50‰), and memory (pre = 80, 9‰, post = 104, 61‰), improved from low average prior to training to average posttraining. Additionally, Jack's pretraining score in reasoning/calculation (pre = 91, 27‰) improved from average to above average (post = 122, 93‰). The QIK™ CPT (Table 11.4) did not reveal any deficits in attention or mental control and was consistent with the MicroCog™ in terms of information processing speed, demonstrating a slight improvement in information processing speed and a significant improvement in consistency of response over pretraining scores.

The computerized power spectral analyses (Figure 11.7) of the patient's EEG 14 months posttraining were deviant from normal with

TABLE 11.4 Posttreatment QIK™ CPT Results

14 Months posttreatment results	Data	Norm ± SD	#SDs	Standard score	Percentile
Sustained attention	**0.2%**	0.2 ± 0.3%	− 0.1	**102**	54
Impulse control	**1.6%**	2.2 ± 1.2%	− 0.5	**107**	67
Speed of response	**293.4 ms**	442.9 ± 46.9 ms	− 3.2	**148**	100
Consistency of response	**34.9 ms**	75.4 ± 11.6 ms	− 3.5	**153**	100

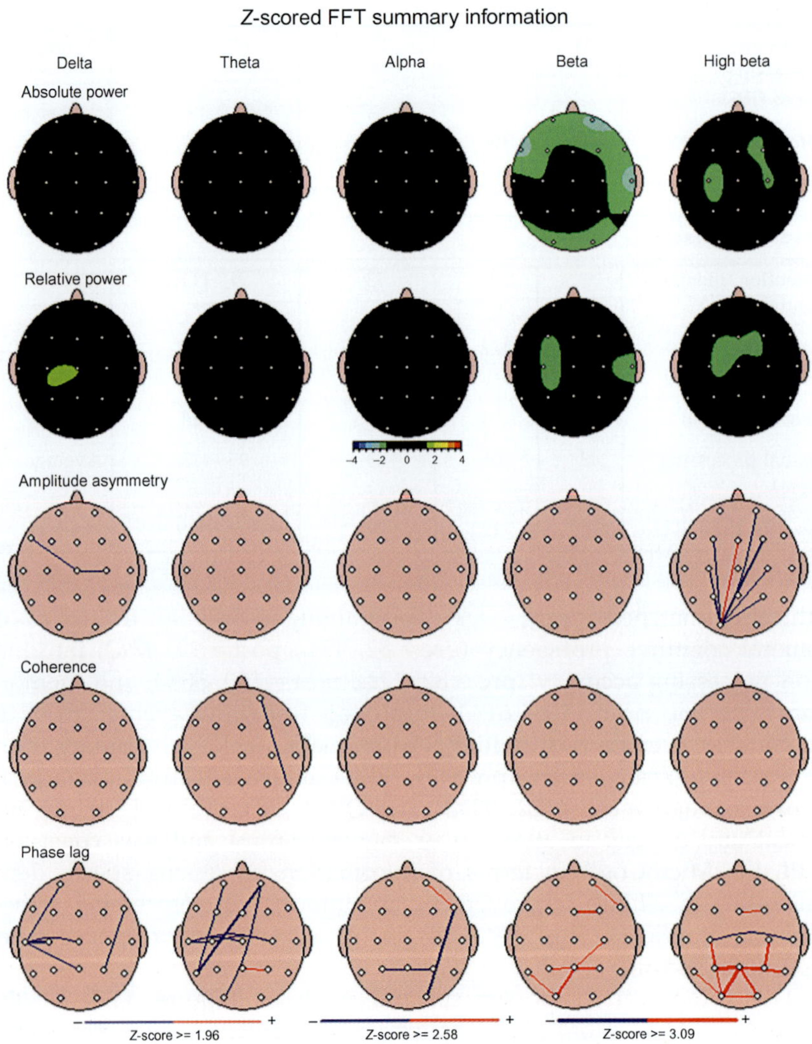

FIGURE 11.7 Posttraining eyes open Z-scored FFT summary.

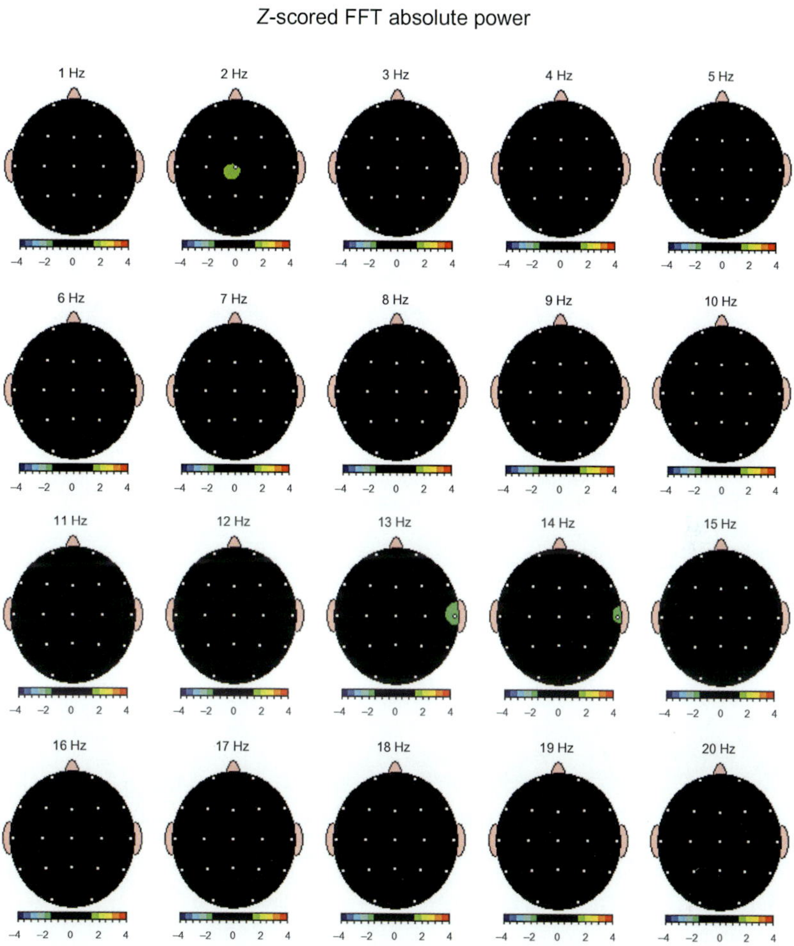

FIGURE 11.8 Posttraining eyes open Z-scored FFT absolute power.

deficient absolute power in total beta (compare to Figure 11.1) in a wide distribution and in high beta (C3 and C4-F4). EEG asymmetry in beta ($> \pm 1.98 < \pm 3.09$ SDs between O1 and bilateral parietal, central, and frontal sites) and phase (all frequencies) were abnormal, though significantly less so than in the pretraining baseline. Inspection of the single herz bins (Figures 11.8 and 11.9) revealed deficient absolute power in 2 Hz at the vertex, at 13 and 14 Hz at T4, and at 29 and 30 Hz at C4.

Analysis of the LORETA three-dimensional sources using NeuroGuide's LORETA Z-scored database was inconsistent with the surface, linked ears, EEG maps (which showed no significant decreases in absolute power in 1–12 Hz activity). The LORETA analysis revealed

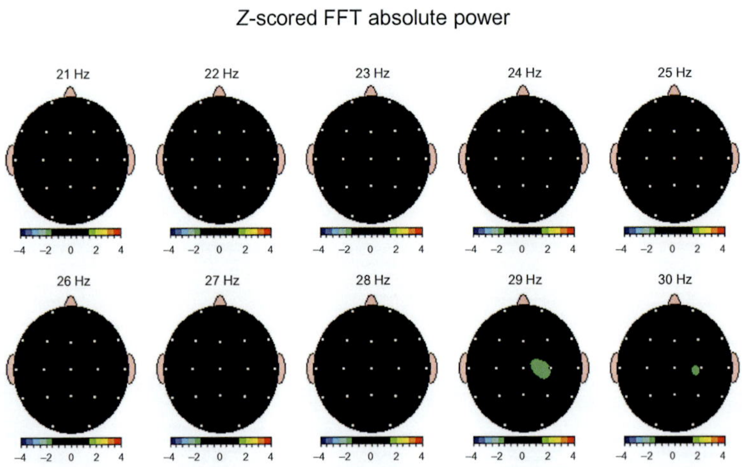

FIGURE 11.9 Posttraining eyes open Z-scored FFT absolute power.

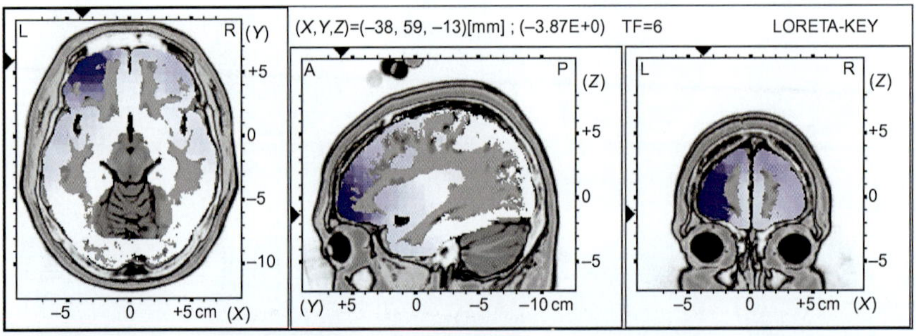

FIGURE 11.10 Posttraining LORETA current source analysis at 5 Hz.

deficient current sources in the left middle and medial frontal gyri with a maximum at 4, 5, 6, and 11 Hz (left Brodmann areas 10 and 11). The deficient current sources were maximal at 5 Hz (−3.87 SDs; $X = -38$, $Y = 59$, $Z = -13$; 1st Best Match ($d = 3$ mm); Brodmann area 11, Middle Frontal Gyrus, Frontal Lobe) (Figures 11.10 and 11.11), but not widely distributed, and mostly confined to left Brodmann areas 10 and 11.

Comparing the pretraining (Figures 11.4 and 11.5) to posttraining (Figures 11.12 and 11.13) LORETA current source and three-dimensional analyses, one can see a significant change (movement toward $Z = 0$) in the low frequency current sources in terms of distribution of deficient current sources, and an overall increase of +3.03 SD in Z-scored current density in 6 Hz (pretraining −4.57 SD, posttraining −1.54 SD). More modest improvements were seen in the maximum current density at 4 Hz

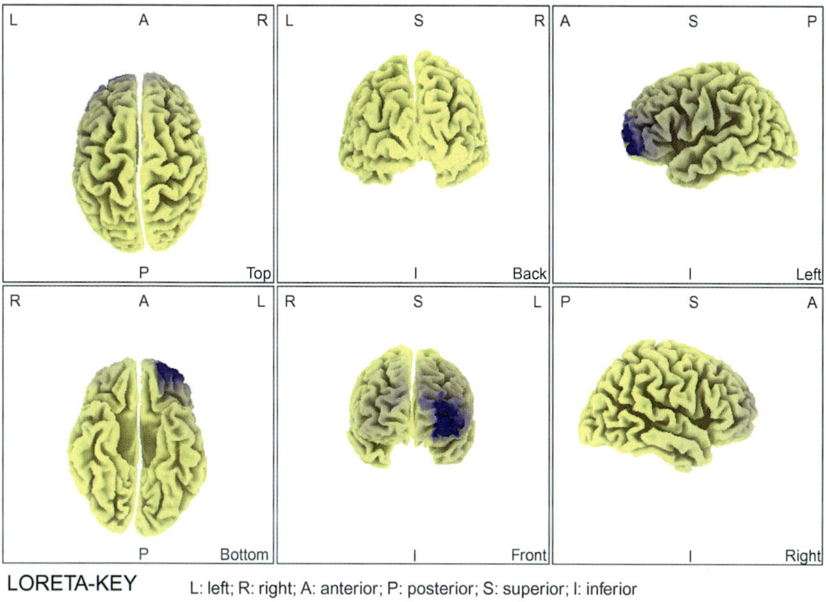

FIGURE 11.11 Posttraining LORETA current source analysis at 5 Hz orthogonal view.

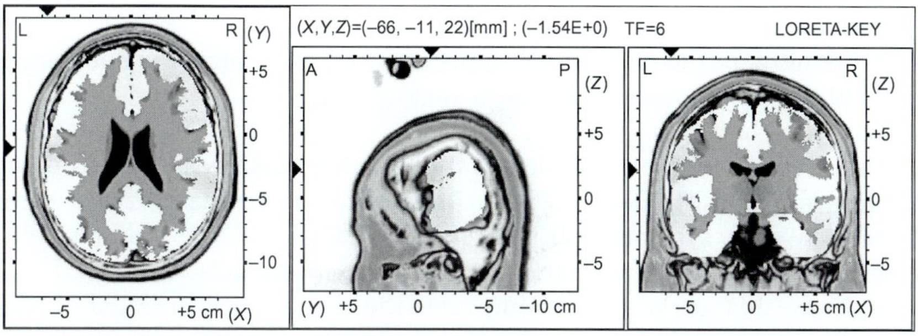

FIGURE11.12 Posttraining LORETA current source analysis at 6 Hz.

(pretraining −4.15 SD, posttraining −3.46 SD), 5 Hz (pretraining −4.47 SD, posttraining −3.87 SD), and 11 Hz (pretraining −4.02 SD, posttraining −3.38 SD). However, even at those frequencies where the increase in slow wave current sources was modest, there was a significant decrease in the amount of affected cortical "real estate." If the assumption that slow wave activity reflects the underlying health of the brain's cognitive, memory, emotion, and regulatory processes (Cannon, 2012, p. 13) is correct, then improvements in slow wave activity should reflect improvements in those processes as this case study indicates.

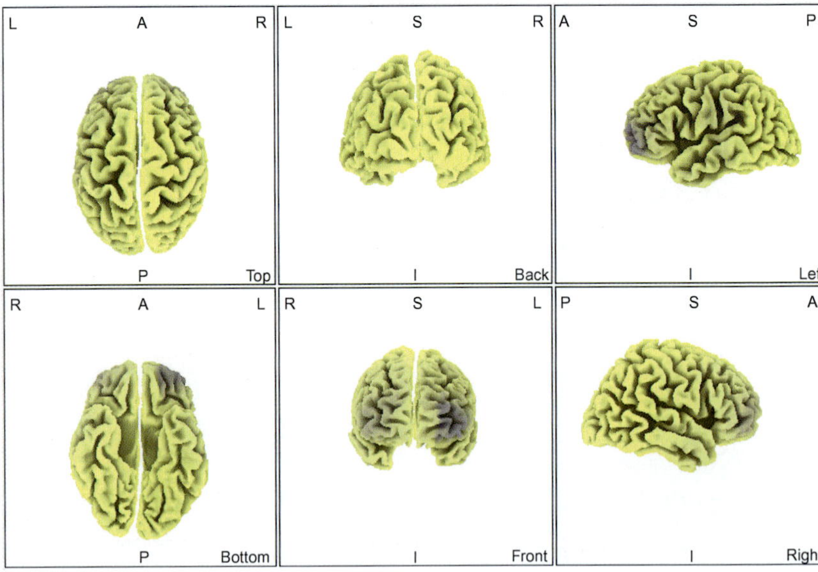

LORETA-KEY L: left; R: right; A: anterior; P: posterior; S: superior; I: inferior

FIGURE 11.13 Posttraining LORETA current source analysis at 6 Hz orthogonal view.

CONCLUSION

Working with the chronic substance abusing population is challenging, particularly given historically high incidences of relapse and comorbid mental health issues. Further, allopathic models and those based in 12-step recovery frameworks do not work for the majority of those seeking treatment (Dodes & Dodes, 2014). Addressing dysregulated brain functional networks, systems, and hubs through LORETA NFB training holds great promise for those who the current treatment models have failed.

Jack met his goals for training over the course of 27 LORETA NFB sessions with minimal intrusion into his life. Significantly, Jack has maintained his gains in LORETA NFB training for over a year with no return to problem drinking and no return of debilitating depression. He continues to report success in employing cognitive restructuring strategies to combat automatic negative thoughts. Importantly, Jack's improvements in executive functions as measured by the MicroCog™, QIK™ CPT, and his own self-report suggest that alcohol-related deficits in memory, information processing speed and accuracy, attention, and mental control are reversible. Our work with Jack suggests that LORETA NFB is a viable adjunct to existing evidence-based treatments, and may have usefulness as a stand-alone treatment though clearly more research is needed.

References

Alcaro, A., Huber, R., & Panksepp, J. (2007). Behavioral functions of the mesolimbic dopaminergic system: An affective neuroethological perspective. *Brain Research Reviews, 56* (2), 283–321.

Aldhous, P. (2010). Prescription: Sobriety. *New Scientist, 205*(2072), 40–43.

Amen, D. G. (1998). *Change your brain, change your life: The breakthrough program for conquering anxiety, depression, oppressiveness, anger, and impulsiveness.* New York, NY: Three Rivers Press.

Amen, D. G. (2004a). *Clinician's brain science toolbox.* Fairfield, CA: MindWorks Press.

Amen, D. G. (2004b). ANT therapy: How to develop your own internal anteater to eradicate automatic negative thoughts (ANTs). In D. G. Amen (Ed.), *Clinician's brain science toolbox.* Fairfield, CA: MindWorks Press.

Antelmi, I., de Paula, R. S., Shinzato, A. R., Peres, C. A., Mansur, A. J., & Grupi, C. J. (2004). Influence of age, gender, body mass index, and functional capacity on heart rate variability in a cohort of subjects without heart disease. *American Journal of Cardiology, 93,* 381–385.

Babor, T. F., La Fuente, J. R., Saunders, J., & Grant, M. (1992). AUDIT, the Alcohol Use Disorders Identification Test: Guidelines for use in primary health care, *Vol. 4.* Geneva: Substance Abuse Department, World Health Organization, WHO/PSA, pp. 1–29.

Bauer, L. O. (1994). Electroencephalographic and autonomic predictors of relapse in alcohol-dependent patients. *Alcoholism, Clinical & Experimental Research, 18*(3), 755–760.

Bauer, L. O. (2001). Predicting relapse to alcohol and drug abuse via quantitative electroencephalography. *Neuropsychopharmacology, 25*(3), 332–340.

Begleiter, H., & Platz, A. (1972). The effects of alcohol on the central nervous system in humans. In B. Kissin, & H. Begleiter (Eds.), The biology of alcoholism. *Vol. 2,* Physiology and behavior. New York, NY: Plenum.

Berridge, K. C., & Robinson, T. E. (1995). The mind of an addicted brain: Neural sensitization of wanting versus liking. *Current Directions in Psychological Science, 4*(3), 71–76.

Brodie, M. S., Pesold, C., & Appel, S. B. (1999). Ethanol directly excites dopaminergic ventral tegmental area reward neurons. *Alcoholism: Clinical and Experimental Research, 23* (11), 1848–1852.

Brody, A. L., Mandelkern, M. A., London, E. D., Childress, A. R., Less, G. S., Bota, R. G., et al. (2002). Brain metabolic changes during cigarette craving. *Archives of General Psychiatry, 59,* 1162–1172.

Brown, T. A., Chorpita, B. F., Korotitsch, W., & Barlow, D. H. (1997). Psychometric properties of the Depression Anxiety Stress Scales (DASS) in clinical samples. *Behaviour Research and Therapy, 35*(1), 79–89.

Buckner, R. L., & Carroll, D. C. (2007). Self-projection and the brain. *Trends in Cognitive Science, 11*(2), 49–57.

Cannon, R. L. (2012). *Low resolution brain electromagnetic tomography (LORETA): Basic concepts and clinical applications.* Corpus Christi, TX: BMED Press.

Center for Substance Abuse Treatment (CSAT) (2005). *Substance abuse treatment for persons with co-occurring disorders.* Rockville, MD: Department of Health and Human Services Publication No. (SMA) 08-3992, Substance Abuse and Mental Health Services Administration, Treatment Improvement Protocol (TIP) Series 42.

Chachamovich, E., Ding, Y., & Turecki, G. (2012). Levels of aggressiveness are higher among alcohol-related suicides: Results from a psychological autopsy study. *Alcohol, 46* (6), 529–536.

Conner, K. R., Hesselrock, M. V. M., Schuckit, M. A., Hirsch, J. K., Knox, H. L., Meldrum, S., et al. (2006). Precontemplated and impulsive suicide attempts among individuals with alcohol dependence. *Journal of Studies on Alcohol, 67,* 95–101.

Costa, L., & Bauer, L. (1997). Quantitative electroencephalographic differences associated with alcohol, cocaine, heroin, and dual-substance dependence. *Drug & Alcohol Dependence, 46* (1–2), 87–93.

Coutin-Churchman, P., & Moreno, R. (2004). Intracranial distribution of diffusely decreased slow EEG activity differs in depressed and non-depressed alcoholic patients. *Clinical EEG and Neuroscience, 35*(4), 229–230.

Coutin-Churchman, P., Moreno, R., Anez, Y., & Vergara, F. (2006). Clinical correlates of quantitative EEG alterations in alcoholic patients. *Clinical Neurophysiology, 117*(4), 740–751.

Cruz, M. T., Bajo, M., Schweitzer, P., & Roberto, M. (2008). Shared mechanisms of alcohol and other drugs. *Alcohol Research & Health, 31*(2), 137–147.

Day, J. J., & Carelli, R. M. (2007). The nucleus accumbens and Pavlovian reward learning. *The Neuroscientist, 13*(2), 148–158.

deBeus, R. J. (2007). Quantitative electroencephalography-guided versus Scott/Peniston neurofeedback with substance use disorder outpatients: A pilot study. *Biofeeback, 35*(4), 146–151.

Demos, J. N. (2005). *Getting started with neurofeedback*. New York, NY: W.W. Norton.

Dehghani-Arani, F., Rostami, R., & Nadali, H. (2013). Neurofeedback training for opiate addiction: Improvement of mental health and craving. *Applied Psychophysiology and Biofeedback, 38*(2), 133–141.

Dodes, L., & Dodes, Z. (2014). *The sober truth: Debunking the bad science behind 12-step programs and the rehab industry*. Boston, MA: Beacon Press.

Drake, R. E., Merrens, M. R., & Lynde, D. W. (2005). *Evidence-based mental health practice: A textbook*. New York, NY: W.W. Norton.

Ehlers, C. L., & Schuckit, M. A. (1990). EEG fast frequency activity in the sons of alcoholics. *Biological Psychiatry, 27*(6), 199–205.

Enoch, M. -A., White, K. V., Harris, C. R., Robin, R. W., Ross, J., Rohrbaugh, J. W., et al. (1999). Association of low-voltage alpha EEG with a subtype of alcohol use disorders. *Alcoholism: Clinical and Experimental Research, 23*(8), 1312–1319.

Ericson, M., Chau, P., Clarke, R. B., Adermark, L., & Söderpalm, B. (2011). Rising taurine and ethanol concentrations in nucleus accumbens interact to produce dopamine release after ethanol administration. *Addiction Biology, 16*, 377–385.

Feltenstein, M. W., & See, R. E. (2008). The neurocircuitry of addiction: An overview. *British Journal of Pharmacology, 154*, 261–274.

Fergusson, D. M., Boden, J. M., & Horwood, J. (2009). Tests of causal links between alcohol abuse or dependence and major depression. *Archives of General Psychiatry, 66*(3), 260–266.

Frierson, R. L., Melakian, M., & Wadman, P. C. (2002). Principles of suicide risk assessment: How to interview depressed patients and tailor treatment. *Postgraduate Medicine, 112*(3), 65–66, 69–71.

Flynn, P. M., & Brown, B. S. (2008). Co-occurring disorders in substance abuse treatment: Issues and prospects. *Journal of Substance Abuse Treatment, 34*(1), 36–47.

Gabrielli, W. F., Mednick, S. A., Volavka, J., Pollock, V. E., Schulsinger, F., & Itil, T. M. (1982). Electroencephalograms in children of alcoholic fathers. *Psychophysiology, 19*(4), 404–407.

Gilpin, N. W., & Koob, G. F. (2008). Neurobiology of alcohol dependence: Focus on motivational mechanisms. *Alcohol Research & Health, 31*(4), 185–195.

Glasner-Edwards, S., & Rawson, R. (2010). Evidence-based practices in addiction treatment: Review and recommendations for public policy. *Health Policy, 97*(2–3), 93–104.

Grant, B. F., Stinson, F. S., Dawson, D. A., Chou, S. P., Dufour, M. C., Compton, W., et al. (2004). Prevalence and co-occurrence of substance use disorders and independent mood and anxiety disorders: Results from the national epidemiologic survey on alcohol and related conditions. *Archives of General Psychiatry, 61*(8), 807–816.

Green, E. E., Green, A. M., & Walters, E. D. (1974). Alpha/theta biofeedback training. *Journal of Biofeedback, 2*, 7–13.

Günther, W., Müller, N., Knesewitsch, P., Haag, C., Trapp, W., Banquet, J., et al. (1997). Functional EEG mapping and SPECT in detoxified male alcoholics. *European Archives of Psychiatry and Clinical Neuroscience, 247*(3), 128–136.

Gusnard, D. A., Akbudak, E., Shulman, G. L., & Raichle, M. E. (2001). Medial prefrontal cortex and self-referential mental activity: Relation to a default mode of brain function. *Proceedings of the National Academy of Sciences, 98*(7), 4259–4264.

Hammer, R. P. (2002). Neural circuitry and signaling in addiction. In G. B. Kaplan, & R. P. Hammer (Eds.), *Brain circuitry and signaling in psychiatry: Basic science and clinical implications*. Washington, DC: American Psychiatric.

Hasen, D. S., & Grant, B. F. (2002). Major depression in 6050 former drinkers. *Archives of General Psychiatry, 59*, 794–800.

Hikosaka, O., Bromberg-Martin, E., Hong, S., & Matsumoto, M. (2008). New insights on the subcortical representation of reward. *Current Opinion in Neurobiology, 18*(2), 203–208.

Hogarth, L., Balleine, B. W., Corbit, L. H., & Killcross, S. (2013). Associative learning mechanisms underpinning the transition from recreational drug use to addiction. *Annals of the New York Academy of Sciences, 1282*, 12–24.

Huebner, R. B., & Kantor, L. W. (2011). Advances in alcoholism treatment. *Alcohol Research & Health, 33*(4), 295–299.

Ikemoto, S. (2007). Dopamine reward circuitry: Two projection systems from the ventral midbrain to the nucleus accumbens–olfactory tubercle complex. *Brain Research Reviews, 56*(1), 27–78.

Johannesson, G., Berglund, M., & Ingvar, D. H. (1982). EEG abnormalities in chronic alcoholism related to age. *Acta Psychiatrica Scandinavica, 65*(2), 148–157.

John, E. R., Prichep, L. S., Alper, K. S., Mas, F. G., Cancro, R., Easton, P., et al. (1994). Quantitative electrophysiological characteristics and subtyping of schizophrenia. *Biological Psychiatry, 36*(12), 810–826.

John, E. R., Prichep, L. S., Fridman, J., & Easton, P. (1988). Neurometrics: Computer-assisted differential diagnosis of brain dysfunctions. *Science, 293*(4836), 162–169.

Jones, A. W. (1996). Biochemistry and physiology of alcohol: Application to forensic sciences and toxicology. In J. C. Garriott (Ed.), *Medicolegal aspects of alcohol* (3rd ed.). Tuscon, AZ: Lawyers & Judges Publishing.

Kahn, M. E., Weiner, R. D., Brenner, R. P., & Coppola, R. (1988). Topographic maps of brain electrical activity- pitfalls and precautions. *Biological Psychiatry, 23*(6), 628–636.

Kauer, J. A., & Malenka, R. C. (2007). Synaptic plasticity and addiction. *Nature Reviews Neuroscience, 8*(11), 844–858.

Kelly, M. J. (1997). Native Americans, neurofeedback, and substance abuse theory: Three year outcome of alpha/theta neurofeedback training in the treatment of problem drinking among Dine' (Navajo) People. *Journal of Neurotherapy, 2*(3), 24–60.

Khalily, M. T., Clarke, L., & Jahangir, F. (2009). Alpha–theta neurofeedback therapy: A non-invasive treatment for addiction and post-traumatic stress disorder. *FWU Journal of Social Sciences, 3*(2), 83–91.

Kiloh, L. G., McComas, A. J., Osselton, J. W., & Upton, A. R. M. (1981). *Clinical encephalography*. Boston, MA: Butterworths.

Knapp, C. M., Ciraulo, D. A., & Kranzler, H. R. (2008). Neurobiology of alcohol. In M. Galanter, & H. D. Kleber (Eds.), *The American Psychiatric Publishing textbook of substance abuse treatment*. Washington, DC: American Psychiatric Publishing.

Knyazev, G. G. (2012). EEG delta oscillations as a correlate of basic homeostatic and motivational processes. *Neuroscience and Biobehavioral Reviews, 36*(1), 677–695.

Koob, G. F. (2008). A role for brain stress systems in addiction. *Neuron, 59*(1), 11–34.

Koob, G. F., Boutrel, B., & Valdez, G. (2013). Addiction is a reward deficit and stress surfeit disorder. *Frontiers in Psychiatry* 34–41.

Koob, G. F., Lloyd, G. K., & Mason, B. J. (2009). Development of pharmacotherapies for drug addiction: A Rosetta Stone approach. *Nature Reviews. Drug Discovery, 8*(6), 500–515.

Koob, G. F., & Valkow, N. D. (2010). Neurocircuitry of addiction. *Neuropsychopharmacology, 35*, 217–238.

Kranzler, H. R., & Ciraulo, D. A. (2005). Alcohol. In H. R. Kranzler, & D. A. Ciraulo (Eds.), *Clinical manual of addiction psychopharmacology*. Washington, DC: American Psychiatric Publishing.

Kropotov, J. D. (2009). *Quantitative EEG, event-related potentials and neurotherapy*. San Diego, CA: Elsevier/Academic.

Lammel, S., Hetzel, A., Haeckel, O., Jones, I., Liss, B., & Roeper, J. (2008). Unique properties of mesoprefrontal neurons within a dual mesocorticolimbic dopamine system. *Neuron, 57*(5), 760–773.

Linden, D. J. (2011). *The compass of pleasure: How our brains make fatty foods, orgasm, exercise, marijuana, generosity, vodka, learning and gambling feel so good*. New York, NY: Penguin.

Little, S. C., & McAvoy, M. (1952). Electroencephalographic studies in alcoholism. *Quarterly Journal of Studies on Alcohol, 13*(1), 9–15.

Lovinger, D. M. (2008). Communication networks in the brain. *Alcohol Research & Health, 31*(4), 196–214.

Michel, C. M., Henggeler, B., & Brandeis, D. (1993). Localization of sources of brain alpha/theta/delta activity and the influence of the mode of spontaneous mutation. *Physiological Measures, 14*(4a), 21–26.

Michel, C. M., Lehmann, D., & Henggeler, B. (1992). Localization of the sources EEG delta, theta, alpha and beta frequency bands using the FFT dipole approximation. *Electroencephalography and Clinical Neurophysiology, 82*(1), 38–44.

Myers, J. E., & Young, J. S. (2012). Brain wave biofeedback: Benefits of integrating neurofeedback in counseling. *Journal of Counseling and Development, 90*(1), 20–28.

Niedermeyer, E., & Lopes da Silva, F. (1982). *Electroencephalography: Basic principles, clinical applications and related fields*. Baltimore, MD: Urban and Schwarzenberg.

Parkitny, L., & McAuley, J. (2010). The Depression Anxiety Stress Scale (DASS). *Journal of Physiotherapy, 56*(3), 204.

Pascual-Marqui, R. D. (1999). Review of methods for solving the EEG inverse problem. *International Journal of Bioelectromagnetism, 1*(1), 75–86.

Pascual-Marqui, R. D. (2002). Standardized low resolution brain electromagnetic tomography (sLORETA): Technical details. *Methods and Findings in Experimental Clinical Pharmacology, 24*(Suppl. D), 5–12.

Pascual-Marqui, R. D., & Biscay-Lirio, R. (1993). Spatial resolution of neuronal generators based on EEG and MEG measurements. *International Journal of Neuroscience, 68*(1–2), 93–105.

Pascual-Marqui, R. D., & Lehmann, D. (1993). Comparison of topographic maps and the reference electrode: Comments on two papers by Desmedt and collaborators. *Electroencephalography and Clinical Neurophysiology, 88*(530/531), 534–536.

Pasqual-Marqui, R. D., Michel, C. M., & Lehmann, D. (1994). Low resolution electromagnetic tomography: A new method to localize electrical activity in the brain. *International Journal of Psychophysiology, 18*(1), 49–65.

Peniston, E. G., & Kulkosky, P. J. (1989). Alpha–theta brainwave training and beta endorphin levels in alcoholics. *Alcoholism Clinical and Experimental Research, 13*, 271–279.

Peniston, E. G., & Kulkosky, P. J. (1990). Alcoholic personality and alpha–theta brainwave training. *Medical Psychotherapy, 2*, 37–55.

Peper, E., & Shaffer, F. (2010). Biofeedback history: An alternative view. *Biofeedback (Online)*, *38*(4), 142–147.

Petrakis, I. L., Gonzalez, G., Rosenheck, R., & Krystal, J. H. (2002). Comorbidity of alcoholism and psychiatric disorders: An overview. *Alcohol Research & Health*, *26*(2), 81–89.

Pollock, V. E., Schneider, L. S., Zemansky, M. F., Gleason, R. P., & Pawluczyk (1992). Topographic quantitative EEG amplitude in recovered alcoholics. *Psychiatry Research: Neuroimaging*, *45*(1), 25–32.

Propping, P. (1983). Pharmacogenetics of alcohol's CNS effects: Implications for the etiology of alcoholism. *Biochemistry and Behavior*, *18*(Suppl. 1), 549–553.

Raichle, M. E., & Snyder, A. Z. (2007). A default mode of brain function: A brief history of an evolving idea. *NeuroImage*, *37*(4), 1083–1090.

Rangaswamy, M., Porjesz, B., Chorlian, D. B., Choi, K., Jones, K. A., Wang, K., et al. (2003). Theta power in the EEG of alcoholics. *Alcoholism: Clinical & Experimental Research*, *27*(4), 607–615.

Reinert, D. F., & Allen, J. P. (2007). The alcohol use disorders identification test: An update of research findings. *Alcoholism: Clinical and Experimental Research*, *31*(2), 185–189.

Robins, J. (2008). A symphony in the brain *(rev. ed.)*. New York, NY: Grove.

Robinson, T. E., & Berridge, K. C. (2003). Addiction. *Annual Review of Psychology*, *54*, 25–53.

Saletu, B., Anderer, P., & Saletu-Zyhlarz, G. (2006). EEG topography and tomography (LORETA) in the classification and evaluation of the pharmacodynamics of psychotropic drugs. *Clinical EEG and Neuroscience*, *37*(2), 66–80.

Saletu-Zyhlarz, G. M., Arnold, O., Anderer, P., Oberndorfer, S., Walter, H., Lesch, O. M., et al. (2004). Differences in brain function between relapsing and abstaining alcohol-dependent patients, evaluated by EEG mapping. *Alcohol & Alcoholism*, *39*(3), 233–240.

Schuckit, M. A. (2005). Alcohol-related disorders. In H. I. Kaplan, & B. J. Sadock (Eds.), *Comprehensive textbook of psychiatry* (8th ed.). Baltimore, MD: Williams & Wilkins.

Schuckit, M. A. (2006). Alcohol and alcoholism. In S. L. Hauser (Ed.), *Harrison's neurology in clinical medicine* (5th ed.). New York, NY: McGraw Hill.

Schuckit, M. A. (2008). Alcohol and alcoholism. In A. S. Fauci, E. Braunwald, D. L. Kaspar, S. L. Hauser, D. L. Longo, J. L. Jameson, et al. *Harrison's principles of internal medicine* (17th ed.). New York, NY: McGraw Hill.

Schultz, W., Dayan, P., & Montague, P. R. (1997). A neural substrate of prediction and reward. *Science*, *275*(5306), 1593–1599.

Scott, W. C., & Kaiser, D. (1998). Augmenting chemical dependency treatment with neurofeedback training. *Journal of Neurotherapy*, *3*(1), 66.

Scott, W. C., Kaiser, D., Othmer, S., & Sideroff, S. I. (2005). Effects of an EEG biofeedback protocol on a mixed substance abusing population. *American Journal of Drug & Alcohol Abuse*, *31*, 455–469.

Selzer, M. L. (1971). The Michigan Alcoholism Screening Test (MAST): The quest for a new diagnostic instrument. *American Journal of Psychiatry*, *127*(12), 1653–1658.

Smith, B. H., Molina, B. S. G., & Pelham, W. E. (2002). The clinically meaningful link between alcohol use and attention deficit hyperactivity disorder. *Alcohol Research & Health*, *26*(2), 122–129.

Sokhadze, E. M., Trudeau, D. L., & Cannon, R. L. (2014). Treating addiction disorders. In D. S. Cantor, & J. R. Evans (Eds.), *Clinical neurotherapy: Application for techniques for treatment*. Waltham, MA: Elsevier/Academic.

Spehr, W., & Stemmler, G. (1985). Postalcoholic diseases: Diagnostic relevance of computerized EEG. *Electroencephalography and Clinical Neurophysiology*, *60*, 106–114.

Substance Abuse and Mental Health Services Administration (SAMHSA) (2013). *National survey on drug use and health (NSDUH)*.

Sutherland, M. T., McHugh, M. J., Pariyadath, V., & Stein, E. A. (2012). Resting state functional connectivity in addiction: Lessons learned and a road ahead. *NeuroImage, 62*, 2281–2295.

Thatcher, R. W. (2012). *Handbook of quantitative encephalography and biofeedback: Scientific foundations and practical applications*. St. Petersburg, FL: Anipublishing.

Thatcher, R. W. (2014). *NeuroGuide Deluxe (Version 2.8) [Software]*. St. Petersburg, FL: Applied Neuroscience, Inc., Available from <www.appliedneuroscience.com>.

Thatcher, R. W., Biver, C. J., & North, D. M. (2002). *Z Tunes: Technical and conceptual foundations*. Unpublished manuscript, NeuroImaging Laboratory, Applied Neuroscience, Inc., Seminole, FL.

Thatcher, R. W., North, D. M., & Biver, C. J. (2005). Evaluation and validity of a LORETA normative EEG database. *Clinical EEG and Neuroscience, 36*(2), 116–122.

Thatcher, R. W., North, D. M., & Biver, C. J. (2012). Diffusion spectral imaging modules correlate with EEG LORETA neuroimaging modules. *Human Brain Mapping, 33*(5), 1062–1075.

Trudeau, D. L. (2005). EEG biofeedback for addictive disorders—The state of the art in 2004. *Journal of Adult Development*, 12(2/3), 139–146.

Trudeau, D. L., Sokhadze, T. M., & Cannon, R. L. (2009). Neurofeedback in alcohol and drug dependency. In T. H. Budzynski, H. K. Budzynski, J. R. Evans, & A. Abarbanel (Eds.), *Introduction to quantitative EEG and neurofeedback: Advance theory and applications* (2nd ed.). Burlington, MA: Elsevier/Academic.

Uddin, L. Q., Clare-Kelly, A. M., Biswal, B. B., Castellanos, F. X., & Milham, M. P. (2009). Functional connectivity of default mode network components: Correlation, anticorrelation, and causality. *Human Brain Mapping, 30*(2), 625–637.

van Sweden, B. (1983). The EEG in alcohol addicts presenting with seizures. *Clinical Neurology and Neurosurgery, 85*(1), 3–11.

Volkow, N. D., & Baler, R. D. (2007). The neural substrates of addiction. *Psychiatric Times, 24*(13), 66.

Wicker, B., Ruby, P., Royet, J. P., & Fonlupt, P. (2003). A relation between rest and the self in the brain? *Brain Research Reviews, 43*(2), 224–230.

Winterer, G., Enoch, M. -A., White, K. V., Saylan, M., Coppola, R., & Goldman, D. (2003). EEG phenotype in alcoholism: Increased coherence in the depressive subtype. *Acta Psychiatrica Scandinavica, 108*(1), 51–60.

Winterer, G., Kloeppel, B., Heinz, A., Ziller, M., Dufeu, P., Schmidt, L. G., et al. (1998). Quantitative EEG (QEEG) predicts relapse in patients with chronic alcoholism and points to a frontally pronounced cerebral disturbance. *Psychiatry Research, 78*(1–2), 101–113.

Yin, H. H., Ostlund, S. B., & Balleine, B. W. (2008). Reward-guided learning beyond dopamine in the nucleus accumbens: The integrative functions of cortico-basal ganglia networks. *European Journal of Neuroscience, 28*, 1437–1448.

Yorgason, J. T., Ferris, M. J., Steffensen, S. C., & Jones, S. R. (2014). Frequency-dependent effects of ethanol on dopamine release in the nucleus accumbens. *Alcoholism: Clinical & Experimental Research, 38*(2), 348–447.

Zohar, A. H., Cloninger, C., & McCraty, R. (2013). Personality and heart rate variability: Exploring pathways from personality to cardiac coherence and health. *Open Journal of Social Sciences, 1*(6), 32–39.

CHAPTER

12

LORETA and SPECT Scans

A Correlational Case Series

Paul Wand[a] *and Gerald Gluck*[b]

[a]Private Practice, Coral Springs, FL, USA [b]Center for Family Counseling and Biofeedback, Coral Springs, FL, USA

INTRODUCTION TO THE CLINICAL USE OF SPECT SCANS

A SPECT scan is a nuclear medicine test which shows the circulation in addition to the anatomy. The acronym stands for single photon emission computed tomography. More specifically, it shows the microcirculation which is of vital interest when looking at disease or trauma to the brain. As any other nuclear medicine test (with the noted exception of certain gastrointestinal (GI) tests), the scan is performed by an intravenous injection of a radioisotope. Currently, there are only two isotopes which are typically used for the brain, which include Ceretec and Neurolite, and come from Technetium 99. In this author's (PW) experience, Ceretec is the superior isotope because it produces consistently superior quality images and less false positive results. It may also be less expensive than Neurolite. The half-life is very limited, approximately 6 h, and therefore coordination of patient scheduling is of vital importance in order not to miss the small window of time within which the scan has to be accomplished. In the case of a brain imaging, almost immediately after the injection, a dynamic flow studies are performed to assess the carotid artery flow. Thus if the patient has a major obstruction and a carotid artery outside of the brain, it may have an impact on the intracranial circulation, see Figure 12.1 which shows the frame by frame uptake of isotope as it passes from the carotid (extra cerebral) to the intracranial circulation.

After an equilibration period, which is a brief (seconds) waiting period after the injection and before the recording, a camera is placed

Z Score Neurofeedback.
DOI: http://dx.doi.org/10.1016/B978-0-12-801291-8.00012-1

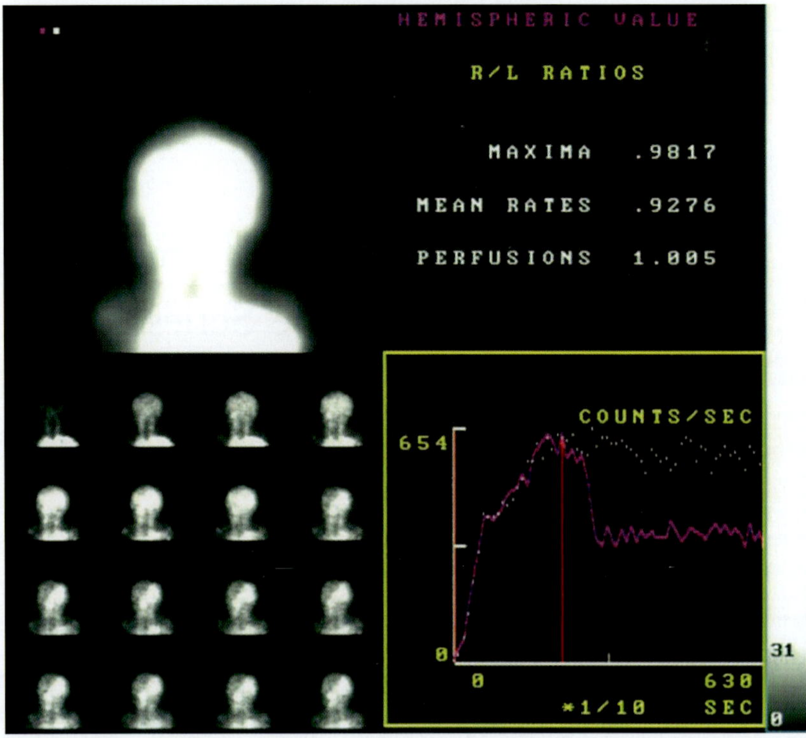

FIGURE 12.1 Dynamic flow of ceretec through the carotids.

very close to the patient's head and records the emitting radioactivity that corresponds to the intracranial blood flow. One can think of the camera as a large and sophisticated Geiger counter capturing evidence of the radioisotope as it exits the person's head. This is then recorded into a computer program. The program then creates images that correspond quantitatively to the blood flow. The images are typically shown as slices of the brain in a two-dimensional (2D) view and also a 3D view of the surface of the cortical flow. The 2D slices are the typical planes as seen in a standard MRI, i.e., coronal, sagittal, and axial, see Figures 12.2–12.4.

The scans are read by assessing the color differences on 10 step scale where a difference of two colors or 20% is considered to be abnormal between the homologous parts of the brain. Since the brain is a highly active metabolic organ, one would expect it to have a high blood flow and indeed it does, measured at approximately 15% of cardiac output, or expressed as 750 ml/min and 50 ml/100 g/min[3]).

One difference between the SPECT scan and MRI is the 3D view. The 3D view is of considerable importance since it reflects the most

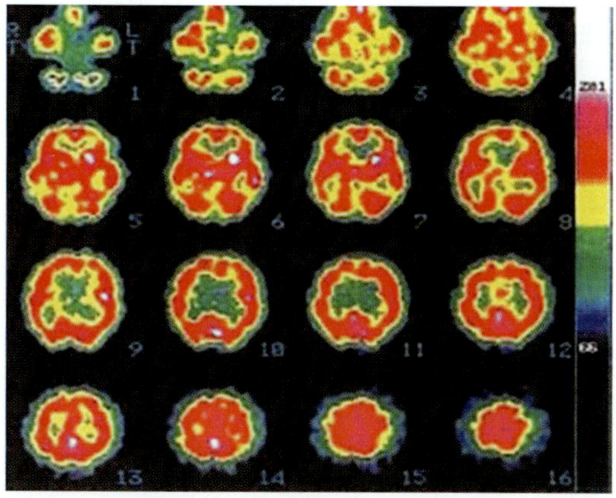

FIGURE 12.2 **2D axial slices of a normal spect scan.** Above: Normal 2D axial slices; note all colors are "hot" at the high/top portion of the color bar.

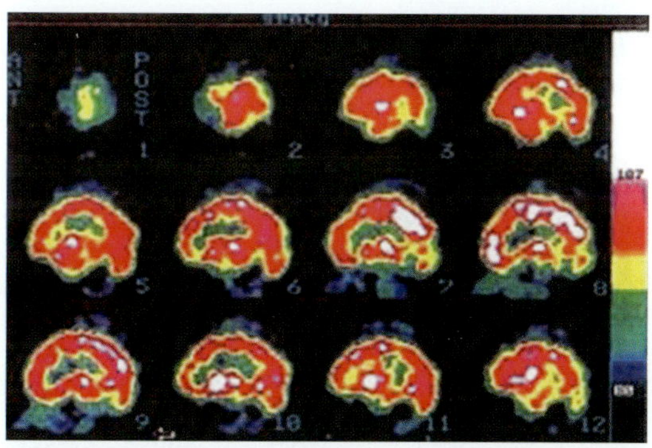

FIGURE 12.3 **2D sagittal slices of a normal spect scan.** Above: Normal 2D sagittal slices; note all colors are "hot" at the high/top portion of the color bar.

superficial blood flow in the brain, i.e., the cerebral cortex. Therefore, any disease or trauma affecting the cerebral cortex is most readily assessed by evaluating the 3D views which are sometimes not able to be detected when viewing the 2D slices. In the case of brain trauma, the 3D views uniquely have the ability to assess the anterior poles of the frontal and temporal lobes' perfusion, which are sites of predilection in the gradient of injury as will be discussed below, see Figure 12.5.

Note the white color indicating flow at the highest end of the flow scale seen in both color and black and white. The cortex appears as all white, smooth, and regular. The first view is the anterior posterior view, and each subsequent view is rotated 22.5° counterclockwise such that

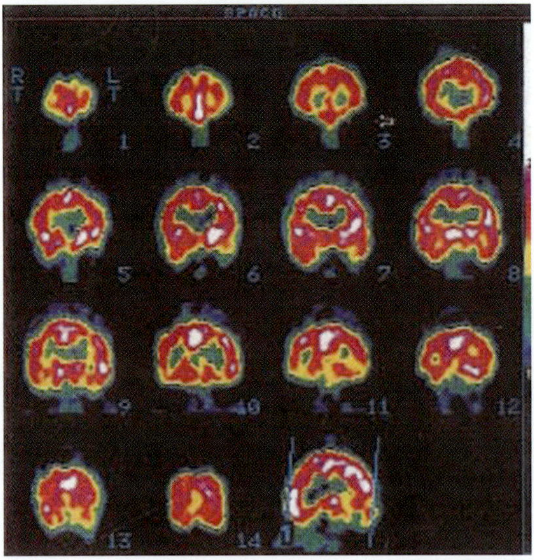

FIGURE 12.4 **2D coronal slices of a normal spect scan.** Above: Normal 2D coronal slices, note all colors are "hot" at the high/top portion of the color bar.

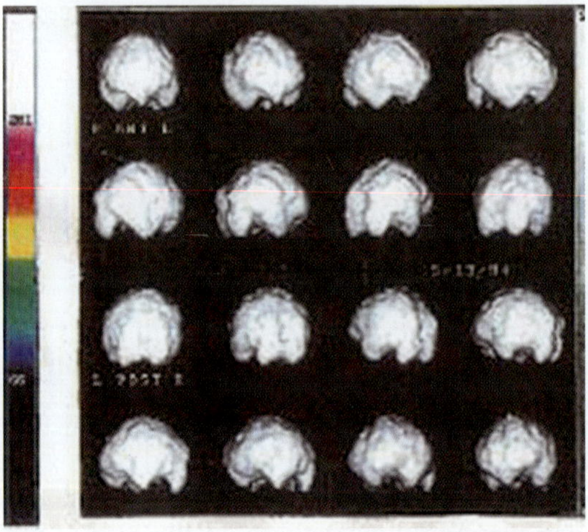

FIGURE 12.5 3D view of a normal spect scan.

all angles of the brain can be evaluated. The images can easily be shown in color, but this author (PW) prefers black and white to the 2D because subtle abnormalities are more easily appreciated as will be seen later in the abnormal examples.

History of Nuclear Imaging

Natural occurring radioactivity was discovered in 1896 by Antoine-Henri Becquerel from the element uranium (Emerson, Pette, & Wright, 2012). Emerson and his colleagues give a good history of SPECT. In 1934, an artificial form of radioactivity was first discovered by Irene Curie and Frederic Joliot with a positron emitting from phosphorous. (Emerson et al., 2012) A positron is a type of radioactive particle. Radioactive isotopes for tracers were not discovered until 1943, and medical applications followed in 1946 at Oak Ridge laboratory. In 1950, Benedict Cassen produce the first automated scanning system that was coupled to a printer, and in 1957, Hal Oscar Anger created the first Anger camera (Emerson et al., 2012) which employed sodium iodine scintillation crystals and vacuum photomultipliers. Later between 1960 and 1970, the most popular radioisotope was developed, technetium 99. In 1963, David Kuhl and Roy Edwards developed emission tomography, which developed into a single photon emission computed tomography or SPECT. Initially there were only 32 detectors, and the images were distorted and not of diagnostic quality (Emerson et al., 2012). By the late 1970s, most organs of the body could be imaged. In the 1980s, applications increased to include a cardiac scan (thallium scan) and to detect cancer cells. Today's modern thallium stress test is based upon SPECT technology applied to the heart. In the 1980s, with the introduction of monoclonal antibodies, and attached to the radioisotope, cancer cells could be detected before other anatomical changes. As each radioisotope has different characteristics, and each organ has a different anatomy and physiology, certain isotopes yield better quality imaging than others. Thus, it has been determined that different radioisotopes are preferred to image different organs, and so it is typical for one isotope to be used for one organ, etc. For example, technetium 99 is used for the brain; xenon 127 for the lungs, and chromium 51 for red blood cells (Emerson et al., 2012). Each isotope has a different half-life and radiation exposure. Modern SPECT scanners are made by the same manufactures as other imaging equipment such as GE, Siemens, Phillips, and Toshiba. First generation of scanners had single heads which limited the resolution and increased the time of scanning because one camera had to move around the entire head. Over time, dual and triple head technology was developed which increased the resolution and decreased (Catafau, 2001) the time of scanning because more parts of the brain were scanned simultaneously. Statistically, there were 17 million nuclear scans performed in 2010, with the majority of scans performed in the outpatient setting (87%), 47% inpatient studies were for cardiac application (thallium stress test), one-third of outpatient locations are physician offices, and only one-third are neurology applications (Emerson et al., 2012).

CLINICAL INDICATIONS FOR BRAIN SPECT SCANS

There are numerous indications to perform a SPECT scan. Two broad categories are distinguished, namely neurological conditions and psychiatric/psychological conditions. The main advantage of a SPECT scan over other imaging techniques such as MRI or CT scan is the functional component, i.e., the cerebral perfusion or more accurately the micro-perfusion data that is provided by the SPECT scan. Microperfusion refers to the smaller vessels or arterioles that provide blood flow to the various parts of the brain. This is of considerable importance when assessing the highly developed cerebral cortex in patients because many pathological states have normal structural imaging yet abnormal SPECT scans. Thus in the typical case of a mild traumatic brain injury, also known as mTBI, the highest resolution MRI scan such as a 3.0 T, performed with diffusion tensor imaging (DTI) is typically normal, whereas the SPECT scan can be significantly abnormal based on the authors' experience. The main disadvantage of the SPECT scan would be the lack of spatial resolution as compared to MRI or CT scan. This is the reason why a SPECT scan should be combined with a CT scan (performed simultaneously) or sequentially or have an MRI scan independently of the SPECT scan. Another disadvantage is the theoretical ionizing radiation which is emitted from the photon, which is offset by not performing frequent SPECT scans on the same patient. A disadvantage that observed in practice is the lack of availability of the radioisotope, which is not commonly manufactured, and from time to time there is an actual shortage, which can create a waiting period to get the scan done. Another disadvantage is the possibility of an allergic reaction to the radioisotope, but this would also be true of all contrast media for CT/MRI scans. In 30 years of performing SPECT scans, this author (PW) has not seen even one allergic reaction.

REVIEW OF THE LITERATURE

In the field of neurology, there are many indications for the application of SPECT scanning. This modality of imaging is of particular interest because the information obtained has functional significance, i.e., blood flow which is typically linked to metabolism. Thus for example in the workup of dementias, when the patient is symptomatic and the structural imaging tests such as MRI/CT are completely normal or may show atrophy, the SPECT scan can show specific areas of hypoperfusion indicating a reduced metabolic capability. In the differential diagnosis of dementia, the SPECT scan can easily demonstrate frontal lobe dementia from Alzheimer type, which typically affects the posterior regions

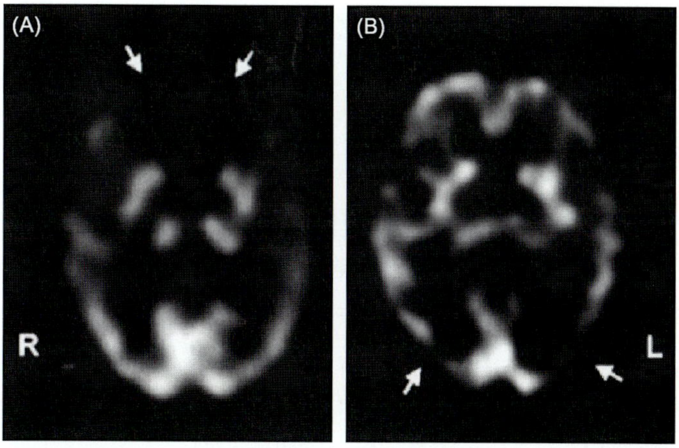

FIGURE 12.6 **SPECT of brain in dementia and Alzheimer's.** "Brain perfusion SPECT patterns in dementia, using ^{99m}Tc-ECD. (A) Frontal lobe dementia: markedly decreased uptake in frontal lobes (arrows). (B) Dementia of Alzheimer's type: hypoperfusion in posterior temporal regions, predominantly in left hemisphere (arrows). Indirect signs of cortico-subcortical atrophy, such as marked separation between hemispheres and between basal ganglia, can be clearly appreciated in both SPECT 2D slices" (Catafau, 2001, p. 260).

such as the temporal parietal lobes, at least early in the course of that disease, see Figure 12.6.

It should be pointed out as well that while the findings on SPECT scans are sensitive to the functional component, they may not be specific for one condition. For example, the frontal lobe hypoperfusion seen in Figure 12.6 may be characteristic for frontal lobe dementia, but it is also characteristic and common in traumatic brain injury. Therefore, the history and other clinical information regarding the patient's diagnosis are crucial to correlate to the SPECT scan findings.

In the case of an ischemic stroke, a common cause for admission to the hospital, structural imaging is always performed to differentiate between ischemic and hemorrhagic-type stroke. In the garden variety stroke, which is of the ischemic type, typically structural imaging is negative, or depending upon when the scan is performed may show cerebral edema. A SPECT scan is advantageous because it will show very early on a defect or area of hypoperfusion which will correspond to the vascular territory of the obstructed artery. It may also show alterations in vascularity, e.g., a paradoxical increase of perfusion known as luxury perfusion syndrome typically seen several days to 1 week after the acute onset, see Figure 12.7.

Other applications include the assessment and evaluation of surgical candidates for epilepsy surgery. In the case of unmanageable or intractable seizures after all conservative treatment has failed, certain patients are selected for resection procedures typically of the temporal

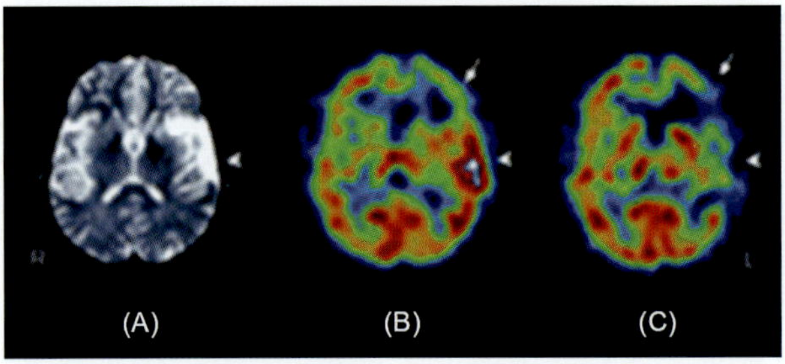

FIGURE 12.7 **Left temporal lobe infarct with luxury perfusion.** "Left temporal lobe infarction in 62-year-old patient. (A) MRI (T2-weighted) at admission shows hyperintensity at site of infarction (arrowhead). (B) ^{99m}Tc-HMPAO SPECT image obtained 1 week after stroke shows increased tracer uptake (hyperperfusion) in left temporal lobe caused by luxury perfusion (arrowhead). Hypoperfusion is also seen in left frontal cortex (*arrow*), interpreted as ischemia in anatomically preserved region. (C) ^{99m}Tc-HMPAO SPECT image obtained 1 month after stroke shows left temporal lobe hypoperfusion (arrowhead) corresponding to initial MRI image of ischemia. Perfusion changes in left frontal lobe are also seen: improvement in anterior and medial aspects caused by recovery of ischemia, as well as perfusion impairment in lateral aspect caused by extension of the infarction (*arrow*)" (Catafau, 2001, p. 262).

lobe. Part of the workup is to assess the ictal versus the inter-ictal site of focal pathology. Typically the ictal pattern is identified as a focal area of hyperperfusion, even any absence of structural pathology with MRI (Van Paesschen, 2004) is resected. In contradistinction, the inter-ictal patterns demonstrate hypoperfusion and are typically areas that are not resected. More sophisticated subtraction methods are available, and overlay with structural-based imaging increases the accuracy of localization and are associated with a better surgical outcome (Goffin, Dedeurwaerdere, & Van Laere, et al., 2008).

SPECT scanning is useful in the case of subarachnoid hemorrhage. This is a type of bleeding in the brain, in the subarachnoid space which is between the linings of the brain, or more accurately the space between the Dura Mata which contains the cerebral spinal fluid and the brain itself. The typical cause of this type of bleeding is related to a cerebral aneurysm that bursts which allows blood to escape into the subarachnoid space, which is in very close proximity to the surface of the cerebral cortex. Blood in this particular area is very irritating to the cortex, and blood vessels, and is known to cause both seizures secondary to irritation of the cortex, as well as vasospasm or narrowing of the arteries/arterioles. In one study, the SPECT scan was used to demonstrate frontal lobe hypoperfusion, which was correlated to loss of executive function in a group of 22 patients (Uchikawa, Inaba, & Kagami, 2014). In another study of 55 patients with subarachnoid bleeding associated with a ruptured

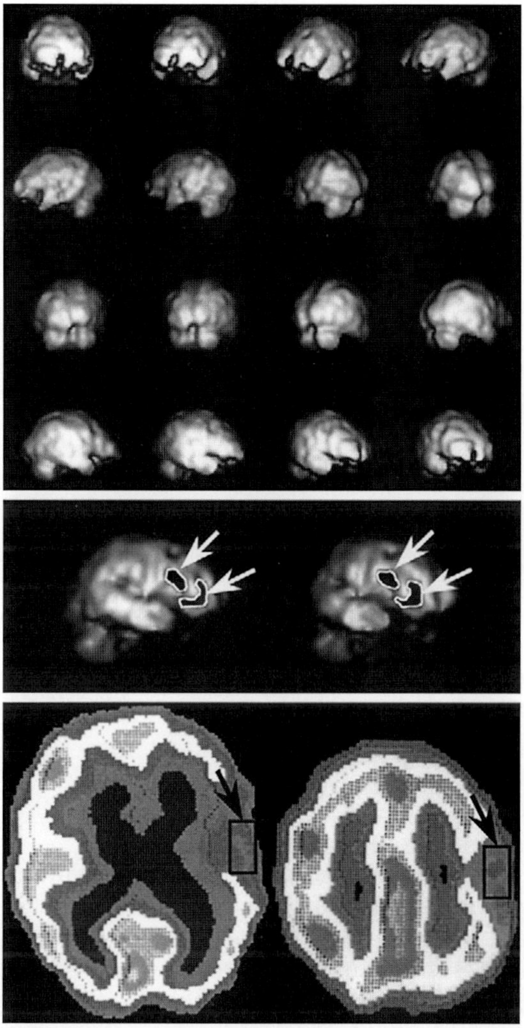

FIGURE 12.8 **3D reconstructed transaxial spect data.** Methods of rCBF assessment. *Top*, 3D images were made by reconstructing the transaxial SPECT data.
Middle, The surface threshold value was set at 30 ml/100 g/min, and the image defects, which indicate the region with rCBF less than 30 ml/100 g/min, were outlined and calculated by using the image-analysis system (*arrows*).

aneurysm, it was determined that SPECT scans could be used as an independent factor of clinical outcome (Mustonen, Koivisto, Vanninen, & Hänninen, 2008). Typical examples of SPECT appearances are seen in Figures 12.8 and 12.9 which also demonstrate the

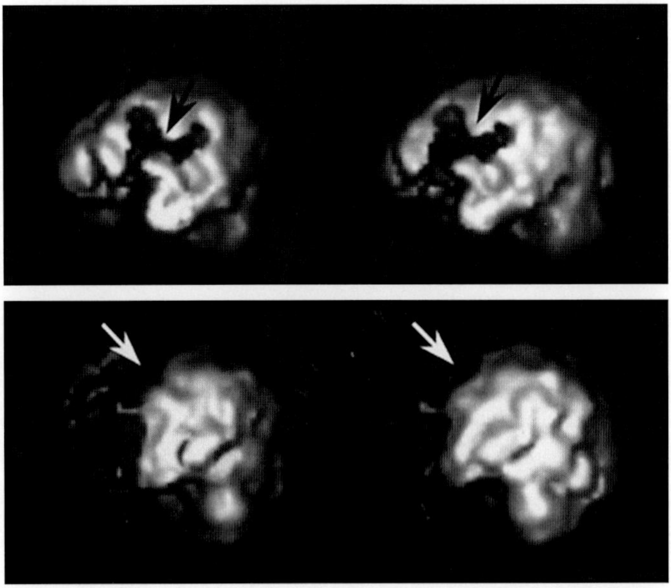

FIGURE 12.9 **Characteristic findings in cases of dind (delayed ischemic neurologic deficit).** Characteristic findings in cases with DIND (Ohkuma, Suzuki, & Kudo, 2003). *Top*, Figure shows widely decreased cortical rCBF at the left MCA region (arrows). *Bottom*, Figure shows widely decreased cortical rCBF at the left ACA region (*arrows*).

superiority of the 3D views to see detailed cortical flow, or the characteristic hypoperfusion (Ohkuma et al., 2003).

The functional outcome after a subarachnoid hemorrhage is dependent upon multiple factors. Some of these factors include the location of the bleeding, whether or not there is blood in the ventricular system or in the parenchyma itself, time of diagnosis, and delay of treatment, which is both medical and surgical. While there has been much advancement in modern times in early diagnosis and treatment resulting in better outcomes, there is still a significant portion of patients that are left with neurocognitive deficits. Therefore, some experts advocate for a complete neuropsychological evaluation (Hütter, Kreitschmann-Andermahr, & Mayfrank, 1999). Numerous studies have documented significant neurocognitive deficits that persist long term after the initial phase of hemorrhage. On the other hand, the mechanism and pathophysiology underlying the reason for persistent deficits is not well understood, although certain experts propose mechanisms such as cerebrovascular spasm and intracranial hypertension (Al-Khindi, Macdonald, & Schweizer, 2010). The relevance and importance of cerebral vasospasm is probably underestimated and will be addressed later in this chapter under the section of traumatic brain injury.

Cerebral concussion is the most common form of brain injury and there are several million new cases diagnosed every year (Slobounov, Gay, Johnson, & Zhang, 2012). This number does not take into consideration the number of cases of concussion that occur but do not present to emergency room for acute evaluation. While there is no clear consensus on the definition of concussion, most would agree with the fact that there is a transient interruption of ongoing cerebral function, with or without a loss of consciousness. The concept that a person does **not** have to lose consciousness to sustain a concussion has evolved over time and has replaced the older definition which did require such a loss. Similarly, it was believed that a person's head had to hit an object in order to sustain a concussion, whereas it is now considered that indirect trauma such as a whiplash can cause a concussion as well. Shaken baby syndrome is another example of indirect trauma causing a concussion which may include hemorrhaging in the brain. What is important is the force applied to the head and/or neck, or the acceleration/deceleration generated. In fact the definition is still evolving over time to reflect a greater knowledge and understanding of the evolving pathophysiology. One hypothesis is that an injury to the cervical spine can activate nociceptive afferents to the parietal lobe (Otte, Ettlin, & Nitzsche, 1997). Another emerging concept is that there are different phases to the condition, and a clearer understanding of acute (concussion) versus chronic symptoms (post-concussion syndrome)/findings based upon more sophisticated testing is being made (Slobounov et al., 2012). While it is true that a SPECT is not typically a first line imaging test that is ordered to assess mTBI, it is in fact more useful than MRI, because even the most sensitive MRI such as 3.0 T with DTI is typically normal in most mTBI cases. This clinical observation was reaffirmed in a correlative study. This author (PW) carried out using neuropsychological testing as "gold standard," and comparing abnormal focal neuropsychological results of one hemisphere with various other diagnostic structural imaging scans. The study was carried out on 38 patients that all underwent MRI scans, SPECT, QEEG, QEP (quantitative evoked response), and the neuropsychological testing. The results showed that MRI (dark blue) was abnormal in approximately 20% of the cases, whereas the SPECT (turquoise) was abnormal in approximately 75%, see Figure 12.10.

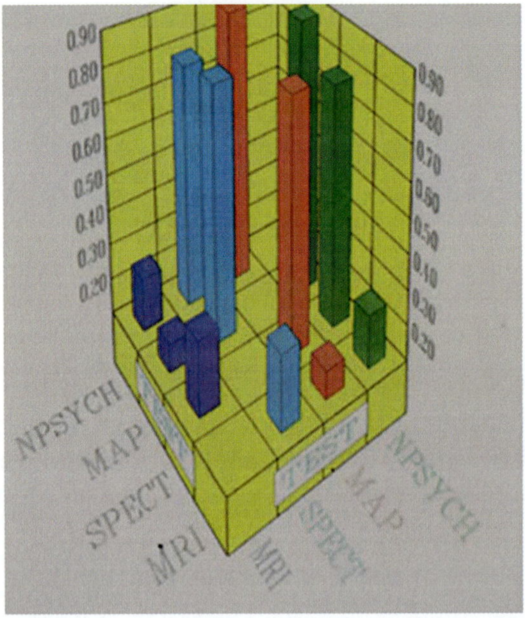

FIGURE 12.10 Comparative measures of patient symptoms in mTBI.

HOW TO INTERPRET THE 3D FIGURE 12.10

The *X* axis is on the left side, the *Y* axis is on the right side, and the *Z* axis is on the back side of the 3D diagram. Both the *X* and *Y* axes contain the type of test used to correlate their coefficient of agreement. The graph is read by comparing one test with another on the *X* and *Y* axes, then correlating the two where they meet on the *Z* axis. Neuropsychological testing is represented by "NPSYCH" in dark blue, and "MAP" in orange represents QEEG/QEP data. Thus correlating "NPSYCH" with MRI yields 0.2 or 20%, and with "MAP" 0.85 or 85% respectively.

Another application of SPECT scans involving trauma/concussion is its use in medico-legal cases where objective data is of paramount importance to prove a brain injury. The author (PW) has testified on numerous occasions that the SPECT did provide objective evidence. A similar conclusion was published by physicians at the Nuclear Medicine Department at the University of Gdansk, Poland of Nuclear Medicine, and they also stressed that SPECT scans are underutilized (Piskunowicz, Krzyzanowski, & Piotr, 2003). In an article in the *Journal of the American Academy of Psychiatry and Law* stressed that SPECT scans are underutilized (Wortzel, Filley, & Anderson, 2008). The authors from

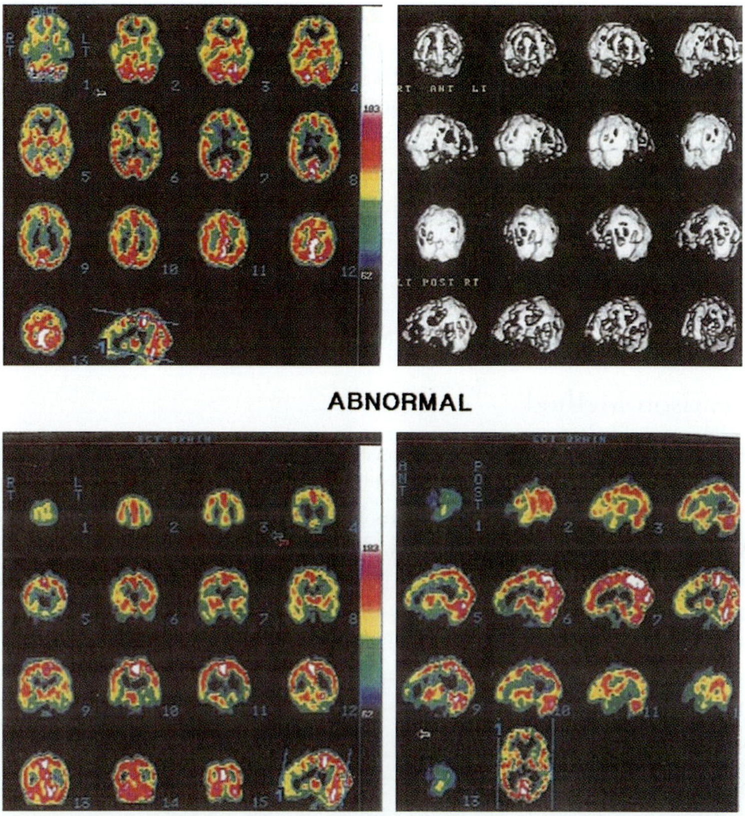

FIGURE 12.11 Abnormal 2D and 3D SPECT scans.

the Department of Psychiatry at the University of Denver Colorado concluded that SPECT scans fulfilled the criteria of *Daubert vs. Merrell Dow Pharmaceuticals*, but that it was not a standalone test and should be used in conjunction with other diagnostic testing such as clinical history and neuropsychological testing (Wortzel et al., 2008).

The common findings in SPECT scans after trauma to the head and/or neck area is a characteristic pattern of decreased blood flow or hypoperfusion seen in a gradient with greater severity in the anterior regions of the brain when compared to the posterior regions. This is seen best on the 3D surfaces images (the top right image in black and white) and easily seen by the untrained eye, but also on the 2D slices, see Figure 12.11.

Often times, classic patterns of "coup contrecoup" can be easily observed, e.g., areas of maximum hypoperfusion in the left frontal and right parieto-occipital lobes respectively. An example of this pattern is seen in the accompanying report (see Appendix).

Other publications have confirmed these findings, e.g., Bonne, Gilboa, and Louzoun (2003) reported similar findings in 28 patients with 20 matched controls. Umile, Sandel, and Alavi (2002) found a similar correlation of 75% using SPECT/PET scans. In another study by Ichise, Chung, and Wang (1994), similar findings were demonstrated; in fact both CT and MRI scans were used to compare, and as predicted the SPECT was abnormal in the highest percentage at 66%, MRI at 45%, and CT the least sensitive at 34% of a total of 29 patients.

CASE STUDIES

Comparison Method

EO LORETA was used for all cases to be compared in this study. The first inspection was of Current Source Density in 1 Hz bins and if similarities were found, that was used as the basis of comparison. However, in most cases, we used FFT generated coherence and phase statistics. The most abnormal 20 pairs, 10 most positive, and 10 most negative Z scored pairs were used. Then they were characterized as right, left, or homologous pairs. Then BA of each pair was counted and classified as being frontal, temporal, parietal, posterior cingulate, central, or occipital.

Areas were classified as follows:

Frontal: 4, 6, 8, 9, 10, 11, 24, 25, 32, 33, 44, 45, 46, 47
Temporal: 20, 21, 22, 27, 28, 34, 35, 36, 37, 38, 41, 42
Posterior cingulate: 23, 29, 30, 31
Parietal: 5, 7, 39, 40
Central: 1, 2, 3, 43
Occipital: 17, 18, 19

Identical pairs in different frequencies that were abnormal were counted only one time.

CASES

Patient KL was a 20-year-old left-handed white male originally seen for evaluation of consideration of stem cell treatment for his underlying diagnosis of anoxic encephalopathy which occurred at the time of birth. He was otherwise healthy. Neurological examination demonstrated a young obese white male otherwise alert and oriented ×3. Language showed significant dysarthria which was severe enough to cause difficulty in understanding his speech. Detailed neurological examination showed evidence of left greater than right frontal and parietal lobe signs (loss of fine motor control, right greater than left, severe impairment of graphesthesia of the right hand, and mild impairment of the left hand). A SPECT scan showed widespread diffuse cortical hypoperfusion, maximum anteriorly in the frontotemporal lobes, and posteriorly, possibly right greater than left but with relative sparing of the parietal lobes.

On QEEG intake, he complained that his most severe problems were poor social and motor skills. He has difficulty recognizing objects by touch (consistent with the impaired graphesthesia above) and difficulty with impulsivity. Other behaviors rated as very severe are:

1. Difficulty calculating
2. Dyslexia, letter reversals
3. Executive functioning
4. Multitasking
5. Poor judgment
6. Slow reader
7. Speech articulation
8. Word finding

The pattern of symptoms are both left and right hemispheric and consistent with a diffuse loss as was given by history (anoxic encephalopathy). Could LORETA find the sources of these symptoms and would it match maximum abnormality in frontal temporal areas?

Absolute power did not show as substantially abnormal. However, coherence and phase did show substantial abnormalities in LORETA. Of the top 20 coherence Z score deviations, 13 involved a frontal area, 3 involved temporal areas for a total of 16 out of the top 20 were frontal/temporal. Eight were shown abnormal in the left hemisphere and 12 of the 20 abnormal in the right hemisphere making the LORETA findings right greater than left. The Hippocampus and the Amygdala were among the areas shown as abnormal in LORETA coherence. In addition, the fusiform gyrus was abnormal as well (Table 12.1).

In LORETA phase 13 of the top 20 pairs involved a frontal BA and 5 of the 20 top pairs involved a temporal BA for a total of 18 out of 20 making this largely a frontal temporal finding. Two additional areas were members of the posterior cingulate. Seven were left hemispheric pairs and 13 were right hemispheric making this right greater than left and therefore in agreement with then SPECT scan (Table 12.2).

Patient LB was a 66-year-old right-handed white male seen for a slip and fall accident at a local target store. He was seen him almost 5 years after his injury and had been seen by multiple physicians. He was diagnosed with post-concussion syndrome and had multiple complaints including headache, poor recent memory, vertigo, tinnitus, trouble

TABLE 12.1 LORETA Coherence Z Score Pairs for KL

32 L–39 L	5.80	Theta
19 L–32 L	5.26	Theta
4 R–24 R	5.07	Theta
18 L–32 L	4.95	Theta
7 L–10 L	4.88	Theta
18 R–32 R	4.79	Theta
9 L–32 L	4.73	Delta
1 L–32 L	4.68	Theta
19 R–24 R	4.65	Theta
5 R–10 R	4.64	Theta
25 R–35 R	− 2.34	H Beta
1 R–4 R	− 2.46	Alpha2
18 R–39 R	− 2.47	Beta3
Amy R–Hip R	− 2.56	Delta
29 R–43 R	− 2.64	Alpha2
4 R–40 R	− 2.67	Alpha2
36 L–Amy L	− 2.68	Delta
41 R–43 R	− 2.71	Beta2
17 L–23 L	− 2.93	Delta
24 L–24 R	− 4.74	Delta

swallowing, poor balance, falling asleep inappropriately, and atypical movement disorder. Detailed neurological examination demonstrated right greater than left frontal lobe dysfunction, and left greater than right parietal lobe dysfunction. The latter topography, coupled with a history of trauma, was suggestive of a coup contrecoup type injury. The SPECT scan showed hypoperfusion in the right greater than left temporal lobe, the right superior frontal lobe, hypoperfusion in the left occipital greater than parietal lobes. The latter topography, coupled with a history of trauma, was suggestive of a coup contrecoup type injury.

LORETA showed right temporal lobe abnormality BA 38 right. The Uncus is found in the ventromedial aspect of the temporal lobe (Clark, Boutros, & Mendez, 2010, p. 181) (Figures 12.12–12.14).

LORETA found abnormality in the right superior frontal lobe, BA 10R and BA 8R.

TABLE 12.2 LORETA Phase Z Score Pairs for KL

9 L–32 L	3.93	Delta
8 L–32 L	3.87	Delta
24 R–45 R	3.72	Delta
18 R–39 R	3.68	Beta3
19 R–44 R	3.62	Delta
6 L–44 L	3.47	Delta
18 R–44 R	3.33	Delta
11 R–44 R	3.28	Delta
25 R–47 R	3.22	Delta
32 R–46 R	3.20	Delta
37 R–39 R	− 2.91	H Beta
10 L–25 L	− 2.96	Delta
38 L–46 L	− 3.00	Delta
7 R–27 R	− 3.07	H Beta
23 R–27 R	− 3.15	H Beta
30 R–31 R	− 3.18	H Beta
46 L–47 L	− 3.19	Delta
27 R–31 R	− 3.25	H Beta
11 L–24 L	− 3.31	Delta
10 R–38 R	− 3.37	Delta

However, more significant abnormality was found in the left parietal lobe more closely corresponding to the neurological examination. In short, LORETA found agreement in abnormalities in both the neurological and the SPECT scan examinations. However, LORETA found parietal abnormality greater than that found on SPECT but more closely related to the neurological examination. LORETA evidence supports coup-contrainjury indication (Figure 12.15).

Patient TS was a 37-year-old right-handed black male who was a former NFL player. He played for 10 years, and his last year was in 2002. He also played football in and prior to college. He played football for a total of 27 of his 37 years of life. He had multiple complaints including difficulty with comprehension of speech at times, right hand tremor, and trouble falling, and staying asleep. He was also requesting evaluation for hormones. He had four known concussions, all without any loss of consciousness. The only neurological workup he had was either

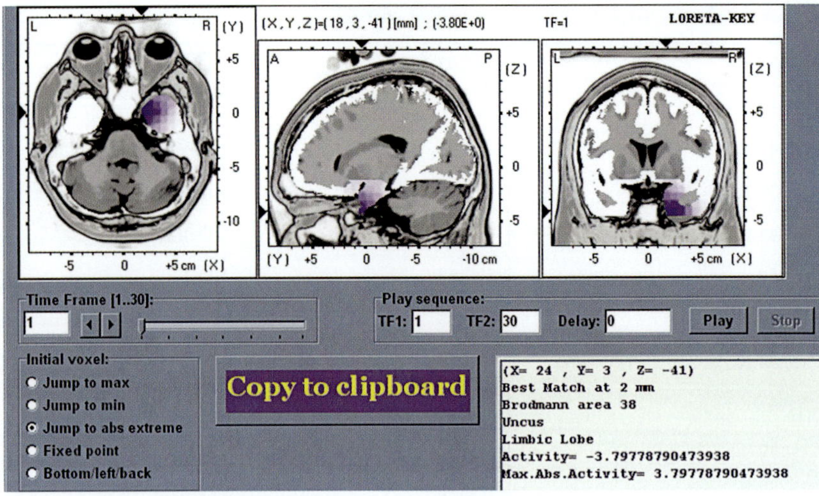

FIGURE 12.12 LORETA Current Source Density for LB BA 38.

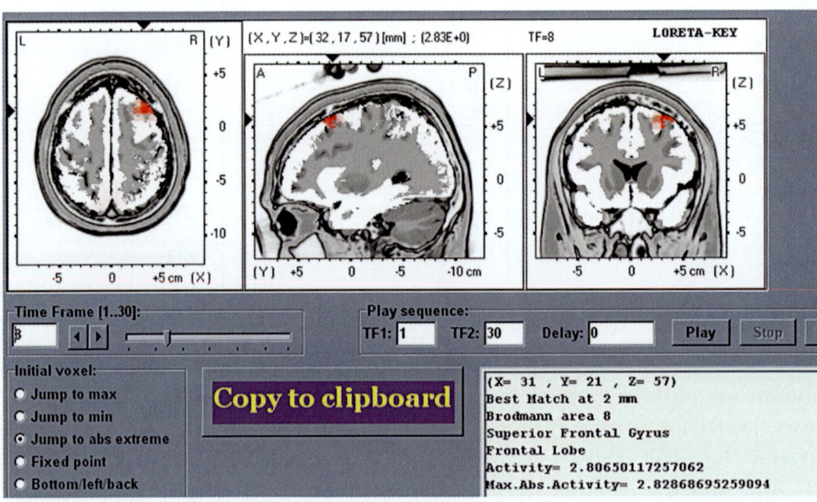

FIGURE 12.13 LORETA Current Source Density LB BA 8 and the left occipital lobe as well as the right.

an MRI or CT of the brain, which he reported was "negative." Most recently he had a quantitative EEG that was abnormal. Detailed neurological examination demonstrated left frontal and right parietal lobe dysfunction. The latter topography, coupled with a history of trauma, was suggestive of coup contrecoup. SPECT scan showed multiple areas of hypoperfusion, but with a gradient of anterior greater than posterior, and right greater than left anteriorly, and left greater than right

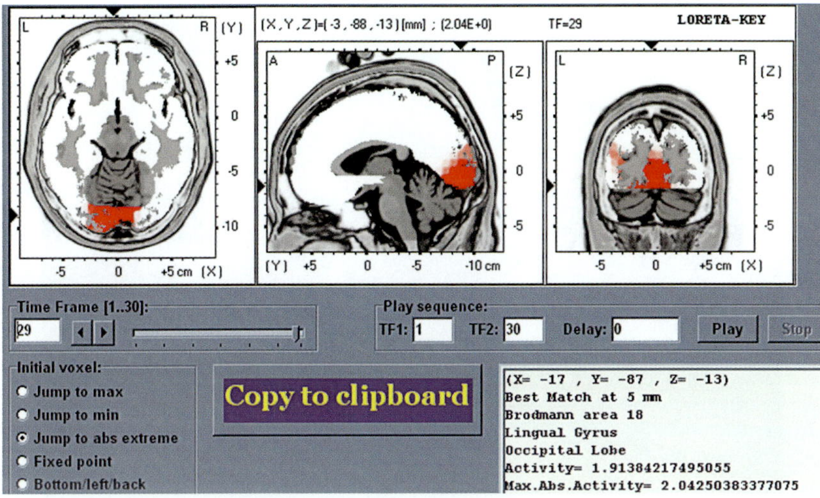

FIGURE 12.14 LORETA Current Source Density BA 18 occipital.

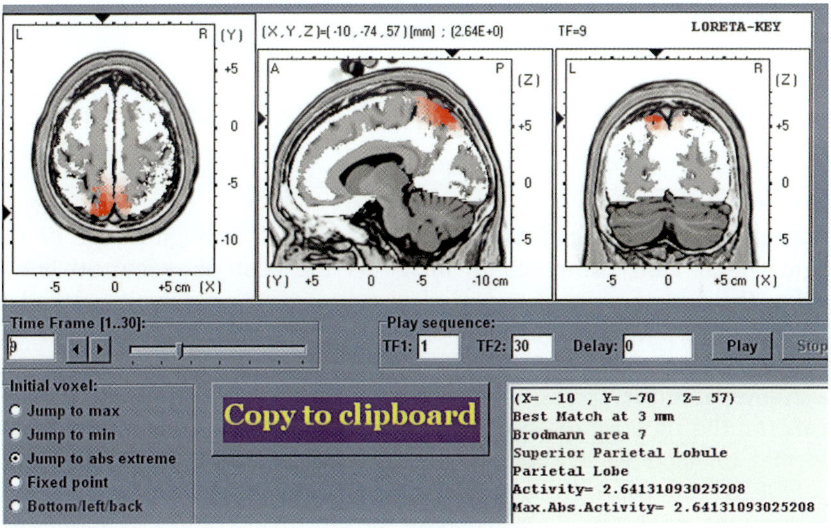

FIGURE 12.15 LORETA Current Source Density BA 7 parietal LOBE.

posteriorly. The latter topography, coupled with a history of trauma, was suggestive of a coup contrecoup injury.

The procedure to read and identify the images is as follows: the numeration is from left to right, top to bottom. Thus, the top left image is #1, the anterior posterior view, and the last image of the top row is image #4, the right lareral view, and so forth. Note the gross irregularity and darker colors in Figure 12.6 at image #1 of line 1 more prominent on the right

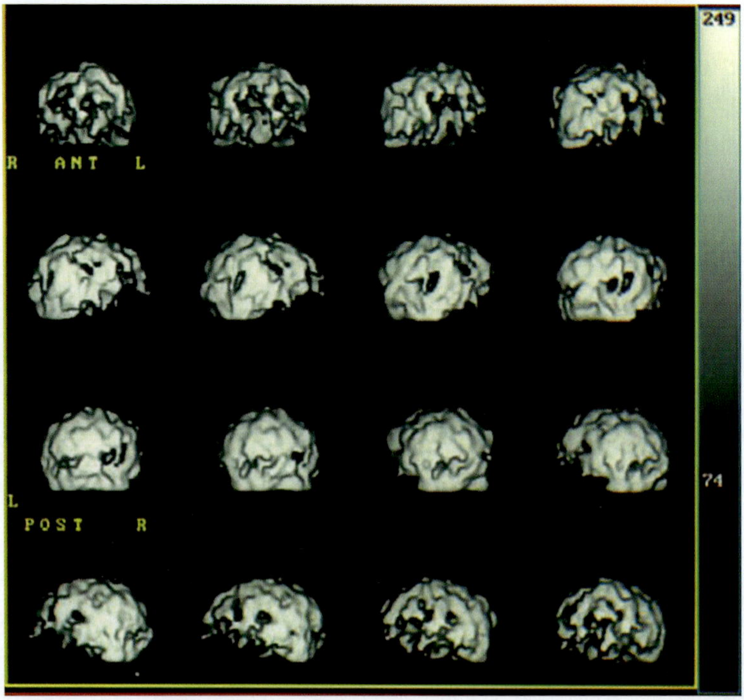

FIGURE 12.16 CASE TS SPECT 3D image.

hemisphere than left and on all images of line 1 through image #4 the right lateral view compared to image #9 the posterior view on line 3 where the darker areas of hypoperfusion are more prominent on the left (also seen on the right posterior obliques of line 2 compared to the left posterior obliques of line 3) (Figures 12.16 and 12.17).

Above note the excessive green colors on the inferior 2D axial especially on the right representing low flow on the color scale at 30–40% of normal, on slices #3, 4, and 5.

LORETA shows right greater than left anterior with nine coherence pairs on the right frontal abnormal (of the top 20) as compared to one pair with a left frontal BA. With nine in the right frontal, the anterior is also greater than posterior because as we move backward toward the temporal lobe, there are six coherence pairs that are abnormal. Thus the gradient is on the right side anterior worse than posterior which matches the SPECT scan. BAs 1, 3, 5, and 40 are also involved in abnormal coherence pairs which the SPECT did not register making the LORETA more sensitive. The right parietal finding on LORETA in coherence closely matches the neurological examination, but of course neither the SPECT nor the neurological examination has the spatial resolution of LORETA (Table 12.3).

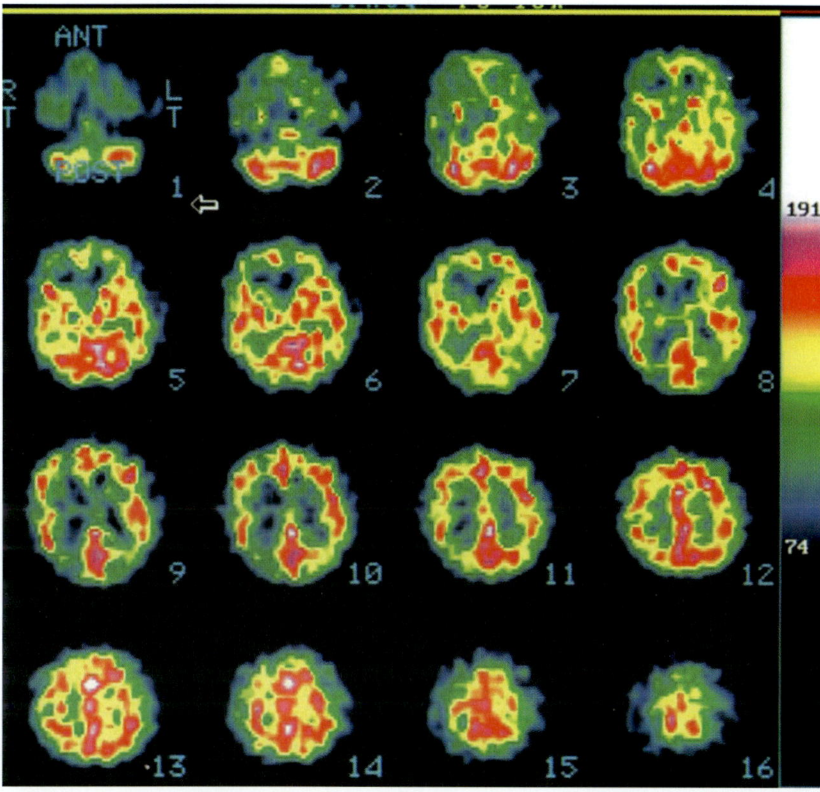

FIGURE 12.17 CASE TS 2D SPECT.

In phase of the top 20 abnormal Z score pairs, 12 are right hemispheric and 8 are left. Of the 12 on the right, 10 involve a frontal BA and 1 involves a temporal area. Of the 8 on the left, 2 are frontal, 1 parietal, 3 temporal, and 3 central (Table 12.4).

The LORETA findings do confirm the SPECT scan results but also yield results of abnormalities not shown in the SPECT, such as central and parietal, but that did show on the neurological examination.

Patient AE was a 41/2-year-old left-handed white male seen for a diagnosis of myoclonic epilepsy which was thought to be due to a genetic aberration. He did however have a long complex history where his first seizure suffered was associated with fever and again after vaccinations. MRI of the brain was somewhat abnormal in that it showed a relative increase of white matter. EEG performed previously at another office was abnormal with focal paroxysmal abnormality seen bilaterally, posteriorly, with bilateral slowing with left greater than right amplitude, and photomyoclonus. The patient was taking Keppra and phenobarbital

TABLE 12.3 LORETA EO Coherence Z Score Values for TS

1 R–5 R	4.68	Beta2
5 R–40 R	4.41	Beta2
8 R–21 R	4.34	Alpha2
9 R–20 R	4.28	Alpha2
3 R–9 R	4.25	Beta1
1 L–9 L	4.25	Alpha2
42 R–Hip R	4.20	Beta1
3 L–37 L	4.10	Alpha2
1 R–9 R	4.04	Beta1
2 L–37 L	4.00	Alpha2
13 R–20 R	−5.25	Beta1
34 R–45 R	−5.29	Alpha2
46 R–47 R	−5.33	Alpha2
38 R–47 R	−5.51	Beta1
34 R–36 R	−5.61	Beta1
38 R–44 R	−5.66	Alpha1
40 L–43 L	−7.06	Alpha2
29 L–41 L	−7.85	Alpha2
45 R–47 R	−7.85	Alpha2
44 R–47 R	−9.13	Alpha2

as an anticonvulsants for his treatment of epilepsy. At the time when he was seen, his seizure frequency was about once a week, lasting between 40 and 60 s. This typically occurs during the transition from waking or going to sleep. Neurological examination was limited since the patient was nonverbal, and he was photosensitive to ambient light. Motor examination showed a generalized hypotonia. He showed a preference to move the left arm and left leg. The plantar responses were difficult to assess. Sensory examination was severely limited to his response to pain, which appeared to be attenuated on the right side of the body. In conclusion the neurological examination was somewhat suggestive of a left focal hemispheric dysfunction, consistent with a previously reported EEG. Clinically he had poorly controlled epilepsy. The patient had a baseline/pretreatment SPECT scan performed on August 10, 2009. The study was significantly abnormal, with marked

TABLE 12.4 LORETA EO Phase Z Score Values for TS

44 R–47 R	6.17	Alpha2
45 R–47 R	5.42	Alpha2
38 R–45 R	5.25	Alpha2
38 R–45 R	5.00	Beta1
34 R–44 R	4.53	Alpha2
40 L–43 L	4.48	Alpha2
36 R–44 R	4.48	Alpha1
36 R–45 R	4.43	Alpha2
38 R–44 R	4.40	Alpha1
44 R–Amy R	4.30	Alpha1
4 R–13 R	−3.97	Alpha1
8 L–9 L	−4.00	Alpha1
8 L–9 L	−4.08	Alpha2
20 L–42 L	−4.21	Alpha2
11 L–11 R	−4.21	Theta
1 L–2 L	−4.25	Alpha1
2 L–3 L	−4.51	Alpha2
21 L–42 L	−4.67	Alpha2
21 R–43 R	−4.75	Alpha2
1 L–2 L	−4.91	Alpha2

hypoperfusion seen in the right greater than left frontal and temporal lobes, left frontal lobe hypoperfusion superiorly and laterally, left posterior parietal/anterior occipital hyperperfusion, thinning of the frontal and parietal cortices, probably responsible for ventriculomegaly/hydrocephalus. The patient's hypoperfusion was treated aggressively, with 65 hyperbaric oxygen treatments (HB OT), and nimodipine (brandname of Nimotop) at a dose of 15 mg twice a day. He was also treated with physical therapy and occupational therapy. Clinically he was more alert and responsive; his motor functions had improved. He was able to comprehend a simple request and able to walk with assistance. His seizure frequency was greatly improved and occurred predominantly if he had fever or he was exposed to light. Posttreatment SPECT scan performed on February 22, 2010, shows significant improvement with an increase of perfusion in the frontal lobes, little change in the temporal lobes, and no change in the parietal occipital lobes. Overall the posttreatment SPECT scan showed improvement predominantly in the frontal lobes.

Although LORETA registered similar findings as the SPECT, it did not register the right greater than left frontal temporal lobe abnormality. In coherence it registers left greater than right hemispheric abnormality with of the 17 pairs on the left one is frontal and 16 are temporal, 5 are posterior cingulate, and 3 occipital.[1] LORETA does register the diffuseness of the findings and shows abnormality in the posterior cingulate that SPECT did not register, yet at the same time shows much greater left than right abnormality and much greater temporal than frontal abnormality (Table 12.5).

TABLE 12.5 LORETA Coherence Z Scores for AE

22 L–23 L	8.05	Beta1
17 L–22 L	7.21	Beta1
23 L–37 L	7.18	Beta2
31 L–37 L	7.14	Beta2
23 L–42 L	6.74	Beta1
22 L–23 L	6.60	Beta2
17 L–37 L	6.26	Beta2
31 L–42 L	5.98	Beta1
21 L–21 R	5.81	Alpha2
20 L–33 L	5.79	Beta1
27 L–35 L	−3.92	Beta3
41 R–43 R	−4.16	Theta
27 L–35 L	−4.20	H Beta
17 L–23 L	−4.23	H Beta
17 R–23 R	−4.95	H Beta
20 L–35 L	−5.28	H Beta
21 L–35 L	−5.29	Beta3
20 L–35 L	−5.44	Beta2
17 R–23 R	−5.53	Beta3
20 L–35 L	−7.45	Beta3

[1]Sum is greater than 20 due to some pairs registering in two lobes.

In phase there are 16 left abnormal pairs and 4 right abnormal pairs of the highest 20. On the left 12 are in the temporal area and 9 frontal. Four are in the central area, 3 in the posterior cingulate, 2 occipital, and one in the parietal. This is left greater than right and does not co-register with the SPECT. On the right, there are four abnormal pairs and one temporal and one central. Added together this makes 13 frontal BAs involved and 14 temporal which makes this a frontal temporal dominant abnormal study. In that LORETA and SPECT agree that this is frontal temporal, but there is hemispheric severity disagreement (Table 12.6).

Patient RD was a 5-year-old male diagnosed with West syndrome visiting from Italy for the purpose of undergoing intensive medical treatment and hyperbaric oxygen therapy. Neurological examination demonstrated a severely impaired child with a weight of only 22 pounds

TABLE 12.6 LORETA Phase Z Scores for AE

17 L–35 L	6.04	Beta2
23 L–35 L	5.45	Beta2
10 R–38 R	5.20	Theta
17 L–37 L	4.94	Beta3
31 L–35 L	4.88	Beta2
10 L–32 L	4.78	Theta
30 L–35 L	4.73	Beta2
3 R–25 R	4.71	Delta
33 L–41 L	4.69	Beta1
23 L–27 L	4.57	Beta3
4 L–7 L	−6.32	Beta2
10 L–42 L	−6.42	Beta2
2 L–32 L	−6.44	Alpha2
11 R–46 R	−6.59	Alpha1
3 L–32 L	−6.60	Alpha2
27 L–47 L	−6.68	Theta
4 L–11 L	−6.89	Alpha2
11 R–46 R	−6.93	Alpha2
10 L–42 L	−7.05	Beta1
11 L–41 L	−7.11	Beta1

and measured 90 cm in height. It was clear the patient demonstrated failure to thrive. Motor examination demonstrated a spastic quadriplegia, worse in the lower than upper extremities, with a tendency to fisting. Frontal signs included positive grasp reflex bilaterally, positive glabellar tap, mildly positive jaw jerk, and probably a mildly positive palmomental reflex. Patient was nonverbal and nonambulatory. The rest of the neurological examination could be performed due to the patient's severely impaired status. MRI of the brain showed severe central and cortical atrophy and hydrocephalus ex vacuo. There was also an increased signal seen in the basal ganglia, which was apparently analyzed by a nuclear magnetic resonance (NMR), and a peak for *N*-acetyl aspartic acid (NAA) was detected. A pretreatment/baseline SPECT scan was performed on March 23, 2009. This was a severely abnormal study with marked hypoperfusion and low-flow state in most of the frontal and temporal lobes, possibly worse on the right. Global hypoperfusion also seen in the basal ganglia and cerebellum. There was relative preservation of perfusion posteriorly in the bilateral parietal and occipital lobes. A follow-up SPECT scan was performed on 15 February, 2010, almost 1 year later from the pretreatment scan. In the interim he was treated with nimodipine to increase cerebral blood flow (CBF) and neurofeedback. He was also treated with growth hormone (rHGH), and testosterone based upon lab values that showed severe deficiency. The repeat SPECT scan showed very significant increase of perfusion in all lobes of the brain, but especially in the frontal lobes, where he had had a low-flow state. Clinically was more alert, more active, and demonstrated some increase of comprehension of speech. He was also treated aggressively with physical therapy between 2 and 4 h a day.

Below see the pretreatment SPECT scan: 2D axial slices #2–16 demonstrating severe hypoperfusion in green which corresponds to almost the lowest flow in the 10 step color scale in all anterior lobes of the brain, as demonstrated by both the 2D and 3D images of Figures of 12.18 and 12.20. Clinically he had poorly controlled epilepsy.

Below see the posttreatment SPECT scan: note the return of flow in the anterior regions of the brain, in particular the frontotemporal lobes on the 2D slices #2–16 with the "hotter colors" in the anterior regions of the brain (Figures 12.19 and 12.20).

Above: Pretreatment 3D views showing massive loss of filling of the frontal lobes anteriority and superiorly, the bilateral central-temporal lobes on the AP view image #1 of line 1, on the right lateral view of image #4, and the left lateral/oblique views of line 4 showing the left frontal lobe, and a rudimentary temporal lobe. Note the relative preservation of perfusion posteriori in the occipital lobes of image #9/line 3. The odd shaped triangular filling is outside of the brain most likely an artifact from uptake of isotope in the midline sinuses.

Below: 3D posttreatment views: note the return of flow represented by the white color, at the highest/top of the flow scale, especially in the anterior regions of the brain, e.g., images #1–4 of line 1, representing the AP view, the right anterior obliques, and the right lateral views; and images #12–16 of line 4 representing the left lateral and left anterior obliques (Figure 12.21).

In LORETA coherence pairs looking at the top twenty the top twenty 11 are in the right hemisphere 3 in the left and there is one homologous pair, BA 24 LR. There are only 14 pairs because 3 pairs on the right and 2 on the left had Z scores which were in different frequencies but in the same pair of BAs. Of the 11 pairs on the right 8 temporal BAs are involved, 3 pairs involving frontal and posterior cingulate BAs and 2 in the occipital and one in the central. On the left, there are two frontal BAs, one of which is the homologous pair BA 24, the anterior cingulate. LORETA indicates that in coherence, there is agreement with the SPECT that right is worse than left but differs in that it is more temporal than frontal temporal (Table 12.7).

In phase there are 15 left BAs that are abnormal in the top 20 and 18 on the left making this slightly more right than left. On the left, 6 are parietal areas, 3 are occipital, two each temporal and central, 1 as part of the

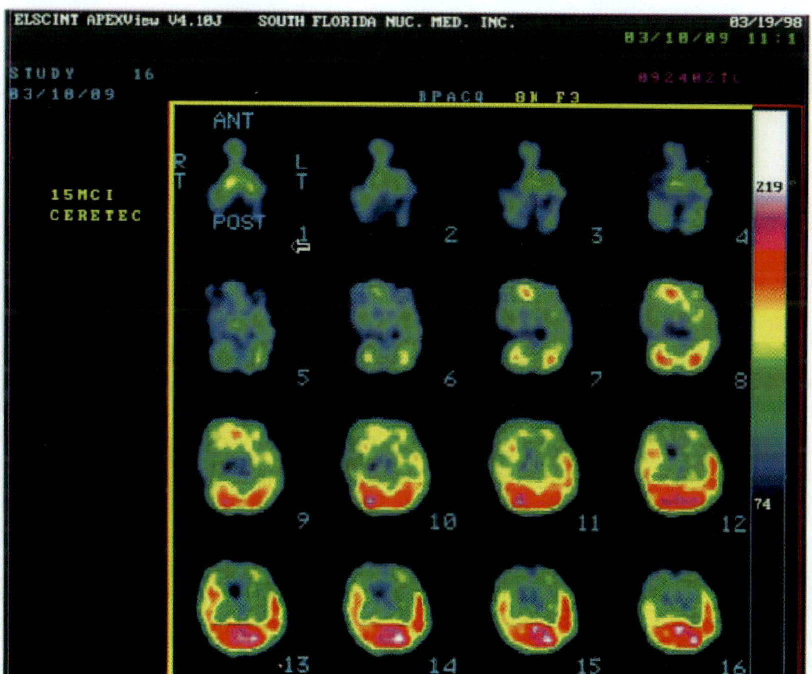

FIGURE 12.18 CASE RD pretreatment 2D spect scan images.

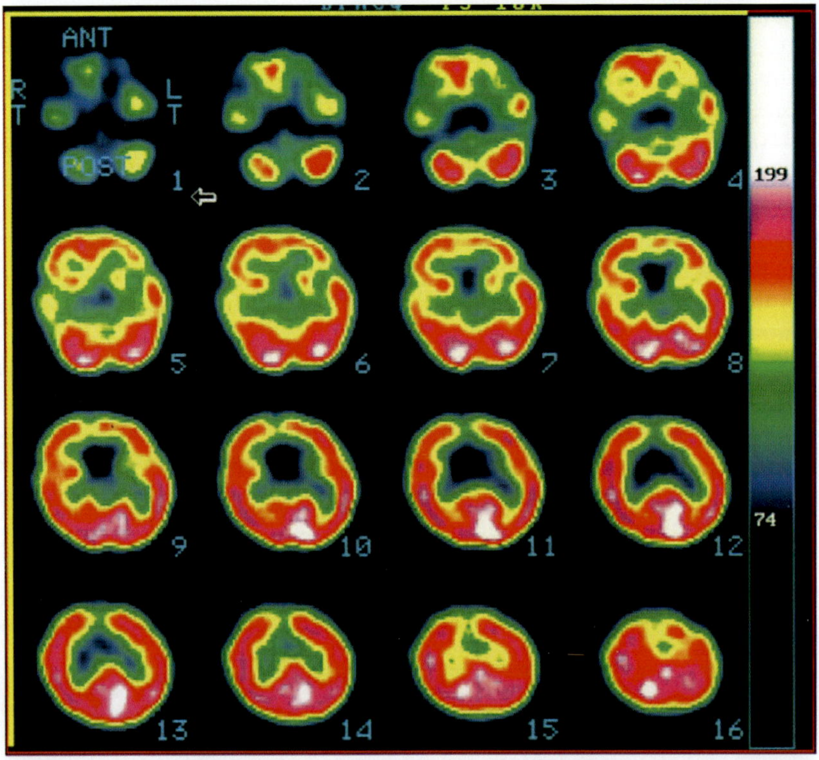

FIGURE 12.19 CASE RD posttreatment 2D spect scan images.

posterior cingulate and one homologous pair, frontal, BA 46. This makes the left hemisphere phase LORETA abnormalities parietal or parietal/occipital. On the right, there are 18 abnormalities of which 7 are frontal, 6 central, 3 parietal, and 2 temporal making the right side frontal/central.

In current source density going frequency by frequency, Figure 12.22 is more representative of all of the 30 frequencies.

Other images show bilateral temporal parietal abnormalities in the higher frequencies as well. This shows frontal temporal to the right with cingulate involvement and is closer to the SPECT.

In comparison to the pretreatment SPECT, there is good agreement that this is more right than left and but is more frontal central than temporal. The Z score values in coherence extend to >8 standard deviations and in both phase and coherence, the Z scores are higher on the right than left indicating a much greater departure from normal on the right than left, again consistent with the SPECT scan. However, current source density using Z scores based on microamperes shows higher correspondence to the SPECT than the FFT coherence and phase though

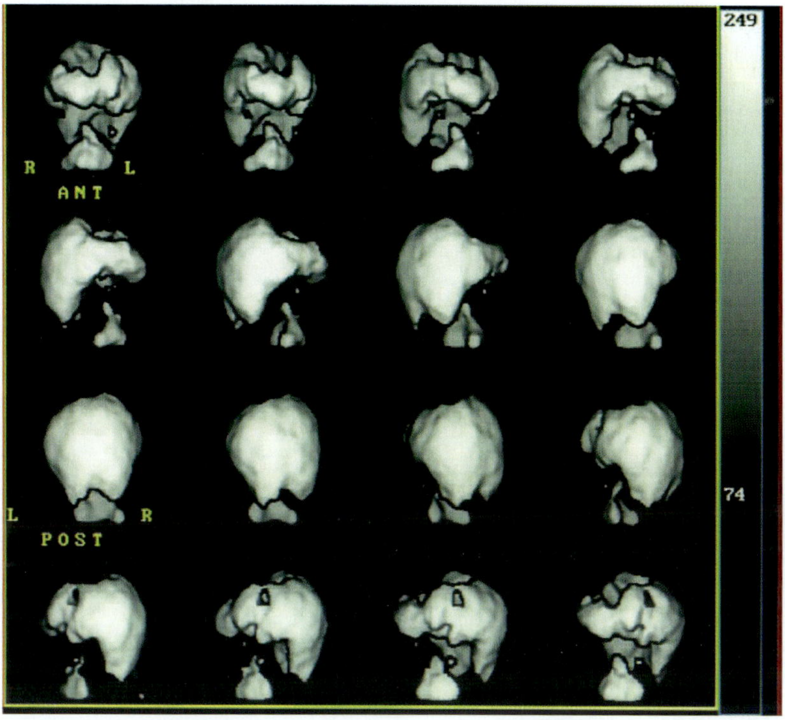

FIGURE 12.20 CASE RD pretreatment 3D spect scan images.

both clearly show agreement in the frontal lobe and right greater than left abnormality. In some cases, the FFT calculations may not register as sensitively to SPECT findings (Table 12.8).

Patient JK was a 32-year-old right-handed white male seen for evaluation of abnormal EEG/QEEG. Clinically he was complaining of headaches, jaw pain, some numbness of the right orbit right hand. Examination suggested that the headache was probably a TMJ related/myofascial pain and dysfunction, carpal tunnel syndrome, and routine EEG showed irritability, and some focal left parietal lobe dysfunction. His history is unusual. He gave a history of seeking neurofeedback treatment for fatigue and anxiety from a practitioner. The history revealed that he received about 20 single channel neurofeedback treatments which were guided by measuring amplitude and then making treatment decisions based on the percentage of a specific frequency that should or should not be at a particular site or lobe. These were a priori judgments not based on a normative database and essentially results in a protocol based on relative power. This patient deteriorated rapidly to the point where he became unemployed and disabled. The practitioner could not be contacted as he had left the country.

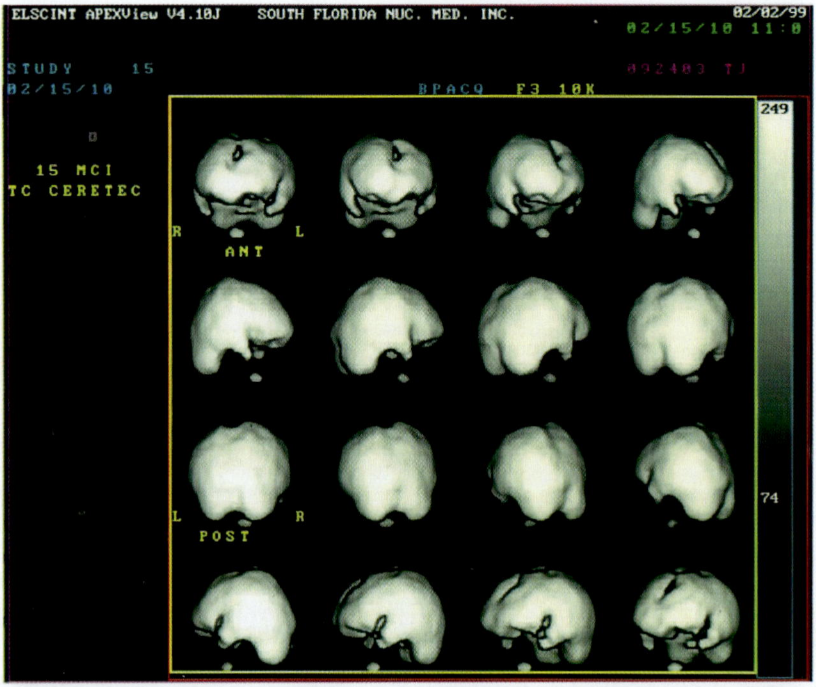

FIGURE 12.21 CASE RD posttreatment 3D spect scan images.

After lengthy neurofeedback treatment, he is reentering the workforce. There is no history of head trauma or seizures. A SPECT scan was abnormal, with widespread hypoperfusion, anterior greater than posterior, and right greater than left frontal, right greater than left temporal, and biparietal bioccipital hypoperfusion.

LORETA coherence reveals: 5 left pairs abnormal, 13 right pairs abnormal and 2 homologous pairs, 7 and 47 abnormal making this bifrontal and biparietal consistent with the biparietal finding of the SPECT. There were (not in the top 20) 6 abnormal findings corresponding to the occipital area, totally in the study, all on the right, O2, so in that sense right > left occipital, not bilateral in the occipital area. The findings as illustrated by Figure 12.23 involved BAs 18, 19, and 37 on the right extending into the temporal lobe.

In a 3D map it is rendered thus:

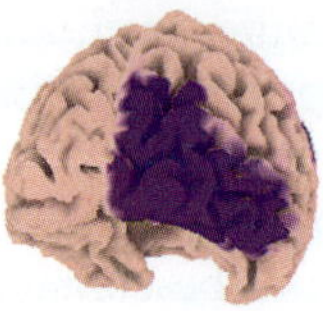

TABLE 12.7 LORETA Coherence Z Score Pairs for RD

36 R–42 R	6.54	Delta
42 R–Amy R	6.41	Delta
28 R–42 R	6.12	Delta
18 L–23 L	5.94	Delta
34 R–42 R	5.84	Delta
22 R–34 R	5.80	Delta
25 R–30 R	5.79	Delta
23 R–37 R	5.78	Delta
17 R–37 R	5.68	Delta
24 R–30 R	5.57	Delta
36 R–Hip R	−3.27	H Beta
2 L–3 L	−3.60	Alpha2
5 L–7 L	−3.77	Delta
24 L–24 R	−4.10	Delta
2 L–3 L	−4.52	Theta
2 L–3 L	−4.82	Delta
2 R–3 R	−5.17	Theta
2 R–3 R	−7.55	Alpha1
2 R–3 R	−8.20	Alpha2
2 R–3 R	−8.56	Delta

Of the 5 left hemispheric pairs, 4 frontal BAs were involved, 3 temporal and 1 parietal. Of the 13 right pairs involved, 12 were frontal, 10 temporal and 4 central, and 1 parietal. LORETA agrees with SPECT that this is a right > left abnormal study and agrees that this is more anterior than posterior. It also agrees right > left frontal and temporal lobe deregulation and biparietal but not bioccipital. This makes this better than a 90% agreement. This case also highlights the risk of a non-Z-score-based protocol based solely on relative power.

In phase 1 left hemisphere pair, 15 right pairs and 4 homologous BAs, 7, 34, 38, and 47 were found abnormal. This makes phase LORETA findings consistent with a biparietal, bifrontal, bi-temporal SPECT study finding. Of the 20 possible pairs (40 possible BAs), 4 were left frontal, 4 left temporal, 1 left posterior cingulate and 17 right frontal, 6 right temporal, 6 right parietal and 1 right occipital, and 1 central.

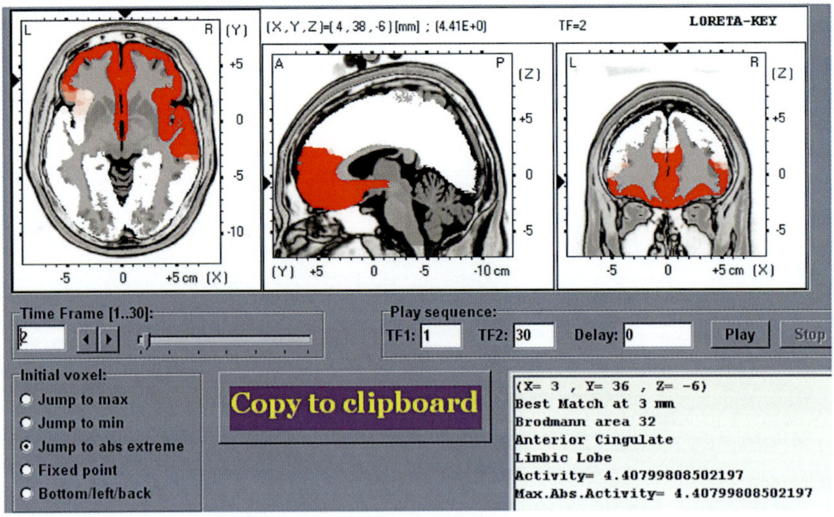

FIGURE 12.22 LORETA Current Source Density case of RD BA 32 anterior cingulate.

Patient GC was a 19-year-old right-handed white male seen for evaluation of known epilepsy and recent abnormal QEEG. He was diagnosed with epilepsy at the age of 10 and had a previous normal MRI of the brain. He did have two previous episodes of head trauma. The first episode at the age of 3 striking the right frontal area without any loss of consciousness. The other at the age of 14 or 15 was running at full speed and ran into a street pole and was unconscious for a brief period of time. Neither episode prompted any medical evaluation. His description of a seizure was quite consistent with a generalized seizure, preceded by an aura, no tonic or clonic movements, and followed by a postictal period, but without incontinence. At the time when he was seen, he did not have any clinical seizures in the last 3 years. Detailed neurological examination showed signs consistent with left frontal and parietal lobe dysfunction, consistent with the EEG, QEEG, and previous neuropsychological testing. SPECT scan did show significant hypoperfusion in the left greater than right frontotemporal lobes and to a lesser extent the bioccipital lobes.

Coherence found 10 left hemispheric pairs abnormal, 7 right pairs and 3 homologous pairs, Amygdala, 36 and 46. Phase found 10 left hemisphere pairs, 9 right hemisphere pairs, and one homologous pair abnormal, BA 36. This shows that LORETA agrees with SPECT of left greater than right by hemisphere. It was probably of significance that BA 36 LR was significantly abnormal in both coherence and phase given the patient's history of head trauma and seizure. BA 36 is associated with social and emotional processing on the right and semantic and episodic memory on the left. The patient had complaints of difficulty with

TABLE 12.8 LORETA Phase Z Score Pairs for RD

5 L–31 L	5.75	Delta
5 R–31 R	5.32	Delta
18 L–39 L	4.39	Delta
46 L–46 R	4.22	Delta
2 R–3 R	3.61	Alpha2
2 R–3 R	3.61	Delta
1 L–4 L	3.35	Theta
1 R–9 R	3.29	Delta
2 L–3 L	3.26	Delta
30 L–39 L	3.24	Delta
17 R–39 R	− 3.42	Delta
19 R–31 R	− 3.44	Delta
4 R–7 R	− 3.53	Theta
11 R–24 R	− 3.57	Theta
11 R–24 R	− 3.63	Alpha1
4 R–7 R	− 3.69	Alpha2
20 R–45 R	− 3.73	Delta
4 R–7 R	− 3.78	Beta1
21 R–44 R	− 4.44	Delta
10 R–44 R	− 4.44	Delta

relationships, especially new ones in particular, and recall and learning in school. Mood and memory improved with neurofeedback. Coherence showed 10 frontal and 3 temporal BAs as abnormal and 5 frontal and 5 temporal areas abnormal on the right. This is consistent with left greater than right frontal temporal abnormality on the SPECT. However, LORETA found no occipital abnormality in coherence.

In phase there were 16 frontal and 1 temporal abnormality, 1 BA in the posterior cingulate and 3 in the occipital area. On the right, there were 10 frontal BAs involved, 5 temporal, and one each in the central, parietal, and occipital areas. BA 36 was abnormal in both left and right hemispheres. This is consistent with the SPECT finding of left greater than right frontal temporal and consistent with the finding in the biocci-pital area suggesting in this case that phase may be more sensitive than coherence.

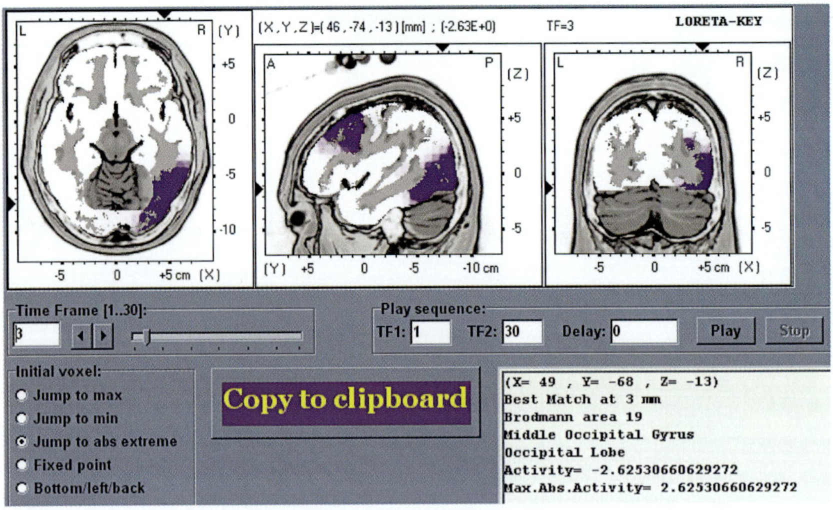

FIGURE 12.23 Illustrative right occipital temporal finding in case JK.

Patient TA was an 11-year-old white left-handed male with the diagnosis of autism and heavy metal intoxication who came to Florida for the purpose of performing intensive neurofeedback. He had been evaluated and treated intensively and was chelated for mercury and lead. He was also treated for some usual infections. He also had a previous SPECT of the brain 6 years before, which was verbally reported to show hypoperfusion in the frontal lobes, according to his father who brought the patient. The father believed it was in the left hemisphere. TA's prior treatment also included 2 weeks of hyperbaric oxygen therapy, but there was no apparent clinical improvement. Neurological examination revealed an alert and cooperative adolescent male who was significantly dysarthric and aphasic for both receptive and motor language. He spoke in short sentences and did appear to have difficulty with comprehension. Motor examination was somewhat limited because of his ability to cooperate, but did show some slowing of the rapid and fine movements. On primary sensory testing, he appeared to be intact. On secondary cortical testing, he appeared to be severely impaired for graphesthesia of the palms, significantly worse in the left hand than the right considering he cannot detect any letters in the left hand, and a few letters in the right hand. He did have extinction of the distal point of stimulation on double simultaneous stimulation, and this finding was bilateral. He was also noted to have some degree of left-right confusion. An updated SPECT scan was abnormal with moderate hypoperfusion seen in the frontal lobes, and anteriorly and inferiorly, and right greater than left. There was also hypoperfusion seen in the temporal lobes, especially inferiorly, medially, laterally, and left greater than right. Hypoperfusion also in the occipital lobes, slightly greater on the right than left and probable hypoperfusion in the left basal ganglia.

LORETA coherence showed 10 left hemisphere abnormalities, 8 right and 2 homologous pairs, Amygdala and BA 36, both in the temporal lobe. The frontal lobe showed 13 BAs on the left and 5 on the right showing left greater than right abnormality, not matching SPECT. Temporal lobe showed 5 abnormalities and the left 4 thus slightly right greater than left also not matching the SPECT. No abnormalities seen in the occipital lobe.

LORETA phase showed overall 10 left and 9 right with one homologous pair making it slightly left greater than right and individual BAs showed 15 left frontal and 8 right frontal again not matching SPECT which showed right greater than left in the frontal lobe. Temporal lobe showed 3 BAs on the right and 2 on the left making it right greater than left by a little and also not matching the SPECT. Phase also showed 4 left occipital BAs abnormal and 1 in the posterior cingulate and 1 right in the parietal lobe. The abnormality in phase in the occipital was 4 on the left and none on the right thus not matching the SPECT.

MS was a 15-year-old right-handed white male seen for evaluation of traumatic brain injury and abnormal QEEG. The patient did sustain multiple injuries as a result of the accident which occurred approximately 3 years prior to the initial consultation. A pediatric neurological examination was said to be normal as well as a routine EEG. He dropped out of high school in the ninth grade because of the above problems. Prior to the accident he was more an A than a B student. After the accident his grades deteriorated. He had episodes of spacing and zoning out which prevented him from focusing and studying and learning. He was treated with stimulants such as Concerta up to 36 mg a day. He complained of memory deficit, long-term greater than short-term. Tingling of both hands, a decrease of dexterity in the hands, cervicogenic headaches, neck and low back pain as well. Detailed neurological examination showed difficulty with optico-kinetic nystagmus with gaze to the right, slowing of fine motor in both hands, impaired balance, was able to stand on the right foot with eyes open, unable to stand on the left foot with eyes closed, and difficulty with tandem gait. Sensory examination showed nonphysiological responses to vibration such as splitting of vibration of the fourth, but classically positive Tinel sign at the carpal tunnel. Secondary cortical testing with graphesthesia of the hand showed a mild impairment of the right palm. The clinical impression was multiple injuries with post-concussion syndrome, left greater than right hemispheric dysfunction, probable posttraumatic partial seizure disorder, and depression. His SPECT scan was abnormal with multiple areas of hypoperfusion as follows: Left greater than right frontal hypoperfusion, right greater

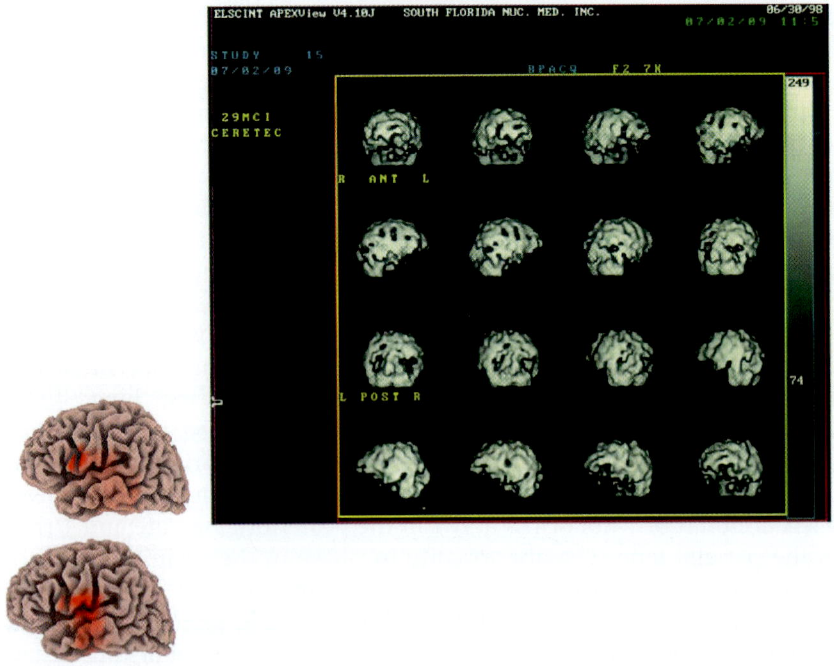

FIGURE 12.24 Case of MS 3D SPECT.

than left temporal hypoperfusion affecting the medial, inferior, and lateral aspects. Right greater than left parietal hypoperfusion. The topography of left frontal, right parietal, coupled with a history of trauma is characteristic of clinical contrecoup type injury.

His SPECT is shown in Figure 12.24 in the 3D views of the typical gradient in TBI of anterior > posterior as seen when comparing the anterior view of image #1 of line 1 to image #9 of the line the posterior view. There are more areas of dark or black on image #9 compared to image #1. There is another gradient here typical of trauma which is the coup contrecoup pattern. When looking at image #1, the left frontal (right side of the image) is darker than the right, and on image #9, the right side (also right side of the image) is darker indicating greater hypoperfusion. This topography as described above is typical of trauma (Figure 12.24).

Note similarity of LORETA topography on left and SPECT topography above in black and white.

LORETA shows left greater than right frontal abnormality (Figures 12.25 and 12.26).

LORETA does show dysfunction in the parietal lobes as well, bilaterally (Figures 12.27 and 12.28).

And on 3D it appears as shown in Figure 12.29.

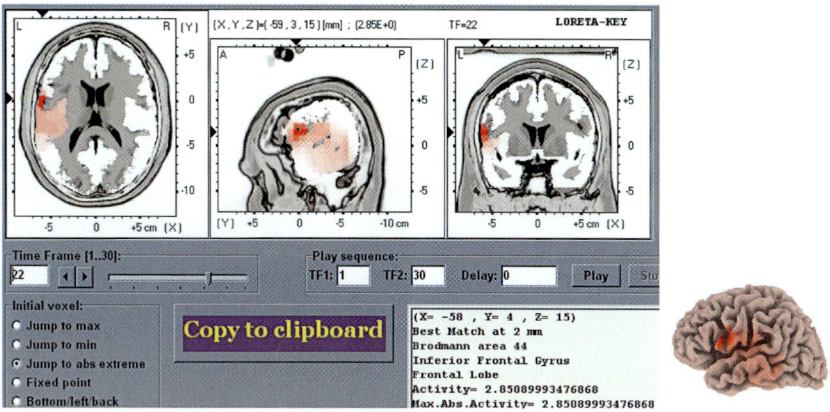

FIGURE 12.25 LORETA in case of MS showing left > right abnormality BA 44.

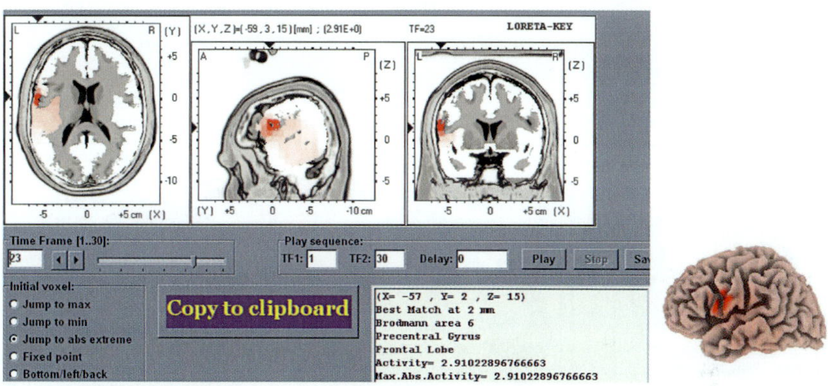

FIGURE 12.26 **LORETA in case of MS showing left > right abnormality BA 6.** This showed left greater than right frontal lobe dysfunction.

Thus LORETA does register the parietal abnormality seen in SPECT but appears that the left is slightly greater than the right in abnormality. Thus there is agreement as to where the deregulation is but disagreement on where it is most severe.

LORETA also shows temporal abnormality but left greater than right (Figure 12.30).

Patient SP was an unfortunate 7-year-old possibly left-handed white male who was born prematurely and sustained an intracerebral hemorrhage which left him permanently impaired. He was previously diagnosed with West syndrome, a severe seizure disorder, and treated with corticosteroids for a prolonged period of time. The patient was maintained on valproic acid and has not had any seizures in several years.

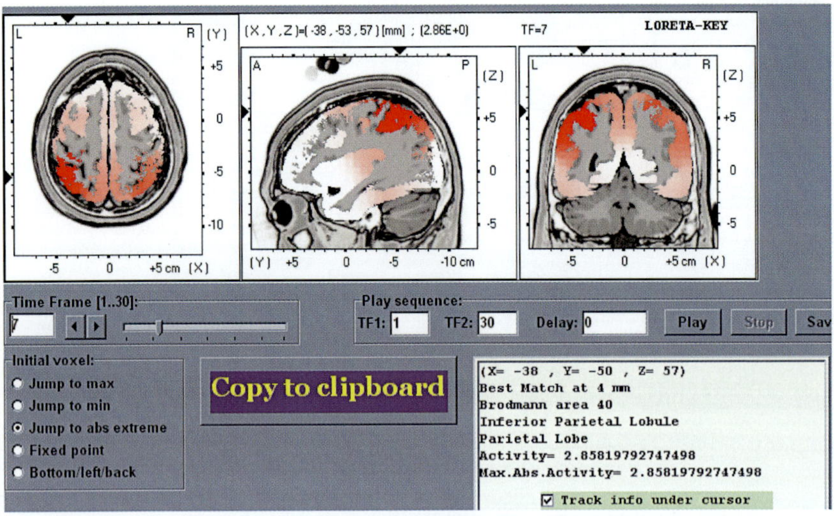

FIGURE 12.27 Case of MS LORETA BI lateral parietal deregulation left.
On the left it shows Z = 2.8
On the right it shows Z = 2.5

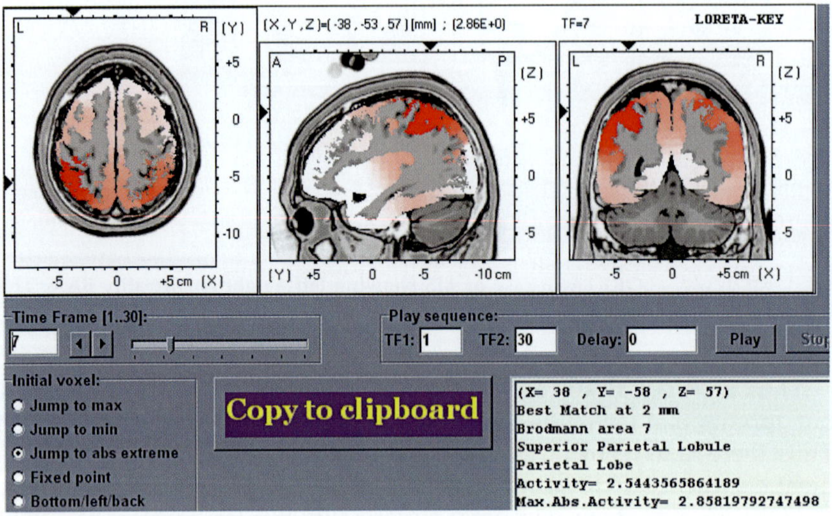

FIGURE 12.28 Case of MS LORETA BI lateral parietal deregulation right.

As other patients described in this report, this patient came to South Florida to undergo HB OT, and aggressive physical therapy in hopes of ameliorating his severe clinical condition. After undergoing a number of HB OT, his valproic acid dosage was reduced. However it was observed that after reduction of the medication, he started to develop jerking of the

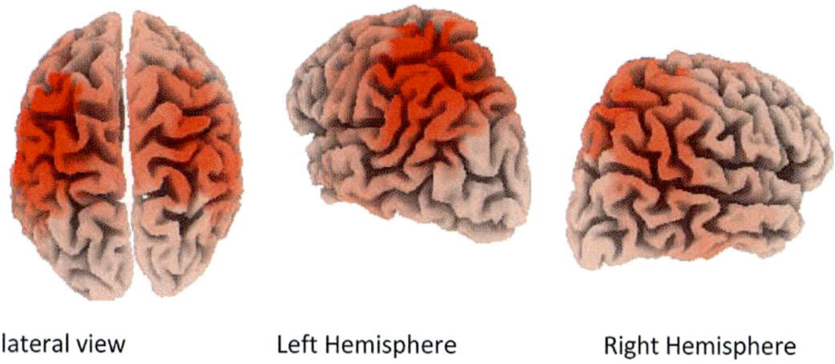

FIGURE 12.29 LORETA 3D images bilateral parietal deregulation case of MS.

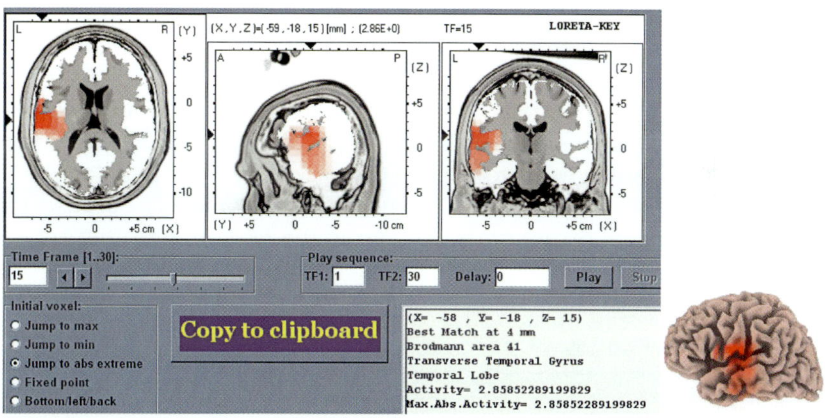

FIGURE 12.30 Case of MS LORETA temporal left > right.

arms which one author (PW) witnessed and it looked like a myoclonic jerk. While undergoing a PET scan, the patient had a combined CT scan of the brain. The PET scan was abnormal and did show hypometabolism in the basal ganglia, specifically the caudate nucleus, but normal metabolism in the cerebral cortex. Some degree of atrophy and hydrocephalus was also noted. Review of the films revealed in addition to the above, widening of the interhemispheric fissure anteriorly suggesting atrophy of the medial anterior frontal lobes, left greater than right. The author (PW) also thought that there was some hypometabolism in the temporal lobes, in particular the medial aspects, and possibly left greater than right. Another possibility was that there was some hypometabolism in the anterior temporal lobes as well. Other pertinent medical records revealed genetic testing indicating a specific mutation called 20210, with a substitution of guanine for adenosine. Routine EEG when he was approximately 4 1/2 years old was significantly abnormal, with evidence of spike wave paroxysmal abnormality posteriorly, and extending into the central and lateral regions. Neurological examination revealed a chronically ill-appearing young male, who was uncomfortable and crying most of the time in a stroller. He was awake alert but uncooperative to examination. He weighed about 50 pounds; head circumference was only 45 cm, and measured about 3 ft tall, indicating failure to thrive. Motor examination demonstrated classic spastic quadriparesis affecting lower greater than the uppers. Reflexes were not pathological. Cerebellar testing showed markedly truncal ataxia, requiring assistance to sit and control the head. The only frontal release sign was a positive glabella tap. The overall impression was spastic tetraplegia consistent with cerebral palsy, history of seizure disorder, and hypometabolism as described. The clinical question at the time was whether or not he needed more HB OT which could be only determined by SPECT scan. The SPECT scan was abnormal to a moderate and severe degree, with marked hypoperfusion seen anteriorly in the frontotemporal lobes, asymmetric worse on the left than right. There is also thinning of the cortical mantle with dilatation of the ventricles, correlation with CT or MRI for hydrocephalus ex vacuo. There is relative preservation of perfusion posteriorly in the parietal and occipital lobes.

LORETA absolute power will be used in this analysis because the Z scores are so extraordinary. Following is the table of absolute power (Table 12.9).

TABLE 12.9 LORETA Absolute Power Z Scores for SP

35 L	14.22
11 L	11.65
6 L	11.48
27 R	10.50
46 R	9.98
11 R	8.37
24 L	8.16
11 L	8.12
5 R	7.81
33 R	7.57
10 R	6.36
5 L	6.35
11 L	5.98
30 L	5.56
5 R	5.35

There are 8 left hemisphere and 7 right hemisphere Z scores of the top 15 that are abnormal. This makes this left greater than right abnormal. There are 9 frontal Z scores compared to 2 temporal Z scores that are abnormal making this frontal greater than temporal matching the SPECT scan.

In coherence, there were 10 nonrepeating BAs in the left frontal and 5 in the right frontal making left greater than right frontal. There were 3 BAs in the left temporal and 7 right temporal making this frontal greater than temporal but temporal right > left. There is agreement with the SPECT that frontal is greater than temporal, left greater than right frontal, but LORETA registers right temporal greater than left temporal. Not registered by SPECT but seen in coherence in LORETA is dysfunction in the right central area, right parietal, left and right posterior cingulate with L > R and left and right equally in the occipital. All of these however are less than the abnormalities seen in the frontal area making this anterior greater than posterior which is in agreement with SPECT. There is relative sparing of posterior areas but it is relative and not absolute as measured by LORETA coherence (Table 12.10).

In LORETA phase, there are 14 left hemisphere pairs and 5 right hemisphere pairs and one homologous pair BA 6 frontal. There are 10 left frontal BAs that are abnormal in Z scores and 4 right frontal making it frontal left greater than right which is in agreement with the SPECT. However, there are 14 BAs in the left temporal that are abnormal and 3 right temporal. The left > right agrees with SPECT but this makes the temporal area greater than the frontal area which is not in agreement with SPECT. Central BAs there is 1 abnormal and right 3 abnormal. In the parietal area there are 3 left and 1 right and 1 abnormal in the posterior cingulate. The occipital area shows 1 abnormal Z scored BA. This shows moderately good agreement with left greater than right generally but phase shows more abnormality than frontal. There is relative sparing of the posterior areas which makes this anterior greater than posterior also in agreement with SPECT (Table 12.11).

DISCUSSION

SPECT scans are a measure of perfusion and availability of oxygen to cells of the brain. The maps themselves are relative measures and are not compared to a database. LORETA on the other hand has a normative database and the conclusions reached about the patient's abnormalities using SPECT were reached by looking at the relative perfusion of areas and not absolute measures.

TABLE 12.10 LORETA Coherence Z Scores for SM

30 L–33 L	8.84	Delta
11 R–27 R	8.55	Delta
27 L–40 L	8.46	Delta
25 R–37 R	8.26	Delta
11 L–30 L	8.18	Delta
24 R–37 R	8.17	Delta
27 R–46 R	8.14	Delta
25 L–30 L	8.10	Delta
24 L–27 L	8.06	Delta
8 R–23 R	8.04	Delta
17 L–17 R	− 3.17	Delta
8 L–9 L	− 3.97	Alpha2
23 L–23 R	− 3.98	Delta
24 L–24 R	− 4.03	Beta2
2 R–3 R	− 4.50	Alpha1
28 R–Amy R	− 4.94	Alpha1
28 R–Amy R	− 5.80	Theta
8 L–9 L	− 6.53	Alpha1
8 L–9 L	− 7.41	Theta
28 R–Amy R	− 15.46	Delta

LORETA showed good to excellent agreement with SPECT as to hemisphere and lobe location though there were some differences in laterality in some lobe findings. This may be due to the following factors:

1. LORETA differences are matched against a database and is an absolute interval measure. SPECT is a relative and ordinal measure and therefore comparisons of the two may be due in part to the differences in level of measurement.
2. LORETA measures were normative and SPECT measures were not.
3. SPECT measures were localized and influenced by the structure of the circulatory system. LORETA measures, coherence, and phase are measures of connectivity and are influenced by network dynamics as well as blood flow and oxygen availability. LORETA measures may therefore be more sensitive to network characteristics and therefore

TABLE 12.11 LORETA Phase Z Scores for SP

27 L–33 L	4.82	Delta
2 R–4 R	4.60	Delta
4 L–40 L	4.59	Delta
3 R–9 R	4.58	Delta
1 L–4 L	4.57	Delta
33 L–35 L	4.30	Theta
13 L–40 L	4.10	Delta
1 R–27 R	4.10	Delta
6 L–6 R	4.02	Delta
27 R–40 R	3.99	Delta
21 L–35 L	− 4.17	Theta
34 L–35 L	− 4.39	Delta
6 R–17 R	− 4.40	Delta
33 L–40 L	− 4.44	Delta
30 L–47 L	− 4.47	Beta1
35 L–38 L	− 4.58	Delta
28 L–Amy L	− 4.62	Delta
35 L–45 L	− 4.84	Theta
27 L–45 L	− 4.87	Theta
27 L–47 L	− 5.19	Beta1

not measuring purely local phenomena, as SPECT is, but actually reflect the areas functional measurement in one or more networks.

4. LORETA measures' unit of analysis are groups of voxels organized categorized into cyto-architecturally homogeneous Brodmann area, a more specialized and precise measurement location/construct than can be seen on SPECT. In short, LORETA spatial resolution is better than SPECT.

This may account for the differences, but what of the large degree of agreement? This demonstrates that LORETA may not only be a measure of functional normality but of structural normality as well. This is consistent with Ghaziri's and colleagues' (Ghaziri, Tucholka, Larue, & Blanchette-Sylvestre, 2013) recent article showing that neurofeedback changes both gray and white matter and that LORETA may be a good measure for that. Indeed, LORETA registered changes not seen on

SPECT and some of those abnormalities were correlated with a thorough neurological exam suggesting LORETA may be more sensitive than the SPECT scan. However, the SPECT is a superior measure of oxygen presence or availability when compared to LORETA.

The next interesting question is what explanation might there be that LORETA coherence and phase were more sensitive to changes than current source density? SPECT is a measure of perfusion and the isotope "tags" the oxygen molecule and it is that emitting radiation that is recorded by the camera. Thus SPECT is a measure of the presence of oxygen, and oxygen presence correlates with SPECT when measuring oxygen extraction fractions in major cerebral artery occlusive disease (Chida et al., 2011). Less perfusion means ischemia or hypoxia. In fact SPECT highly correlates with PET/CT and was found to be equally useful, and therefore a lower cost alternative in detection of recurrent glioma (Karunanithi et al., 2014).

After trauma there is swelling and edema, sometimes microscopic, which would put pressure on local vessels and restrict blood flow. Gray and white matter relaxation times have been linked to EEG coherence (Thatcher, Biver, & Salazar, 1998). This early seminal article is reinforced most recently in Thornton's review of this area where he gives a good description of some of the trauma mechanics when he writes:

> A neurochemical cascade develops immediately following the biomechanical trauma to the brain and involves a multitude of cellular changes. The biomechanical effects are the stretching and tearing of the axons. Edema (fluid) and leakage occur in the axon as a result of the physical trauma. ... The neuronal membranes are negatively affected. The axonal stretching leads to an increase in extracellular potassium which is then followed by subsequent depolarization and then a release of excitatory neurotransmitters...This sequence includes a loss of ionic gradients, apoptosis (cell death), cell depolarization, cytotoxic edema (swelling of the cell elements), glutamate release, and many other biochemical effects. ... the neuron breaks down, the axon splits into two sections, a retraction ball (collection of cytoplasm) is formed at the end of the axon and Wallerian degeneration occurs which result in axonal collapse and ***resultant disconnection effects***... (emphasis added) (Thornton, 2014, p. 348).

Connectivity measures are crucial measures and sensitive to damage caused by trauma because they reflect network connections. Networks are disrupted by this process, i.e., the effects of the insults are not merely focal or local though one may be able to localize them using SPECT or LORETA. Coherence and phase are measures of network regulation and are affected by trauma (Thatcher, 2006). Coherence has been specifically used to measure effects of ischemia and with the use of Granger causality analysis can also indicate direction of information flow (Chen, Maybhale, Israel, Thakor, & Jia, 2013). Ischemia in cardiac cases showed altered synchronous gamma (phase) and anterior posterior connectivity (Borjigin et al., 2013), and coherence changes in network patterns in ischemic stroke (Zhu et al., 2009). But this is not related to trauma as coherence in current source density and LORETA is found in psychiatric disorders as well (Velikova, Locatelli, Insacco, Comi, & Leocani, 2010). Trauma can cause vasospasm and vasospasm can affect phase (Otite et al., 2014) and coherence (de Vico Fallani et al., 2009).

In general both increase and decrease in CBF influences neuronal activity though decrease and increase CBF may originate from different mechanisms, they both affect neuronal activity, correlate with it, (Mullinger, Mayhew, Bagashaw, Bowtell, & Francis, 2014) thus further linking SPECT and LORETA conceptually and empirically. And, blood flow is linked to coherence even in neonates (Simpson, BoteroRosas, & Infantosi, 2005). Ischemia not only affects activity of pyramidal cells but also astrocytes and thus their role in regulating calcium increases. Their increased presence was correlated with "neuronal anoxic depolarization... [and] altered gap junction mediated intercellular network ..." under conditions of oxygen deprivation (Shinotsuka, Yasui, & Nuriya, 2014, p. 171).

It would appear then, subject to additional research and confirmation, that LORETA coherence and phase highly correlate with SPECT results because the damage to cells secondary to hypoperfusion and thereby oxygen deprivation affects metabolically and structurally the ability of neurons to participate in networks and to communicate with other neurons and to so consistently over time when they are connected.

Confirmation of, and extension of, these findings would be helped by replication of SPECT LORETA analysis using LORETA phase reset statistics such as LORETA Phase Shift Duration and LORETA Phase Lock Duration.

These correlations between SPECT and specifically LORETA coherence and LORETA phase demonstrate both concurrent and construct validity for LORETA measures and thus lend a solid basis for the results clinicians obtain using LORETA Z score feedback.

CONCLUSION

The data in this chapter demonstrates that LORETA has very good to excellent concurrent validity, construct validity and coregistration with SPECT scans. It further suggests that LORETA may not only a good functional but also possibly a structural measure of change in the brain. The data further suggests that the usefulness of SPECT could be improved by the development of a normative database which would provide an easier set of comparisons to other measures and possibly improve spatial resolution of the SPECT scan. LORETA appears therefore to be a sound measure to guide treatment and correlate with other measures for diagnosis (Table 12.12).

TABLE 12.12 Summary Results Table

Case	SPECT	Agreement Hemisphere	Agreement Lobe	Disagree Lobe	LORETA only
1.KL	DIFFUSE, FT SYMMETRIC; POST? R > L	100% match.	LORETA found 16/20 = 80% in coherence and 18/20 = 90% in phase highest as FT match.		POST CINGULATE consistent with symptoms.
2.LB	R > L TEMPORAL, RIGHT SUP FRONTAL L OCCIPITAL > LEFT PARIETAL (TBI, COUP CONTRECOUP)	100% match.	100% LORETA		PARIETAL > OCCIPITAL
3.TS	DIFFUSE, ANT > POST, R > L ANT, L > R POST (TBI, COUP CONTRECOUP)	Right > Left match in coherence; ANT > POST match.	Anterior > Posterior match.	L > R Phase.	AREAS CONSISTENT WITH SYMPTOMS, NEURO EXAM, and COHERENCE.
4.AE	SEVERE R > L FRONTOTEMPORAL, LEFT SUP FRONTAL SUP, LAT; LEFT POST PARIETAL/ANT OCCIPITAL	Left > right match			DIFFUSE, CONSISTENT WITH HISTORY.
5.RA	SEVERE, ANT > POST, FRONTOTEMPORAL,? R > L, BASAL GANGLIA, CEREBELLUM	Match, R > L.	Match, R > L FT on Current Source density; Match R Frontal.		

6.JK	DIFFUSE, ANT > POST, R > L FRONTAL TEMPORAL, BIPARIETAL/ OCCIPITAL	Match at 95%, R > L.	95% agreement by lobe. Major difference is in the Occipital in coherence and phase.	Bioccipital in coherence and phase	
7.GC	L > R FRONTOTEMPORAL > BIOCCIPITAL	Match at 100% L > R.	Match at 100%, L > R FT in phase and coherence; Match BIOCC in phase only. Coherence did not disagree		
8.TA	R > L FRONTAL, ANT, INF; L > R TEMPORAL; R > L OCCIPITAL	Match, L > R TEMPORAL	Matches the same lobes as abnormal.	R > L FRONT, OCCIPITAL	
9.MS	L > R FRONTAL, L > R TEMPORAL;R > L PARIETAL (TBI, COUP CONTRECOUP)	Match L > F Frontal.	Match in L > R Frontal, and shows L > R other lobes except temporal,? parietal both hemispheres	? R > L Temp. ? Parietal	
10.SP	L > R FRONTOTEMPORAL, THINNING OF CORTEX, HYDROCEPHALUS	Match L > R Frontal in absolute power.	Match Frontal and Temporal, but Temporal lobe hemisphere disagreement. Absolute power lobe matches SPECT with Frontal > Temporal.	Temporal Coherence and phase. F > T in absolute power.	

SUMMARY OF TABULAR FINDINGS

1. Hemispheric agreement is 10/10 = 100%.
2. Lobar agreement is 9/10 = 90%.

TABLE OF FIGURES

References

Al-Khindi, T., Macdonald, R., & Schweizer, T. (2010). Cognitive and functional outcome after aneurysmal subarachnoid hemorrhage. *Stroke, 41*(8), e519–e536.

Bonne, O., & Gilboa, A. (2003). Cerebral blood flow in chronic symptomatic mild traumatic brain injury. *Psychiatry Research, 124*(3), 141–152.

Bonne, O., Gilboa, A., & Louzoun, Y. (2003). Cerebral blood flow in chronic symptomatic mild traumatic brain injury. *Psychiatry Research, 124*(3), 141–152.

Borjigin, J., et al. (2013). Surge of neurophysiological coherence and connectivity in the dying Brain. *PNAS*14432–14437.

Catafau, A. (2001). Brain SPECT in clinical practice. Part I: Perfusion. *Journal of Nuclear Medicine, 42*(2), 259–271.

Chen, C., Maybhale, A., Israel, D., Thakor, N., & Jia, X. (2013). Assessing thalamocortical functional connectivity with granger causality. *IEEE Transactions on Neural Systems and Rehabilitation Engineering*, 725–733.

Chida, K., et al. (2011). Central benzodiazepine receptor binding potential and CBF images on SPECT correlate with oxygen extraction fractio images on PET in the cerebral cortex with unilateral major cerebral artery occlusive disease. *Journal of Nuclear Medicine*, 511–518.

Clark, D., Boutros, N., & Mendez, M. (2010). *Brain and behavior*. New York, NY: Cambridge University Press.

Fabrizio De, Vico Fallani, Laura, Astolfi, Febo, Cincotti, Donatella, Mattia, Daria la, Rocca, Elira, Maksuti, et al. (2009). Evaluation of the Brain Network Organization from EEG signals. *The Anatomical Record*, 2023–2031.

Emerson, C., Pette, C., & Wright, D. (2012). *<http://web.eng.fiu.edu/godavart/bme4531-sp12/spect_student_ppt_spring2012.pdf>*. Retrieved march 2014, from fiu.edu: <http://ebook-browsee.net/gdoc.php?id = 357618525&url = cd6bd687f06d12d251f364701d3101d0>.

Ghaziri, J., Tucholka, A., Larue, V., & Blanchette-Sylvestre, M. (2013). Neurofeedback training induces changes in white and gray matter. *Clinical EEG and Neuroscience*, 1–8.

Goffin, K., Dedeurwaerdere, S., Van Laere, K., et al. (2008). Neuronuclear assessment of patients with epilepsy. *Seminars in Nuclear Medicine*, *38*(4), 227–239.

Hütter, B., Kreitschmann-Andermahr, I., & Mayfrank, L. (1999). Functional outcome after aneurysmal subarachnoid hemorrhage. *Acta Neurochirurgica Supplement*, *72*, 157–174.

Ichise, M., Chung, D., & Wang, P. (1994). *Journal of Nuclear Medicine*, *35*(2), 217–226.

Karunanithi, S., et al. (2014). Prospective comparison of (99m)Tc-GH SPECT/CT and (18)F-FDOPA PET/CT for detection of recurrent Glioma: A Pilot study. *Clinical Nuclear Medicine*, 121–128.

Mullinger, K., Mayhew, S., Bagashaw, A., Bowtell, R., & Francis, S. (2014). Evidence of negative BOLD response is neuronal in origin: A simultaneous EEG-BOLD-CBF study in humans. *Neuroimage*, 263–274.

Mustonen, T., Koivisto, T., Vanninen, R., & Hänninen, T. (2008). Heterogeneity of cerebral perfusion 1 week after haemorrhage is an independent predictor of clinical outcome in patients with aneurysmal subarachnoid haemorrhage. *Journal of Neurology Neurosurgery and Psychiatry*, *79*(10), 1128–1133.

Ohkuma, H., Suzuki, S., & Kudo, K. (2003). Cortical blood flow during cerebral vasospasm after aneurysmal subarachnoid hemorrhage: Three-dimensional *N*-isopropyl-*p*-[(123)I] iodoamphetamine single photon emission CT findings. *AJNR American Journal of Neuroradiology*, *24*(3), 444–450.

Otite, F., et al. (2014). Impaired cerebral autoregulation is associated with vasospasm and delayed cerebral ischemia in subarachnoid hemorrhage. *Stroke*, 677–682.

Otte, A., Ettlin, T., & Nitzsche, E. (1997). PET and SPECT in whiplash syndrome: A new approach to a forgotten brain? *Journal of Neurology Neurosurgery and Psychiatry*, *63*(3), 368–372.

Piskunowicz, M., Krzyzanowski, M., & Piotr, L. (2003). The usefulness of CBF brain SPECT in forensic medicine: The civil law code cases. A description of four cases. *Nuclear Medicine Review*, *6*(1), 45–47.

Shinotsuka, T., Yasui, M., & Nuriya, M. (2014). Astrocytic gap NJunctinal networks suppress cellular damage in an in vitro model of ischemia. *Biochemical and Biophysical Research Communications*, 171–176.

Simpson, D., BoteroRosas, D., & Infantosi, A. (2005). Estimation of coherence between blood flow and spontaneous EEG activity in neonates. *IEEE Transactions on Bio-Medical Engineering*, 852–858.

Slobounov, S., Gay, M., Johnson, B., & Zhang, K. (2012). Concussion in athletics: Ongoing clinical and brain imaging research controversies. *Brain Imaging and Behavior*, *6*(2), 224–243.

Thatcher, R. (2006). Electroencephalography and mild traumatic brain injury. In S. Slobounov, & W. Sebastianelli (Eds.), *Foundations in sports related brain injuries* (pp. 241–266). New York, NY: Springer.

Thatcher, R., Biver, C. M., & Salazar, A. (1998). Biophysical linkage between MRI and EEG coherence in closed head injury. *Neuroimage*, 307–326.

Thornton, K. (2014). The role of quantitative EEG in the diagnosis and rehabilitation of traumatic brain injury patients. In S. Slobounov, & W. Sebastianelli (Eds.), *Concussion in athletes* (pp. 345–362). New York, NY: Springer.

Uchikawa, K., Inaba, M., & Kagami, H. (2014). Executive dysfunction is related with decreased frontal lobe blood flow in patients with subarachnoid haemorrhage. *Brain Injury*, *28*(1), 15–19.

Umile, E., Sandel, M., & Alavi, A. (2002). Dynamic imaging in mild traumatic brain injury: Support for the theory of medial temporal vulnerability. *Archives of Physical Medicine and Rehabilitation*, *83*(11), 1506–1513.

Van Paesschen, W. (2004). Ictal SPECT. *Epilepsia*, *45*(Suppl. 4), 35–40.

Velikova, S., Locatelli, M., Insacco, C. E., Comi, G., & Leocani, L. (2010). Dysfunctional brain circuitry in obsessive compulsive disorder: Source and coherence analysis of EEG rhythms. *Neuroimage*, 977–983.

Wortzel, H., Filley, C., & Anderson, C. (2008). Forensic applications of cerebral single photon emission computed tomography in mild traumatic brain injury. *The Journal of the American Academy of Psychiatry and the Law*, *36*(3), 310–322.

Zhu, C., Guo, X., Wu, W., Jin, Z., Qiu, Y., & Tong, S. (2009). Influence of subcortical ischemic stroke on cortical neural network. *Conference Proceedings IEEE Engineering in Medicine and Biology Society*, 18–21.

APPENDIX

Typical SPECT Scan Report

PROCEDURE: Technetium 99 mm Ceretec SPECT Brain Scan

INDICATION: TBI with post-concussion syndrome, rule out hypoperfusion.

Performed at Boca Nuclear Medicine.

Multiple time sequential scintophotos of the head were performed following the IV bolus injection of Technetium 99 mm Ceretec. There is prompt bilateral symmetric visualization of the carotids. Bilateral symmetric uptake in the middle cerebral arteries and anterior cerebral arteries is seen. There is normal diffusion of tracer seen within the capillary phase throughout both hemispheres. These findings are consistent with a normal CBF study. The washout phase cannot be evaluated when using Technetium 99 mm Ceretec, which crosses the blood–brain barrier and remains bound.

Single photon emission computerized tomography (SPECT) imaging was performed following the injection of Technetium 99 mm Ceretec. Imaging was begun 50 min following the IV injection, allowing the Ceretec to localize in the brain. Tomographic reconstruction was performed in the axial, coronal, and sagittal planes. Technetium 99 mm Ceretec acts as a "chemical microsphere," crossing the blood–brain barrier and remaining trapped in brain tissue with a distribution that is proportional to blood flow. Ceretec does cross the blood–brain barrier by passive diffusion by merging with the lipid molecules that make up the membranes of the capillaries and brain tissue. Ceretec cannot diffuse back across the blood–brain barrier into the capillaries. More than 70% of initial brain uptake remains fixed in the brain up to 24 h postinjection, allowing enough time to perform SPECT imaging. Ceretec does not exhibit intracellular redistribution patterns over time.

In all image planes, cerebral white matter shows notably less intense Technetium 99 mm Ceretec uptake and therefore shows a light gray appearance on SPECT images. Blood flow to gray matter is approximately four times greater than to white matter. Therefore, there is a higher Ceretec activity in the periphery which corresponds to the cortical gray matter than there is centrally in the SPECT images.

(*Continued*)

PATIENT:

DATE: January 29, 2014

PROCEDURE: Technetium 99 mm Ceretec SPECT Brain Scan

INDICATION: TBI with post-concussion syndrome, rule out hypoperfusion.

PAGE: 2

Following the injection of intravenous Ceretec, there is prompt and symmetric uptake of the carotid extra cranial blood flow. The intracranial blood flow appears symmetric except for a possible decrease in the left inferior frontal lobes seen best on image #5. On the 2D images, there is some relative decrease or hypoperfusion seen in the left greater than right superior frontal lobes. This does continue high over the convexity of the frontal lobes, seen best on the axial slices 14 through 16. In addition, the temporal lobes are not well perfused, as demonstrated best on the coronal slices. In particular, slice 11 shows some perfusion of the right temporal lobe and less perfusion of the left temporal lobe. Finally on the 3D reconstructed images, there is more clear hypoperfusion seen in the left frontal lobe, both inferiorly, continuing superiorly, and seen best on Figure 12.1 which is the AP view of line 1. The left temporal lobe hypoperfusion is confirmed on the left lateral view which is image #13 of line 4, and on the left anterior obliques, which shows some widening of the Sylvian fissure. The PA view which is image #9 of line 3 clearly demonstrates a decrease of flow on the right side, in the occipital and parietal lobes. This is seen again on the right posterior obliques of line 2 including Figures 12.5–12.8 respectively. The right temporal lobe hypoperfusion is also seen on the right lateral view which is Figure 12.4 of line 1 and the right anterior obliques of line 1 as well. Incidental note is made up of uptake of isotope outside of the brain, bilaterally and inferior to the temporal lobes, most likely representing incidental sinus disease.

Impression: Abnormal Ceretec brain SPECT.

1. **Hypoperfusion seen in the left frontal temporal lobes.**
2. **Hypoperfusion seen in the right occipital parietal temporal lobe.**
3. **The latter topography, coupled with a history of trauma, is characteristic of a coup contrecoup.**
4. **Normal dynamic flow study.**
5. **Correlation with ancillary diagnostic testing suggested.**

CHAPTER

13

Brainsurfer and Brain Computer Interface Z-Score Biofeedback

Robert W. Thatcher, Carl J. Biver and Duane M. North

NeuroImaging Laboratory, Applied Neuroscience, Inc., Seminole, FL, USA

The term brain–computer interface (BCI) is a type of electroencephalogram (EEG) biofeedback or neurofeedback (NFB) procedure in which particular EEG activity is detected, and then, subjects are trained to increase the probability of that EEG activity linked to a device like a computer display or robot or prosthesis. BCI uses the same physiological principles of operant conditioning as with EEG biofeedback to increase the probability of occurrence of a particular EEG event or feature. However, BCI differs from EEG biofeedback by the use of a continuous control loop between the brain and physical device or prosthesis and focusing primarily on modifications of motor cortical–subcortical networks. For example, in NFB, when a given brain event reaches threshold, then a feedback signal is delivered (sound or visual display or DVD) to reinforce the brain event at that moment in time. The goal is to modify the synapses involved in producing a given brain event, and when a threshold is met, a discrete feedback signal is delivered to achieve increased stability in networks linked to symptoms. BCI also involves modification of a selected brain event but differs by a continuous feedback loop between the subject and the subject's own brain directly instead of turning on or off a feedback signal if a threshold criteria is met. Thus, both involve operant conditioning but with a different emphasis on the way that an external device is controlled by the brain. BCI is continuous and intimate by a real-time loop involving a real-time view of the subject's own brain, while NFB involves a discrete threshold being met that turns on or off a feedback signal like a DVD or video.

BCI was developed in the 1990s to help locked-in and paralyzed patients gain control over an external device (Birbaumer, Ghanayim, &

Z Score Neurofeedback.
DOI: http://dx.doi.org/10.1016/B978-0-12-801291-8.00013-3

Hinterberger, 1999). In contrast, NFB began with simple alpha rhythm operant conditioning in the 1940s and then was more fully developed using digital computers in the 1960s to modify the firing rate of single neurons or groups of neurons. From the 1970s to today, modification of the EEG is designed to improve functioning in individuals with various psychological problems and also patients with epilepsy (Fox & Rudell, 1968; Lubar & Shouse, 1976; Sterman & Friar, 1972). Therefore, the applications and the neurophysiology of instrumental learning are shared, but currently, BCI is mostly used as a type of prosthesis for severely impaired patients, whereas NFB is used more in less severe clinical disorders and also in a wider range of clinical disorders. Both BCI and NFB use frequency domain EEG signals such as sensorimotor rhythms (SMRs) or event-related synchronization and desynchronization or instantaneous Z scores. Also, both involve operant or instrumental learning in which synapses and networks are altered in order to increase the probability of occurrence of the threshold event.

Figure 13.1 is an example of EEG biofeedback or NFB. The top of Figure 13.1 is standard non-Z-score NFB in which an arbitrary threshold

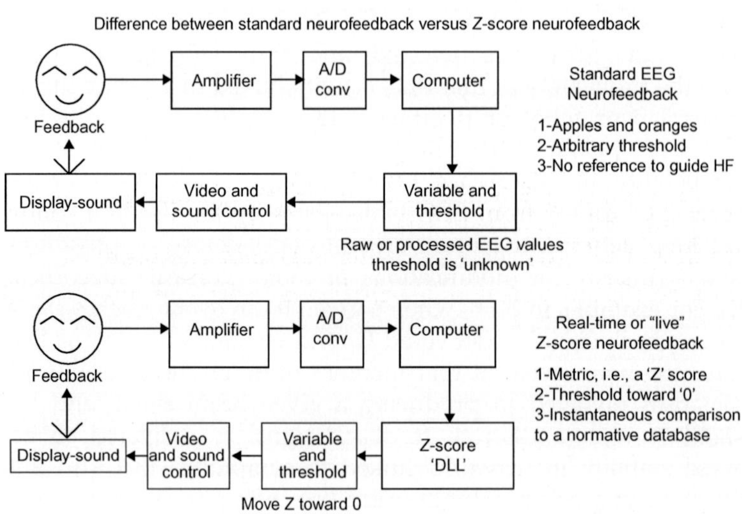

FIGURE 13.1 Top row is conventional or standard EEG biofeedback in which different units of measurement are used in an EEG analysis (e.g., μV for amplitude, theta/beta ratios, relative power 0–100%, coherence 0–1, phase in degrees or radians), and the clinician must "guess" at a threshold for a particular electrode location and frequency and age to when to reinforce or inhibit a give measure. The bottom row is Z-score biofeedback in which different metrics are represented by a single and common metric, i.e., the metric of a Z score and the guess work is removed, because all measures are reinforced to move Z scores toward Z = 0, which is the approximate center of an average healthy brain state based on a reference age-matched normative database in real time.

is set by a clinician by guessing at a threshold. Once the threshold is met, a sound or visual signal is delivered to the patient as a reinforcer or prediction of a future reward.

The absolute threshold shown in the top for Figure 13.1 is arbitrary, because the clinician must use subjective judgment to decide on an absolute EEG value based on his or her personal experiences or "rumors" without the support of scientific publications nor the support of physics and statistics. Instead, the clinician must use subjective judgment and decide, "Do I reinforce alpha rhythms if they are greater than 5 μV or maybe 10 μV or 15 μV or 25 μV?" or "Do I inhibit theta if it is greater than 5 μV or 10 μV or whatever?" In other words, unlike with Z scores, there is no standardization when using absolute values, because the skull thickness and brain of each individual are different. However, the fact is that all physical attributes including subatomic particles in physics are Gaussian distributed or can be transformed to Gaussian. Because essential physical attributes are Gaussian distributed, therefore, the science of statistics and physics can be applied, and it is not necessary to "guess" or use subjective "insights" or "dreams" to decide on a threshold. The bottom of Figure 13.1 illustrates the use of a Z score as a statistical reference based on Gaussian statistics and the physics of the EEG. The real-time Z score simplifies BCI and NFB by providing an instantaneous "guide" or "reference" with respect to a group of healthy functioning individuals with no history of neurological or psychological disorders. This means that statistics and physical principles allow one to apply modern neuroscience to an energetic 2.5 pounds of mass that is continually modifying itself called "neuroplasticity." The science of synapse growth and operant conditioning when combined with modern physics and statistics can successfully replace "guessing" about how a clinician can modify the brain to help reduce symptoms without medications and with low risk of an abreaction (Thatcher, 2012).

Figure 13.2 shows a general schema for BCI systems.

BCI involves an instantaneous feedback loop between the patient's brain, consciousness/subconsciousness, and a device. Conscious strategies and willful acts are a part of BCI as well as subconscious processes, because there is an immediate and continuous feedback between the brain and a device. NFB differs, because it involves a threshold that triggers a discrete feedback signal (e.g., a DVD or video) that is linked back in time like a memory trace. Often, conscious or willful attempts to receive more feedback signals fail, and instead, subjects relax and subconscious process (basal ganglia–limbic–brain stem) are involved and not the frontal cortex and cognitive strategies. In summary, BCI is continuous emphasizing cognitive strategies, while NFB is discrete emphasizing subconscious (nonwillful) processes.

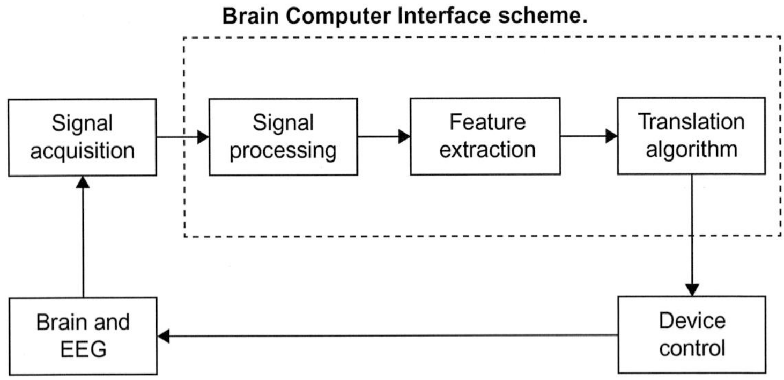

FIGURE 13.2 General technical scheme for BCI systems. Note that this scheme is also the same for EEG biofeedback or NFB by placing a threshold box between the translation algorithm and the device control (see Figure 13.1). That is, with NFB, when a threshold is reached, a discrete feedback event occurs such as a sound, visual display, or turning on or off a DVD player. BCI involves a continuous closed loop between the patient's brain and a device in real time.

An example of BCI that involves continuous feedback but is used for similar purposes as discrete NFB is the Brainsurfer program. Brainsurfer is the patient's own brain rendered by a magnetic resonance imaging (MRI) that provides real-time and continuous feedback about the stability of nodes and connections between nodes in networks of the brain linked to the patient's symptoms. A discrete feedback signal is not used, instead, a moment-to-moment continuous closed loop between the patient and the patient's brain is used as the feedback signal, and the goal is to modify the brain to reach increased levels of stability and information processing efficiency in particular networks. Brodmann areas are considered as nodes, and the cortico–cortical white matter axons are the connections between the nodes. Reinforcement of increased stability in dysregulated nodes and connections between nodes is achieved by real-time low-resolution electromagnetic tomography (LORETA) Z scores. As explained previously, extinction of extreme Z scores that indicate dysregulation and reinforcement of increased stability and efficiency is likely to result in increased information processing in modules and hubs linked to the patient's symptoms. A clinician can zoom inside of the 3D-rendered brain to a specific node or a specific connection between nodes to increase specificity of instrumental learning, in particular Brodmann areas or functional connections between Brodmann areas in real time. Both conscious strategies and subcortical unconscious processes are involved in BCI and NFB.

Figure 13.3 illustrates the brain-to-brain aspect of BCI, when nodes and connections of nodes are the "devices" to be controlled.

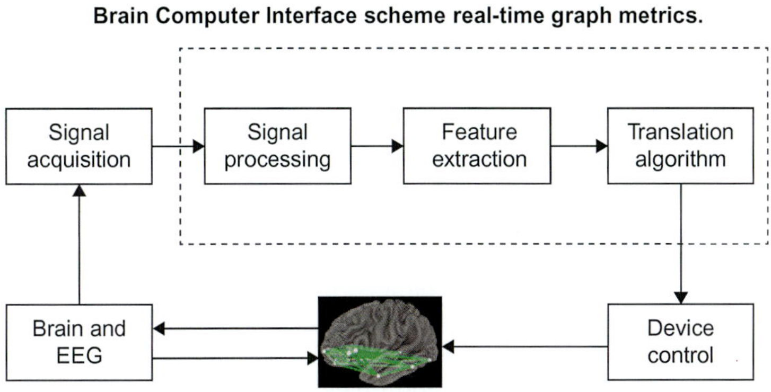

FIGURE 13.3 The scheme is the standard BCI scheme as shown in Figure 13.2. However, the device controls are real-time brain node current density and functional connections between nodes that involve a feedback loop between the patient and the instantaneous state of the patient's brain nodes and functional connections. *From the Neuroguide Brainsurfer program. A You Tube video is a good method to understand this example of BCI at http://youtu.be/wBy0iI0ugBI.*

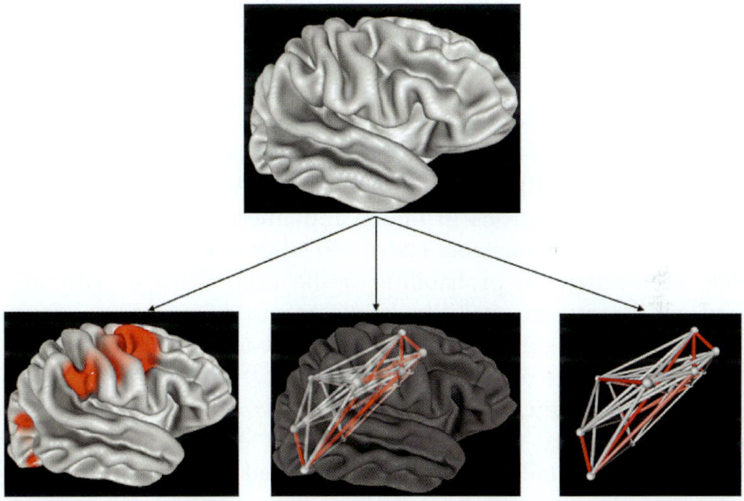

FIGURE 13.4 Example of the Brainsurfer. Top middle is the fully rendered MRI, lower left is the LORETA current source projections to the scalp surface of Z scores greater than two standard deviations of the dorsal executive attention network. Lower middle is real-time Z scores of coherence between the nodes or Brodmann areas of the dorsal attention network in which the red color is Z scores greater than two standard deviations. The brain was made 50% transparent so that the patient can view his or her own dorsal attention network and the connections between Brodmann areas that make up the attention network. Lower right is the same as the lower middle, but transparency is 100%. The goal of the closed loop continuous feedback is for the patient to make the connections between Brodmann areas and/or connections that are white or green when threshold is met.

CONSCIOUS VERSUS UNCONSCIOUS OPERANT CONDITIONING IS NEUROPHYSIOLOGICALLY THE SAME

There are three important facts that must be recognized: (1) Human subjects are not aware of their own EEG, (2) even single neurons can be operantly conditioned, and (3) human subjects can modify the EEG by imagining objects and movements and memories. This means that the human EEG can be consciously changed by will and thought and also that EEG can be changed by unconscious processes, and BCI versus NFB is a procedural difference that achieves the same outcome, i.e., an improved clinical condition by synaptic modification in networks. The difference between BCI and NFB is made even more irrelevant by the fact that the two share the same molecular and synaptic processes. That is, EEG biofeedback and BCI share the same Nobel Prize neuroscience of synapse modification and long-term potentiation processes of operant conditioning of loops of neurons also called instrumental learning (Kandel, 2006). This means that the difference between frontal lobe strategies to change the EEG or basal ganglia and subcortical learning is a matter of emphasis or focus on iterations in a particular network or module or hub with brief phase shift and lock of millions of neurons in small collections for brief periods of time. Dopamine and other neuromodulators reinforce and select circuits and loops that adaptively mediate a stable and reinforced outcome. The brain stem–limbic–cortical structure of the brain with cortex and subcortex adaptively coordinated and controlled by metastable phase shifts between groups of neurons in nodes and hubs of networks is a never-ending sequence of metastable states. Whether conscious or unconscious or both, increasing the probability of the occurrence of synchrony or reduced synchrony and stability between particular groups of neurons linked to symptoms is the goal of EEG biofeedback and BCI.

BCI provides more opportunity for cognitive strategies to change particular nodes and functional connections between nodes than standard EEG biofeedback that involves a secondary feedback signal such as a DVD or video or sound. For example, a patient with generalized anxiety disorder and/or posttraumatic stress disorder (PTSD) can focus on his or her own amygdala and lateral and medial frontal lobes in real time and then by cognitive strategy or by evoking memories of events can monitor his or her own brain nodes and connections by continuous feedback and thereby modify these brain regions in real time.

References

Birbaumer, N., Ghanayim, N., Hinterberger, T., Iversen, I., Kotchoubey, B., Kubler, A., et al. (1999). A spelling device for the paralysed. *Nature, 398*, 297–298.

Fox, S. S., & Rudell, A. P. (1968). Operant controlled neural event: Formal and systematic approach to electrical coding of behavior in brain. *Science, 162*(3859), 1299–1302.

Kandel, E. R. (2006). *In search of memory*. New York, NY: W.W. Norton.

Lubar, J. F., & Shouse, M. N. (1976). EEG and behavioral changes in a hyperkinetic child concurrent with training of the sensorimotor rhythm (SMR): A preliminary report. *Biofeedback and Self-Regulation, 1*(3), 293–306.

Sterman, M. B., & Friar, L. (1972). Suppression of seizures in an epileptic following sensorimotor EEG feedback training. *Electroencephalography and Clinical Neurophysiology, 33*(1), 89–95.

Thatcher, R. W. (2012). *Handbook of quantitative electroencephalography and EEG biofeedback*. St. Petersburg, FL: Ani Publishing.

CHAPTER

14

LORETA Neurofeedback in College Students with ADHD

Scott L. Decker, Alycia M. Roberts and Jessica J. Green

University of South Carolina, Barnwell College, Columbia, SC, USA

Attention deficit hyperactivity disorder (ADHD) is a psychiatric disorder characterized by behavioral symptoms in three main areas—hyperactivity, impulsivity, and inattention. Per the fifth edition of the Diagnostic and Statistical Manual of Mental Disorders (DSM-V), there are three subtypes of ADHD—predominately hyperactive/impulsive, predominately inattentive, and combined type—each of which is classified based on a number of behavioral symptoms (APA, 2013). One of the key factors in diagnosing and understanding ADHD is that the symptoms are pervasive across multiple settings. Additionally, the comorbidity between ADHD and other psychiatric disorders is high, with learning disabilities, depression, and anxiety frequently codiagnosed conditions (Decker, McIntosh, Kelly, Nicholls, & Dean, 2001). ADHD is also a neurodevelopmental disorder, which suggests that while the symptoms change as an individual develops, the disorder continues to affect those individuals across their lifespan (Das, Cherbuin, Easteal, & Anstey, 2014; Fredriksen et al., 2014).

Symptomatology in ADHD is multifactorial; thus, ADHD is a heterogeneous disability. Some research has suggested that the subtypes currently used do not fully encompass the spectrum of the disorder (i.e., Barkley, 2001, 2003; Milich, Balentine, & Lyman, 2001). Diagnosis is still highly dependent on behavioral observations and testing. In part, symptomatology is related to normative standards of development. For instance, being "driven as a motor" and difficulty inhibiting behavior is typical for children at a certain developmental level. However, when these difficulties

Z Score Neurofeedback.
DOI: http://dx.doi.org/10.1016/B978-0-12-801291-8.00014-5

continue into late childhood and early adolescence, they become problematic. Additionally, inattentive behaviors often go unnoticed, particularly in younger children when cognitive demands are kept low. Furthermore, the presentation of ADHD can change across development. Regardless of the exact presentation of the disorder, these difficulties with classification have resulted in significant heterogeneity of how individuals are identified as having ADHD. Consequently, research studies that use participants with a previous diagnosis of ADHD likely involve significant confounds involving the origins of symptomatology. As an inevitable consequence, treatment plans for many individuals with ADHD will be ineffective because most treatment options are based on a categorical diagnosis of behavioral symptomatology without specification of individualistic factors or determination of the underlying causes.

Developmentally, ADHD symptoms are present from preschool to adulthood (Guldberg-Kjar & Johansson, 2013; Scholtens, Rydell, & Yang-Wallentin, 2013; Washbrook, Propper, & Sayal, 2013). However, symptom manifestation may differ across developmental ages. For instance, hyperactivity may be the primary symptom in childhood; whereas working memory (WM) deficits may be the primary symptoms in adulthood (Kim, Liu, Glizer, Tannock, & Woltering, 2013). Children with ADHD are often distinguished by an inability to inhibit their behavior despite an awareness of appropriate behavioral standards (Nigg, 2013). Disruptive behavior, which is typically the primary reason for referral, may be paramount despite having an understanding of the appropriate behaviors within a given context. Although they may be able to verbally explain what they "should" do, they may still be unable to actually complete the motor act. Although children with ADHD do not have significant deficits in language, with possible exceptions in language pragmatics (Green, Johnson, & Bretherton, 2014), they may have significant difficulty in using language to regulate their own behavior (Petersen et al., 2013).

CHALLENGES IN TREATING ADHD IN COLLEGE-AGED POPULATIONS

The transition to early adulthood is often tumultuous for individuals with ADHD. In part, life outcomes depend on the environmental and contextual demands for the person. Individuals in fairly structured and repetitive occupations with low cognitive demand may have little interference from ADHD symptoms, once habits are established. However, individuals attempting to enter new environments with new or complex cognitive demands—a common experience in early adulthood—may experience significant distress and difficulty adapting.

The college years are a particularly vulnerable time for young adults with ADHD. Inherently, matriculating to a university is a highly unstructured task. Routines and habits cultivated from adapting to local high school conditions, in which many students had support from teachers and parents, as well as legal protection from an Individualized Educational Program (IEP), are no longer available. Although hyperactive symptoms may persist, WM and executive function (EF) deficits are more prominent (Barkley, 2010). Indeed, WM and EF deficits have been hallmark symptoms of individuals with ADHD (Barkley, 2006; Das et al., 2014), although these symptoms are also prominent in other disability conditions (Englund, Decker, Allen, & Roberts, 2014; Kofler, Rapport, Bolden, Sarver, & Raiker, 2010; Raiker, Rapport, Kofler, & Sarver, 2012). Such deficits become a struggle as complex course content places high demands on cognitive ability. These increased demands on WM and EF are often overwhelming and insurmountable for college students with ADHD, often leading to destructive emotional states. Misuse of prescription, and recreational drugs are a predictable consequence (Culpepper, 2013). Success or lack thereof, in adapting to the demands of higher education will have a tremendous impact on the life trajectories of individuals with ADHD.

Theoretical Explanations

Theoretical approaches are important for understanding and treating the core deficits of the disorder. There are various theoretical approaches to understanding ADHD and different approaches have different consequences. For example, school-based services view ADHD as a medical condition and require identification as Other Health Impaired, similar to other medical disabilities. Unfortunately, this approach places undue emphasis on medical treatments (i.e., medication) despite the fact that ADHD is no more "medical" than other behavioral disabilities (Wodrich & Schmitt, 2006). Historically, minimal brain dysfunction (MBD) was a precursor classification to ADHD as the symptoms of ADHD are similar to individuals with mild brain injuries. However, subsequent research found that many children with MBD did not have any documented evidence of brain injury, which provided the impetus to find the underlying causes of the disability. Hyperkinetic Reaction of Childhood in the DSM-II (1968), and Attention Deficit Disorder with the specifier "with or without hyperactivity" in the DSM-III (1980) were subsequent classifications that have also been discarded. The therapeutic use of stimulant medication, discovered by chance rather than scientific investigation (Baumeister, Henderson, Pow, & Advokat, 2012), is attributed to increases in dopamine in the frontal regions of the brain (del Campo et al., 2013). Because increases in dopamine alleviate symptoms, "neurochemical" theories have postulated ADHD is caused by a deficiency in neurotransmitters. However, just as migraines are not caused by a deficiency of aspirin in the brain, drugs that increase dopamine may be therapeutic but not necessarily causal of ADHD. Other conceptual approaches range from parenting to food additives (Barkley, 2006).

Without discounting the significant heterogeneity in ADHD causes, contemporary evidence has supported a link between ADHD symptoms and disruptions in specific brain networks, mainly in the prefrontal and subcortical areas of the brain (Silvetti, Wiersema, Sonuga-Barke, & Verguts, 2013; Volkow et al., 2007). Neuropsychological theories (see Sergeant, Geurts, Huijbregts, Scheres, & Oosterlaan, 2003 for a comparison of different models) have emphasized response inhibition and WM deficits as core constructs in explaining ADHD (Barkley, 1997, 2003). Although contemporary models continue to support disruptions in specific brain networks, there has been a shift in the neuropsychological constructs. Indeed, self-regulation (Barkley, 2013) and cognitive control (Nigg, 2010) have increased in importance as core constructs to integrate and unify various symptoms characteristic of ADHD. In contrast to traditional models, these more contemporary models recognize the role of internalized mental processes that regulate goal-oriented behavior. More specifically, self-regulatory process are viewed not as the cognitive functions involved with goal pursuit and obtainment (e.g., goal state representations), but rather as the cognitive processes influencing other cognitive processes that are more directly involved in specific behaviors. Although somewhat undefined, deficits in this area could include self-awareness, inhibition, WM, motivation, and/or innovation (Barkley, 2013).

Self-regulation may provide an important mediating construct to explain treatment outcomes in ADHD. Both behavioral (Pelham & Fabiano, 2008) and psychopharmacological interventions (i.e., stimulant medication) (Bitter, Angyalosi, & Czobor, 2012; Castells et al., 2011; Faraone & Biederman, 2002; Faraone, Spencer, Aleardi, Pagano, & Biederman, 2004) have demonstrated effectiveness in treating ADHD. However, the effect sizes for most of these interventions are modest, few generalize to an ecological context (Van der Oord, Prins, Oosterlaan, & Emmelkamp, 2008), and it is unpredictable why some individuals with ADHD respond to some treatments and not others. Such inconsistency may be a result of unknown, or uncontrolled, mediating variables. Self-regulation is a viable mediating construct that may account for inconsistencies across studies. That is, diverse ADHD interventions work sporadically because each, implicitly, facilitates or sets the occasion for the individual to initiate self-regulation processes, which likely occurs in some individuals and not others. Tasks and situations that require the flexible shifting of attention toward the regulation of internal mental processes enhance cognitive control, which promote response inhibition and enhance WM. Unfortunately, these interventions indirectly train self-regulation, rather than directly, and result in unpredictable outcomes.

ADHD, Self-Regulation, and Neurofeedback

Neurofeedback may be useful to explicitly treat self-regulation deficits in ADHD. The effectiveness of quantitative electroencephalography (qEEG) in both assessment and treatment of ADHD is well supported (Chabot et al., 1996). Meta-analytical research has concluded qEEG measures are capable of differentiating individuals with ADHD from individuals without ADHD (Arns, Conners, & Kraemer, 2013; Chabot, Merkin, Wood, Davenport, & Serfontein, 1996; Snyder & Hall, 2006). Indeed, the American Academy of Pediatrics, which has historically solely supported behavioral and psychopharmacological interventions for ADHD, has recently added EEG biofeedback as a Level 1 Best Supported intervention for ADHD (American Academy of Pediatrics, 2012). Electroencephalographic methods also have the added benefit of being less expensive and more accessible than other neuroimaging techniques.

Like other ADHD treatments there are inconsistencies in treatment outcomes using NF. For example, some studies have found NF to be superior to stimulant medication (Meisel, Servera, Garcia-Banda, Cardo, & Moreno, 2013) and other studies have found NF to be less effective (Ogrim & Hestad, 2013). Like other treatments, NF may provide an opportunity for an individual to engage in self-regulation. Progress monitoring provides self-relevant feedback that rewards self-referential thought processes and increases self-efficacy in cognitive control. As demonstrated by recent studies, control beliefs, defined as the individual's expectancy for contingent result of an action, influences NF performance (Witte, Kober, Ninaus, Neuper, & Wood, 2013), as do implicit learning strategies used during NF (Kober, Witte, Ninaus, Neuper, & Wood, 2013). Furthermore, as indicated in an fMRI NF study, effortful attempts to self-modulate brain activity, in both real and sham conditions, bilateral insula, anterior cingulate, and prefrontal regions of the brain became activated (Ninaus et al., 2013), all of which are brain areas involved in attention. Interestingly, there is a high degree of overlap between brain networks involved in attention and self-regulation, which will be discussed next.

Brain Networks Involved in Self-Regulation

In a meta-analysis of 27 MRI studies that incorporated self-referential tasks, three broad brain regions were identified as consistently activated during self-oriented tasks using both factor analysis and then reanalyzed using cluster analysis (Northoff et al., 2006). These regions include the Ventral Medial Prefrontal, Dorsal Medial Prefrontal, and Precuneus areas of the brain. Together these regions are referred to as the midline cortical structures (MCS) and appear to be a network involved with self-referential cognitive processes (D'Argembeau et al., 2008; Holt et al., 2011; Kim, 2012; Kjaer, Nowak, & Lou, 2002; Northoff & Bermpohl, 2004).

Notably, there is substantial overlap between MCS and brain areas involved with other networks such as the default mode network (Otti et al., 2012; Travis et al., 2010) and attentional control networks (Zhang & Li, 2012). Indeed, a recent study implicated symptoms of ADHD as involving brain areas that are in common to the MCS, default, and attention networks (Posner, Park, & Wang, 2014). Despite the overlap in brain networks, these areas are typically described as attention networks in ADHD research although self-regulation processes, or the lack thereof, could be an alternative viable hypothesis. For example, the anterior cingulate (AC) is repeatedly implicated in both attention and self-regulation studies (Rothbart, Sheese, Rueda, & Posner, 2011). Functionally, the AC has been described as providing a cost-benefits analysis of effortful cognition as mediated by dopamine (Kurniawan, Guitart-Masip, & Dolan, 2011), and is critical for translating intention to motor action (Paus, 2001). Presumably, effortful cognition is metabolically expensive and engaged when there is a mismatch between expected outcomes or rewards and actual outcomes, which is indicated with dopamine signaling.

Increasing activation in brain networks involved in self-referential cognitive processes is thought to increase attentional flexibility, which allows for better allocation of attentional resources across different networks. Thus, the engagement of "self" brain networks may be a critical prerequisite for positive therapeutic outcomes in individuals with ADHD. Neurofeedback may directly amplify self-referential cognitive processes but also directly target the brain networks involved with self-referential thinking. In turn, these brain networks may provide the basis for cognitive control, which in turn leads to changes in brain activity. Mechanistically, the general variables involved with self-regulation NF may involve (i) providing physiological (body related) self-relevant information, (ii) self-awareness of control of cognition and brain activity, and (iii) learning opportunities to facilitate and strengthen strategies for self-regulation to control cognition.

Application and Demonstration of LORETA Neurofeedback in Treating College ADHD

Understanding the role of self-regulation as applied to NF may improve treatment of individuals with ADHD. Certainly, improving

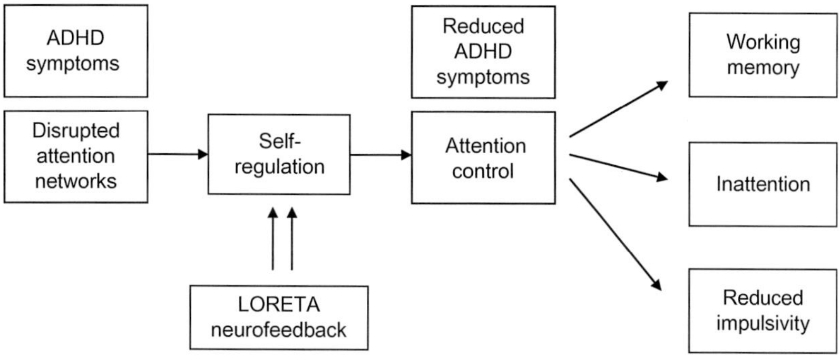

FIGURE 14.1 Theoretical model of LORETA mechanisms of change.

self-regulation skills would benefit college students with ADHD, and should be an integral aspect of treatment.

Figure 14.1 provides a working model of using LORETA NF as a self-regulatory intervention to address ADHD symptoms. As illustrated in the diagram, NF is used as an interactive process to facilitate self-regulation. Effectiveness is determined by linear trends in score change which demonstrate associated contingencies between self-regulatory control and changes in brain activity in prescribed brain networks. The individual's awareness in contingencies between self-regulation cognition and feedback from LORETA estimates provides stabilization and changes in broad attention networks. This "awareness" is a precursor to behavioral change.

LORETA and sLORETA Z-score Neurofeedback

Low-resolution electromagnetic tomography (LORETA)- and standardized LORETA (sLORETA)-based NF approaches are essential for estimating brain areas beyond surface EEG (i.e., areas involving self-regulation). LORETA does so via a mathematical solution to the EEG inverse problem. That is, it provides an estimate of current density in the 3D brain volume, thus providing an estimate of where in the brain the scalp-recorded EEG is being generated. sLORETA is a similar method, wherein the current density estimates are standardized with an estimation of the variability in the data, thus providing pseudo-F statistics as output rather than raw current density estimates. Although source accuracy is not perfect with low-density recordings, mislocalization tends to happen in consistent and predictable ways. Furthermore, LORETA results are consistent. Similar to EEG and quantitative EEG (qEEG), which have been shown to be highly reliable (Burgess & Gruzelier, 1993;

Corsi-Cabrera, Galindo-Vilchis, del-Río-Portilla, Arce, & Ramos-Loyo, 2007; Corsi-Cabrera, Solis-Ortiz, & Guevara, 1997; Gudmundsson, Runarsson, Sigurdsson, Eiriksdottir, & Johnsen, 2007; Roberts, 2012), LORETA results are highly reliable (Cannon et al., 2012).

LORETA Z-score Brodmann areas for attention networks overlap with regions involving the self, as previously identified. For example, selecting attention problems and executive functioning deficits in the symptoms checklist includes 12 Brodmann areas: 7, 8, 9, 10, 11, 19, 23, 24, 33, 45, 46, and 47. Many of these (i.e., Brodmann areas 7, 19, 23) overlap with the default network, and MCS, such as the anterior cingulate and precuneus (i.e., Brodmann areas 23, 24, 33). As previously mentioned, this overlap in "self" and attentional networks forms a core network integrating self-regulation with motivational states involving self-control of cognition. Improving functionality of this core system, although not curative, may mediate symptomatology of most psychiatric conditions, including ADHD.

Applications and Demonstration of LORETA Z-score NF

Case demonstrations will be reviewed from a research project examining the efficacy of LORETA Z-score neurofeedback in college-aged students with ADHD to demonstrate the general approach. We will provide information on ADHD symptomatology as well as neuropsychological test results. Additionally, preliminary results from two individuals who have been treated with LORETA Z-score neurofeedback training will be presented.

Consistent with guidelines for treating ADHD, multiple assessment approaches are used in diagnosing the disorder (American Academy of Pediatrics, Subcommittee on Attention-Deficit/Hyperactivity Disorder & Committee on Quality Improvement, 2001; Chatfield & American Academy of Pediatrics, 2002; Valente, 2001). Such guidelines often specify the need for parent and teacher ratings, which are often irrelevant, or unavailable for college-aged students. Students also often come to college previously identified as having ADHD.

Additionally, consistent with our conceptualization of ADHD as involving self-regulatory deficits, neurofeedback is viewed as an interactive learning process in which a person becomes aware of his or her brain functioning as mediated through EEG technology. The brain–computer interface used in neurofeedback provides the opportunity for an individual to learn and practice self-regulatory skills. However, for this research project, no attempts were made to engage the students in self-regulation.

Performance-based behavioral measures, as well as self-report rating scales, were administered for several reasons. First, such measures provide a baseline for initial functioning status. Baseline scores can then be used as a comparison for judging treatment success posttherapy. Additionally, ADHD is behaviorally diagnosed disorder. As such, using behavioral measures can provide direct evidence of changes in symptom severity on a clinically relevant scale. For the case studies described below, preintervention baseline behavioral measures included three measures of short-term/WM, and a computerized attention task, which assessed omission and commission errors to provide measures of inattention and impulsivity (i.e., self-regulatory behaviors).

Consistent with the guiding theoretical model presented in this chapter and previous discussion on ADHD, a guiding treatment model for ADHD is to divide the individuals into two broad groups. One group involves individuals with ADHD symptoms who have identifiable disruptions in attention networks in the brain as indicated by atypical neurophysiological measures. This could be operationalized by specific Z-scores beyond a set alpha (typically two or three standard deviations from the mean). The other group represents individuals with ADHD who either have symptomatology not due to dysfunction in brain networks (i.e., typical neurophysiological test performance) or have dysfunction, which is not detected by standard clinical EEG measures.

For diagnostic purposes, it is important that clinical symptoms match the underlying neurophysiological problems causing the symptoms. As a preliminary guideline, the following specific steps are offered to guide the treatment of individuals with ADHD using LORETA Z-score neurofeedback:

1. Perform standard qEEG with eyes open and eyes closed
2. Determine if there are disruptions in attention networks that match symptomatology
3. Administer behavioral measures to quantify the degree of attention dysfunction (inhibition, inattention, etc.)
4. Teach and administer neurofeedback procedures and monitor progress
5. Readminister behavioral measures to determine the extent of progress
6. Readminister standard qEEG measures with eyes open and eyes closed to determine the extent of change in attentional dysfunction.

CASE STUDIES

In order to more fully demonstrate the utility of LORETA Z-score neurofeedback with a college population, cases from a study examining the effectiveness of LORETA Z-score neurofeedback training are

TABLE 14.1 Case Study Scores

	Numbers Reversed			Auditory Working Memory			Memory for Words		
	Pretest	**Session 10**	**Posttest**	**Pretest**	**Session 10**	**Posttest**	**Pretest**	**Session 10**	**Posttest**
Student A	18	19	22	27	34	34	20	20	19
Student B	14	15	16	29	31	32	17	19	19
	Omissions			**Commisions**			**Reaction Time**		
	Pretest	**Session 10**	**Posttest**	**Pretest**	**Session 10**	**Posttest**	**Pretest**	**Session 10**	**Posttest**
Student A	44.87	47.96	44.87	62.87	62.87	61.32	34.64	32.26	30.20
Student B	47.31	52.21	47.31	65.96	70.61	52.04	35.12	35.98	39.48

Note: NR, AWM, MW = Woodcock Johnson Tests of Cognitive Abilities, 3rd Edition; omissions, commisions, reaction time = Conners' Continuous Performance Test, 2nd Edition.

presented below. The study employed a delayed treatment design such that for the first 10 sessions, participants were randomly assigned to either a sham or treatment condition. After the completion of those 10 sessions, all participants received neurofeedback training. As such, two case studies are provided. The first is an individual who received neurofeedback training for the entire study, and the second, an individual who first received the sham condition, followed by LORETA *Z*-score training. Both individuals were 20-year-old female university students. Both were diagnosed in late adolescence by a general physician, and were prescribed stimulant medication to alleviate their symptoms. As the study took place during the academic year, students were not asked to stop their current medication regimen. The results described below were found in spite of their medication use.

Pre- and posttest behavioral data was collected at three time points—prior to session one, after session 10, after the final session—in addition to EEG data. Given that deficits in WM and self-regulatory processes are common in individuals with ADHD, the behavioral measures selected include three measures of short-term and WM—numbers reversed (NR), auditory working memory (AWM), memory for words (MW)—from the Woodcock Johnson Tests of Cognitive Abilities, Third Edition (WJ III) and the Connor's Continuous Performance Test, Second Edition (CPT-II), which includes measures of inattention and impulsivity. Both behavioral data and EEG data are presented (see Table 14.1) and discussed below.

CASE 1

TREATMENT CONDITION

Student A was a 20-year-old female who was diagnosed with ADHD at age 18. At pretest she reported symptoms of inattention and hyperactivity/impulsivity, though the latter was more prevalent. In terms of her short-term/WM performance, she obtained the following raw scores on the WJ III subtests: NR = 18, AWM = 27, and MW = 20. Raw scores were used because WJ III measures were constructed using item response models and there were minimal sources of developmental variation (Decker, 2008). Student A was also administered the CPT-II at pretest and obtained the following T-scores: omission errors (i.e., measure of inattention) = 44.87 commission errors (i.e., measure of impulsivity) = 62.87, and hit reaction time = 34.64. T-scores were used for this measure, as the raw scores obtained on the CPT are not directly interpretable.

continued

CASE 1 (*cont'd*)

The first posttest was conducted after 10 sessions of NF. Student A's performance on the WJ III measures was as follows, NR = 19, AWM = 34, and MW = 20. This suggests that her performance stayed fairly consistent on two of the three measures, while she made a substantial improvement on the third measure, AWM. Her raw score of 27 at pretest corresponds to a standard score of 97 (M = 100, SD = 15). The 7-point increase in her raw score (AWM = 34) corresponds to a 16-point increase in standard score (SS = 113), which is greater than one standard deviation of change. In terms of the CPT-II, her midpoint scores were as follows, omissions = 47.96, commissions = 62.87, and hit reaction time = 32.26, suggesting that her performance remained fairly consistent, though she was a little faster at responding. At the second posttest (i.e., after the final session), her performance remained fairly consistent on both the WJ III (NR = 22, AWM = 34, MW = 19) and CPT-II (omissions = 44.87, commissions = 61.32, hit RT = 30.20), suggesting she reached a plateau, though the improvements she did make from pretest to the first posttest were maintained.

CASE 2

DELAYED TREATMENT CONDITION

Student B was also a 20-year-old female, who was diagnosed with ADHD at age 17. At pretest, she too reported symptoms of inattention and hyperactivity/impulsivity. However, per self-report, her distress was more equally distributed across the two domains. In terms of her short-term/WM performance, Student B obtained the following raw scores on the WJ III subtests: NR = 14, AWM = 29, and MW = 17. She also obtained the following T-scores on the CPT-II pretest: omission errors = 47.31, commission errors = 65.96, and hit reaction time = 35.12.

At midpoint, Student B obtained the following scores on the WJ III measures, NR = 15, AWM = 31, and MW = 19. This suggests that her performance stayed fairly consistent across all three measures, as would be expected given that she was receiving sham treatment. In terms of the CPT-II, her midpoint scores were as follows, omissions = 52.21, commissions = 70.61, and hit reaction time = 35.98, suggesting that her performance remained fairly consistent as well. While it is of note that her commission errors increased from Time 1 to

Time 2, her scores fell within the clinically significant range at both time points. As such, it is likely this was due to random variation, rather than suggesting that her performance worsened, especially considering the other measures were commensurate with her earlier performance. Given the delayed treatment design of the study, Student B was not expected to make significant gains from pretest to the first posttest measurement. However, it was hypothesized that she would begin to demonstrate changes by the end of the study.

At posttest 2, Student B's scores on the WJ III were as follows, NR = 16, AWM = 32, and MW = 19, suggesting little change in her WM as a result of the training. However, her performance on the CPT-II suggested the opposite. Her posttest 2 scores on the CPT-II were as follows, omissions = 47.31, commissions = 52.04, and hit RT = 39.48. Commission errors are indicative of impulsivity and her performance on this measure decreased from the clinically significant range into the "average" range after beginning the training.

Figures 14.2A and B illustrate the significant change from pretest to midpoint for Students A and B respectively. As shown below, Student A demonstrated significant change in alpha and posterior beta and high beta after completing 10 sessions of neurofeedback. As a caveat, it is possible that the full scalp alpha change could be due to nonspecific changes in alertness between the two sessions. However, the consistency in this change at both posttests suggests that the changes are likely due to more than chance. For example, as suggested by our theoretical model, self-regulation may produce nonspecific effects that account for changes in brain activity. Student B also demonstrated some significant change (i.e., theta, and some bilateral delta and high beta) during the sham condition, suggesting there was somewhat of a placebo effect as well. However, it is prudent to remember that these are individual cases, and as such, individual variation can have an immense impact on analyses such as these.

Figure 14.3A and B illustrates the significant change from posttest 1 to posttest 2 (end of the study) for both individuals. As expected, Student A showed significant changes in theta, alpha, beta, and high beta, as well as some highly localized change in prefrontal delta by the end of the study. This suggests that Student A continued to experience change following the first 10 sessions, likely building on the changes that occurred at the start of the study. This is most notable in the theta and beta (including high beta) ranges, which are often associated with ADHD. Student B also demonstrated additional significant change after receiving the real treatment. Specifically, this change was evident in

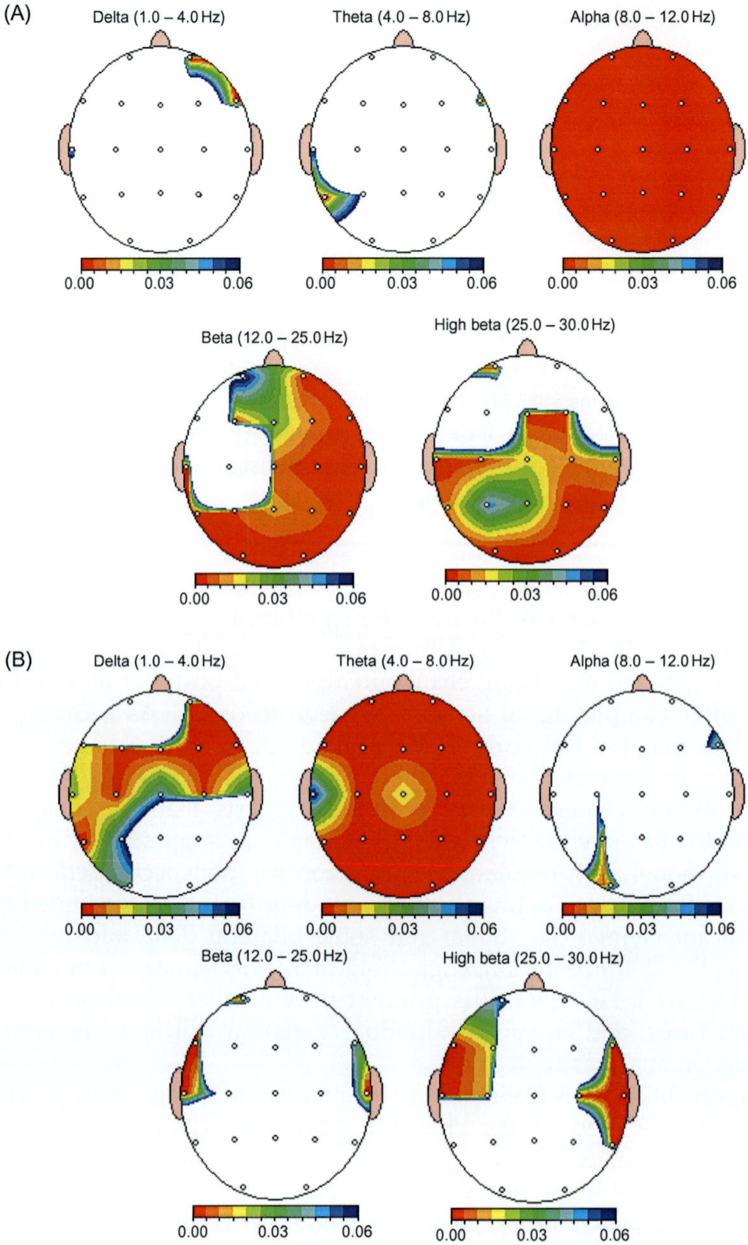

FIGURE 14.2 (A) Changes in absolute power from pretest to session 10 following NF treatment for Student A. (B) Changes in absolute power from pretest to session 10 following NF treatment for Student B. *Note*: Scales at the bottom designate *p*-values.

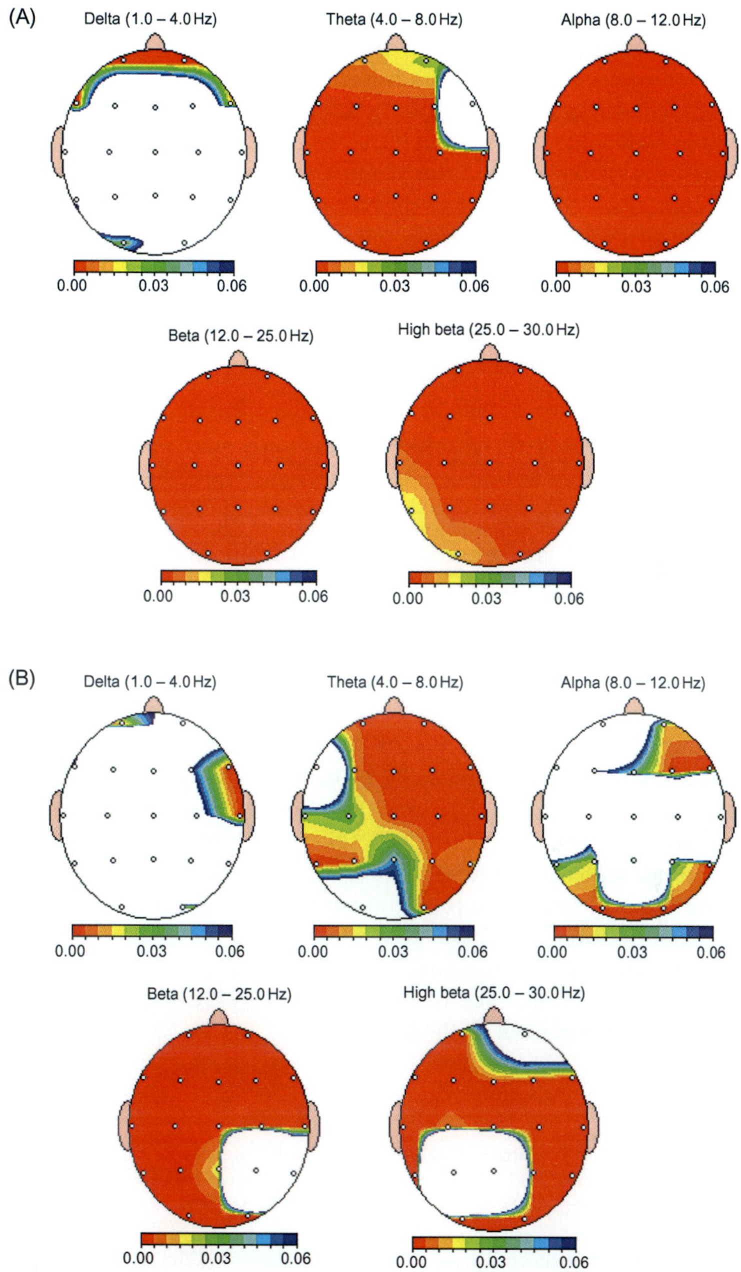

FIGURE 14.3 (A) Changes in absolute power from session 10 to posttest following NF treatment for Student A. (B) Changes in absolute power from session 10 to posttest following NF treatment for Student B. *Note*: Scales at the bottom designate *p*-values.

theta, beta, and high beta, as well as some posterior and right frontal alpha. Again, it seems as though the treatment impacted the theta and beta wavelengths the most, which is consistent with previous and current research, suggesting that the ratio of theta and beta waves is often atypical in individuals with ADHD.

The results of these two case studies are promising, as both demonstrated change in the expected directions. More interesting still, is that the impact of LORETA Z-score training was able to indirectly affect the students' performance on more commonly used behavioral measures as well. The implications of this are far reaching as many psychological disorders are diagnosed through the use of such tools, rather than through the use of neuroimaging techniques.

CONCLUSION

ADHD is a developmental disability that impacts individuals through adulthood. However, core deficits from ADHD are different in adulthood than in childhood. A core deficit in college-aged students with ADHD, and as specified in recent theories of ADHD, are deficits in self-regulation. Neurofeedback may not only provide a vital role in addressing self-regulation deficits but may also be viewed as a self-regulation treatment. Although there are terms to describe individuals with reduced sensitivity to visual input (visually impaired), and for individuals with reduced auditory sensitivity (hearing impaired), there is not a term to describe individuals who have reduced sensitivity to internal thought processes. In part, self-regulation fills this void. Case studies of college-aged students with ADHD were provided to demonstrate the general approach to demonstrating the use of LORETA NF to target core attention networks. It is the authors' hope that this chapter, and the presentation of the case studies, provides a basic overview of the use of this technique for those interested in the use of LORETA NF with a college population with ADHD.

References

American Academy of Pediatrics. (2012). *SharpBrains.org*. Retrieved from: <http://www.sharpbrains.com/blog/2012/10/05/biofeedback-now-a-level-1-best-support-intervention-for-attention-hyperactivity-behaviors/>. Accessed May 26, 2014.

American Academy of Pediatrics, Subcommittee on Attention-Deficit/Hyperactivity Disorder & Committee on Quality Improvement (2001). Clinical practice guideline: Treatment of the school-aged child with attention-deficit/hyperactivity disorder. *Pediatrics, 108*(4), 1033–1044.

APA (2013). *Diagnostic and statistical manual of mental disorders* (5th ed.). Washington, DC: American Psychiatric Association.

Arns, M., Conners, C. K., & Kraemer, H. C. (2013). A decade of EEG Theta/Beta Ratio Research in ADHD: A meta-analysis. *Journal of Attention Disorders, 17*(5), 374–383.

Barkley, R. A. (1997). Behavioral inhibition, sustained attention, and executive functions: Constructing a unifying theory of ADHD. *Psychological Bulletin, 121*(1), 65.

Barkley, R. A. (2001). The inattentive type of ADHD as a distinct disorder: What remains to be done. *Clinical Psychology: Science and Practice, 8*(4), 489–493.

Barkley, R. A. (2003). Attention-deficit/hyperactivity disorder. In E. J. Mash, & R. A. Barkley (Eds.), *Child psychopathology* (2nd ed.). New York, NY: Guilford Press.

Barkley, R. A. (2006). *Attention-deficit hyperactivity disorder: A handbook for diagnosis and treatment*. New York, NY: Guilford Press.

Barkley, R. A. (2010). Differential diagnosis of adults with ADHD: The role of executive function and self-regulation. *Journal of Clinical Psychiatry, 71*(7), e17.

Barkley, R. A. (2013). *Taking charge of ADHD: The complete, authoritative guide for parents*. Guilford Press.

Baumeister, A. A., Henderson, K., Pow, J. L., & Advokat, C. (2012). The early history of the neuroscience of attention-deficit/hyperactivity disorder. *Journal of the History of the Neurosciences, 21*(3), 263–279.

Bitter, I., Angyalosi, A., & Czobor, P. (2012). Pharmacological treatment of adult ADHD. *Current Opinion in Psychiatry, 25*(6), 529–534.

Burgess, A., & Gruzelier, J. (1993). Individual reliability of amplitude distribution in topographical mapping of EEG. *Electroencephalography and Clinical Neurophysiology, 86*(4), 219–223.

Cannon, R. L., Baldwin, D. R., Shaw, T. L., Diloreto, D. J., Phillips, S. M., Scruggs, A. M., et al. (2012). Reliability of quantitative EEG (qEEG) measures and LORETA current source density at 30 days. *Neuroscience Letters, 518*(1), 27–31.

Castells, X., Ramos-Quiroga, J. A., Rigau, D., Bosch, R., Nogueira, M., Vidal, X., et al. (2011). Efficacy of methylphenidate for adults with attention-deficit hyperactivity disorder: A meta-regression analysis. *CNS Drugs, 25*(2), 157–169.

Chabot, R. J., Merkin, H., Wood, L. M., Davenport, T. L., & Serfontein, G. (1996). Sensitivity and specificity of QEEG in children with attention deficit or specific developmental learning disorders. *Clinical EEG (Electroencephalography), 27*(1), 26–34.

Chatfield, J., & American Academy of Pediatrics (2002). AAP guideline on treatment of children with ADHD. *American Family Physician, 65*(4), 726–728.

Corsi-Cabrera, M., Galindo-Vilchis, L., del-Río-Portilla, Y., Arce, C., & Ramos-Loyo, J. (2007). Within-subject reliability and inter-session stability of EEG power and coherent activity in women evaluated monthly over nine months. *Clinical Neurophysiology, 118*, 9–21.

Corsi-Cabrera, M., Solis-Ortiz, S., & Guevara, M. A. (1997). Stability of EEG inter-and intrahemispheric correlation in women. *Electroencephalography and Clinical Neurophysiology, 102*(3), 248–255.

Culpepper, L. (2013). Recognizing and addressing barriers to the effective management of ADHD in college students. *Journal of Clinical Psychiatry, 74*(7), e13.

D'Argembeau, A., Feyers, D., Majerus, S., Collette, F., Van der Linden, M., Maquet, P., et al. (2008). Self-reflection across time: Cortical midline structures differentiate between present and past selves. *Social Cognitive and Affective Neuroscience, 3*(3), 244–252.

Das, D., Cherbuin, N., Easteal, S., & Anstey, K. J. (2014). Attention deficit/hyperactivity disorder symptoms and cognitive abilities in the late-life cohort of the PATH through life study. *PLoS One, 9*(1), e86552.

Decker, S. L. (2008). Intervention psychometrics: Using norm-referenced methods for treatment planning and monitoring. *Assessment for Effective Interventions, 34*(1), 52–61.

Decker, S. L., McIntosh, D. E., Kelly, A. M., Nicholls, S. K., & Dean, R. S. (2001). Comorbidity among individuals classified with attention disorders. *The International Journal of Neuroscience, 110*(1–2), 43–54.

del Campo, N., Fryer, T. D., Hong, Y. T., Smith, R., Brichard, L., Acosta-Cabronero, J., et al. (2013). A positron emission tomography study of nigro-striatal dopaminergic mechanisms underlying attention: Implications for ADHD and its treatment. *Brain, 136*(11), 3252–3270.

Englund, J. A., Decker, S. L., Allen, R. A., & Roberts, A. M. (2013). Common cognitive deficits in children with attention-deficit/hyperactivity disorder and autism: Working memory and visual-motor integration. *Journal of Psychoeducational Assessment, 32*(2), 95–106.

Faraone, S. V., & Biederman, J. (2002). Efficacy of adderall for attention-deficit/hyperactivity disorder: A meta-analysis. *Journal of Attention Disorders, 6*(2), 69–75.

Faraone, S. V., Spencer, T., Aleardi, M., Pagano, C., & Biederman, J. (2004). Meta-analysis of the efficacy of methylphenidate for treating adult attention-deficit/hyperactivity disorder. *Journal of Clinical Psychopharmacology, 24*(1), 24–29.

Fredriksen, M., Dahl, A. A., Martinsen, E. W., Klungsoyr, O., Faraone, S. V., & Peleikis, D. E. (2014). Childhood and persistent ADHD symptoms associated with educational failure and long-term occupational disability in adult ADHD. *Attention Deficit Hyperactivity Disorder, 6*, 87–99.

Green, B. C., Johnson, K. A., & Bretherton, L. (2014). Pragmatic language difficulties in children with hyperactivity and attention problems: An integrated review. *International Journal of Language & Communication Disorders, 49*(1), 15–29.

Gudmundsson, S., Runarsson, T. P., Sigurdsson, S., Eiriksdottir, D., & Johnsen, K. (2007). Reliability of quantitative EEG features. *Clinical Neurophysiology, 118*, 2162–2171.

Guldberg-Kjar, T., & Johansson, B. (2013). ADHD symptoms across the lifespan: A comparison of symptoms captured by the wender and barkley scales and DSM-IV criteria in a population-based Swedish sample aged 65 to 80. *Journal of Attention Disorders*. Available from: http://dx.doi.org/doi:10.1177/1087054713514853.

Holt, D. J., Cassidy, B. S., Andrews-Hanna, J. R., Lee, S. M., Coombs, G., Goff, D. C., et al. (2011). An anterior-to-posterior shift in midline cortical activity in schizophrenia during self-reflection. *Biological Psychiatry, 69*(5), 415–423.

Kim, H. (2012). A dual-subsystem model of the brain's default network: Self-referential processing, memory retrieval processes, and autobiographical memory retrieval. *NeuroImage, 61*(4), 966–977.

Kim, S., Liu, Z., Glizer, D., Tannock, R., & Woltering, S. (2013). Adult ADHD and working memory: Neural evidence of impaired encoding. *Clinical Neurophysiology*.

Kjaer, T. W., Nowak, M., & Lou, H. C. (2002). Reflective self-awareness and conscious states: PET evidence for a common midline parietofrontal core. *NeuroImage, 17*(2), 1080–1086.

Kober, S. E., Witte, M., Ninaus, M., Neuper, C., & Wood, G. (2013). Learning to modulate one's own brain activity: The effect of spontaneous mental strategies. *Frontiers in Human Neuroscience, 7*, 695.

Kofler, M. J., Rapport, M. D., Bolden, J., Sarver, D. E., & Raiker, J. S. (2010). ADHD and working memory: The impact of central executive deficits and exceeding storage/rehearsal capacity on observed inattentive behavior. *Journal of Abnormal Child Psychology, 38*(2), 149–161.

Kurniawan, I. T., Guitart-Masip, M., & Dolan, R. J. (2011). Dopamine and effort-based decision making. *Frontiers in Neuroscience, 5*, 81.

Meisel, V., Servera, M., Garcia-Banda, G., Cardo, E., & Moreno, I. (2013). Neurofeedback and standard pharmacological intervention in ADHD: A randomized controlled trial with six-month follow-up. *Biological Psychology, 94*(1), 12–21.

Milich, R., Balentine, A. C., & Lyman, D. R. (2001). ADHD combined type and ADHD predominantly inattentive type are distinct and unrelated disorders. *Clinical Psychology: Science and Practice, 8*, 463–488.

Nigg, J. T. (2010). Attention-deficit/hyperactivity disorder endophenotypes, structure, and etiological pathways. *Current Directions in Psychological Science*, *19*(1), 24–29.

Nigg, J. T. (2013). Attention deficits and hyperactivity-impulsivity: What have we learned, what next? *Development and Psychopathology*, *25*(4 Pt 2), 1489–1503.

Ninaus, M., Kober, S. E., Witte, M., Koschutnig, K., Stangl, M., Neuper, C., et al. (2013). Neural substrates of cognitive control under the belief of getting neurofeedback training. *Frontiers in Human Neuroscience*, *7*, 914.

Northoff, G., & Bermpohl, F. (2004). Cortical midline structures and the self. *Trends in Cognitive Sciences*, *8*(3), 102–107.

Northoff, G., Heinzel, A., de Greck, M., Bermpohl, F., Dobrowolny, H., & Panksepp, J. (2006). Self-referential processing in our brain—A meta-analysis of imaging studies on the self. *NeuroImage*, *31*(1), 440–457.

Ogrim, G., & Hestad, K. A. (2013). Effects of neurofeedback versus stimulant medication in attention-deficit/hyperactivity disorder: A randomized pilot study. *Journal of Child and Adolescent Psychopharmacology*, *23*(7), 448–457.

Otti, A., Gundel, H., Wohlschlager, A., Zimmer, C., Sorg, C., & Noll-Hussong, M. (2012). Default mode network of the brain. Neurobiology and clinical significance. *Nervenarzt*, *83*(1), 16. 18–24. doi:10.1007/s00115-011-3307-6.

Paus, T. (2001). Primate anterior cingulate cortex: Where motor control, drive and cognition interface. *Nature Reviews Neuroscience*, *2*(6), 417–424.

Pelham, W. E., Jr., & Fabiano, G. A. (2008). Evidence-based psychosocial treatments for attention-deficit/hyperactivity disorder. *Journal of Clinical Child and Adolescent Psychology*, *37*(1), 184–214.

Petersen, I. T., Bates, J. E., D'Onofrio, B. M., Coyne, C. A., Lansford, J. E., Dodge, K. A., et al. (2013). Language ability predicts the development of behavior problems in children. *Journal of Abnormal Psychology*, *122*(2), 542–557.

Posner, J., Park, C., & Wang, Z. (2014). Connecting the dots: A review of resting connectivity MRI studies in attention-deficit/hyperactivity disorder. *Neuropsychology Review*, *24*(1), 3–15.

Raiker, J. S., Rapport, M. D., Kofler, M. J., & Sarver, D. E. (2012). Objectively-measured impulsivity and attention-deficit/hyperactivity disorder (ADHD): Testing competing predictions from the working memory and behavioral inhibition models of ADHD. *Journal of Abnormal Child Psychology*.

Roberts, A. M. (2012). *Test-retest reliability of coherence measures of qEEG during resting state*. Retrieved from ProQuest, UMI Dissertations Publishing (1531752).

Rothbart, M. K., Sheese, B. E., Rueda, M. R., & Posner, M. I. (2011). Developing mechanisms of self-regulation in early life. *Emotion Review*, *3*(2), 207–213.

Scholtens, S., Rydell, A. M., & Yang-Wallentin, F. (2013). ADHD symptoms, academic achievement, self-perception of academic competence and future orientation: A longitudinal study. *Scandinavian Journal of Psychology*, *54*(3), 205–212.

Sergeant, J. A., Geurts, H., Huijbregts, S., Scheres, A., & Oosterlaan, J. (2003). The top and the bottom of ADHD: A neuropsychological perspective. *Neuroscience & Biobehavioral Reviews*, *27*(7), 583–592.

Silvetti, M., Wiersema, J. R., Sonuga-Barke, E., & Verguts, T. (2013). Deficient reinforcement learning in medial frontal cortex as a model of dopamine-related motivational deficits in ADHD. *Neural Networks*, *46*, 199–209.

Snyder, S. M., & Hall, J. R. (2006). A meta-analysis of quantitative EEG power associated with attention-deficit hyperactivity disorder. *Journal of Clinical Neurophysiology*, *23*(5), 440–455.

Travis, F., Haaga, D. A., Hagelin, J., Tanner, M., Arenander, A., Nidich, S., et al. (2010). A self-referential default brain state: Patterns of coherence, power, and eLORETA sources during eyes-closed rest and transcendental meditation practice. *Cognitive Processes*, *11*(1), 21–30.

Valente, S. M. (2001). Treating attention deficit hyperactivity disorder. *Nurse Practitioner, 26*(9), 14–15. 19–20, 23–27; quiz 27–29.

Van der Oord, S., Prins, P. J., Oosterlaan, J., & Emmelkamp, P. M. (2008). Efficacy of methylphenidate, psychosocial treatments and their combination in school-aged children with ADHD: A meta-analysis. *Clinical Psychology Review, 28*(5), 783–800.

Volkow, N. D., Wang, G. J., Newcorn, J., Fowler, J. S., Telang, F., Solanto, M. V., et al. (2007). Brain dopamine transporter levels in treatment and drug naive adults with ADHD. *Neuroimage, 34*(3), 1182–1190.

Washbrook, E., Propper, C., & Sayal, K. (2013). Pre-school hyperactivity/attention problems and educational outcomes in adolescence: Prospective longitudinal study. *The British Journal of Psychiatry, 203*, 265–271.

Witte, M., Kober, S. E., Ninaus, M., Neuper, C., & Wood, G. (2013). Control beliefs can predict the ability to up-regulate sensorimotor rhythm during neurofeedback training. *Frontiers in Human Neuroscience, 7*, 478.

Wodrich, D. L., & Schmitt, A. J. (2006). *Patterns of learning disabilities.* New York, NY: Guilford Press.

Zhang, S., & Li, C. S. (2012). Functional networks for cognitive control in a stop signal task: Independent component analysis. *Human Brain Mapping, 33*(1), 89–104.

CHAPTER

15

19-Channel Z-Score Training for Learning Disorders and Executive Functioning

Rachael M. Little, Brianna H. Bendixsen and Richard D. Abbey

Abbey Neuropsychology Clinic, Palo Alto, CA, USA

We are a neuropsychology clinic specializing in neuropsychological assessment and interventions for children and adults. Whereas quantitative electroencephalography (QEEG) brain mapping allows us to see how the client is using their brain, neuropsychological assessment reveals the functioning of the brain. In other words, neuropsychological assessment identifies the phonotype (i.e., symptoms), whereas QEEG brain mapping reveals the weaknesses of the regions of the brain and their networks that are contributing to the symptoms. This is especially important in identifying the primary cause of learning disorders and executive functioning deficits because there can be a wide range of reasons for these difficulties. Combining neuropsychological assessment with QEEG brain mapping allows a detailed analysis that ultimately reveals the underlying causes of the areas of weakness revealed in a neuropsychological assessment.

The assessment begins with a detailed clinical interview. A thorough history is taken, including developmental, medical, family, and educational history. Early signs of symptoms are often revealed in teacher concerns to the parents. The earlier learning disorders are correctly identified and treated, the better their prognosis. The traditional model of providing skill-based academic interventions is limited. Although neurofeedback is not typically a frontline treatment of choice for learning disorders, it can be a helpful adjunct therapy. Our experience has

Z Score Neurofeedback.
DOI: http://dx.doi.org/10.1016/B978-0-12-801291-8.00015-7

been that combining traditional learning disorder interventions with neurofeedback provides far more favorable outcomes.

We have also developed interventions for executive functioning deficits. As with learning disorders, early intervention improves prognosis. We have found that children respond better to our executive functioning interventions and skill building programs when they have first completed neurofeedback. The demands on executive functioning tend to be low prior to 6th grade; however, there are often early signs of executive functioning deficits. This is most pronounced in the case of autism, where children present difficulties with cognitive flexibility, a narrow focus, cognitive rigidity, difficulties making transitions, and perseveration. Some of these traits may also be seen in children who are not on the spectrum, and it is important to know about them when creating comprehensive treatment plans.

Our neuropsychological assessments are comprehensive. We begin with assessing intellectual functioning, which provides a comparative metric against which to compare academic skills. The assumption is that with adequate exposure to instruction, one's academic skills should be reasonably consistent with their intellectual functioning. However, a discrepancy between intellectual functioning and academic skills may indicate a specific learning disorder depending on the magnitude of this discrepancy. In addition, neuropsychological abilities are assessed, including language, visuospatial, learning and memory, attention, executive functions, motor, and emotional functioning. Synthesizing the assessment results with the client's history reveals a more detailed analysis of the client's symptoms. These findings are then used to link the client's symptoms to the QEEG to develop protocols.

Protocols are created and then updated as the client moves through neurofeedback therapy. Changing the protocols is often necessary depending on the client's response to treatment. We provide two case studies below to illustrate the process of assessment, QEEG brain mapping, and protocol creation in treating learning disorders and executive functioning deficits.

CASE 1

Background Information and Symptom History

Kim is a 12-year-old girl who initially came to our clinic for neuropsychological assessment due to concerns that she was struggling to keep up with the other students in her class. She was previously diagnosed with a reading disorder (i.e., dyslexia) and had undergone reading interventions with limited progress. After conducting a clinical interview, it became clear that her case was much more complex than a simple case of dyslexia. Kim's developmental history is largely unknown, as she was adopted. From what little is known, she likely suffered from malnutrition and a severely impoverished environment. She has always been underweight and has always had trouble maintaining an appropriate weight.

Her parents ensured that she received early interventions to help correct speech deficits, word decoding problems, and motor skills. Many of these interventions proved unhelpful, and while intensive reading tutoring helped to improve her decoding skills, her comprehension and retention remained very poor. She was unable to retain both the overall gestalt and smaller details of her reading material. She also struggled to make inferences from the text but was able to understand concrete concepts. By the time she came to our clinic, she had completed over 100 sessions of reading remediation and had gained very little benefit. Other learning disabilities persisted as well. Kim was unable to understand how to break mathematics problems down into their component pieces, or how to organize an essay into logical chunks. Her language skills were well below grade level, and she often strained to find the appropriate word or phrase in conversations and when writing.

Additionally, Kim's struggles were exacerbated by her poor working memory. She was unable to hold more than a few pieces of information in her mind, which had a significant impact on her academic performance. This was particularly evident in her expressive language skills. Kim found it very difficult to piece together information which she wanted to verbalize and often would simply give up and remain silent out of frustration.

Consistent with her other executive function deficits, Kim found it difficult to maintain her focus and attention in the classroom. Of greater interest was her inability to sustain mental stamina. Kim would become easily fatigued from any small amount of mental effort, and then any information processing became much more difficult for her. She was briefly placed on Adderall to help manage these symptoms, but it had little effect. Rather than a more classical case of inattention due to ADHD, it was felt that her symptoms of inattention were more likely due to her malnutrition and impoverished environment during key formative years. Kim was also receiving several hours of tutoring per week, to little avail. She had started to experience anxiety and moderate depression over her classroom struggles, knowing

continued

CASE 1 *(cont'd)*

that she was unable to keep up with her peers, yet so badly wanting to be a good student. Her parents were at a loss for what to do next.

Assessment

Kim underwent a full neuropsychological battery in order to tease apart the nature of her weaknesses. This was especially important to her overall treatment, as conventional methods for strengthening learning disabilities had proved largely ineffective. Kim was given standardized tests, including an IQ test, and measures examining academics, learning, memory, attention, executive functions, and others. It was important to understand Kim's strengths and her weaknesses as compared to *herself*.

Figure 15.1 details Kim's intelligence domains. This belies the importance of examining each individual's strengths and weaknesses against their innate abilities. One might suspect, given Kim's host of challenges, that her intelligence might in some way be compromised. However, she is indeed of high average intelligence, with, interestingly, strong perceptual reasoning skills, and unsurprisingly, relatively weaker information processing. Already, a clearer picture of her neurocognitive profile begins to emerge.

Kim's academic profile on standardized measures was scattered, with many weaknesses across the board. When her attention was tested, a pattern began to emerge which coincided with her sluggish cognitive tempo and poor mental stamina.

In Figure 15.2, Kim's attention states were measured using the Quotient® ADHD System continuous performance test. Her response times to specific targets were graphed over the 15 min duration of the test. It is easy to see that Kim is able to sustain a reasonable amount

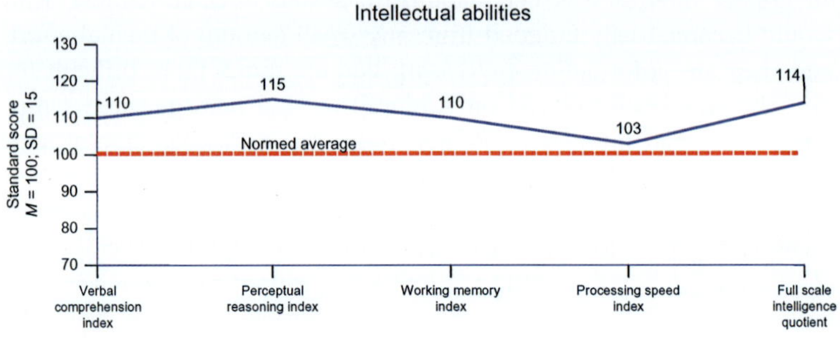

FIGURE 15.1 Kim's intellectual profile compiled from composite scores on the Wechsler Intelligence Scale for Children—4th Edition, December 3, 2012.

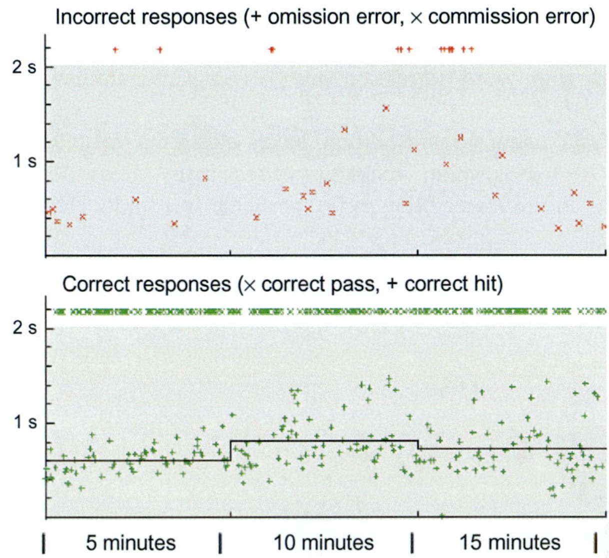

FIGURE 15.2 Kim's responses on her initial Quotient ADHD System continuous performance test, November 11, 2012.

of effort for the first 5 min, but then both her attention and stamina quickly dwindle, and she is unable to recover for the remainder of the test.

Interventions

It was clear that Kim would require a set of interventions to address these cognitive weaknesses from a bottom-up perspective. Neurofeedback training would help to strengthen her neurophysiological foundation, and then other interventions could be added in order to build specific areas of weakness, such as attention and memory. Only then could formal tutoring be successful to introduce specific skills and concepts.

Stage 1: QEEG Analysis

Kim's initial QEEG was conducted on April 27, 2013, using a Nexus amplifier and 19 leads. Eyes open and eyes closed conditions were obtained. The data was then artifacted and the eyes open condition was used to generate the following quantitative analyses.

Surface maps revealed glaringly obvious problems throughout power, phase, and coherence, with the most serious deviations in areas

continued

CASE 1 (*cont'd*)

involved with word formation and language generation, as shown in Figure 15.3.

Analysis using low-resolution brain electromagnetic tomography (LORETA) tomographic imaging yielded many areas of significant deviance. In the lower frequencies, particularly 1 and 2 Hz, Brodmann

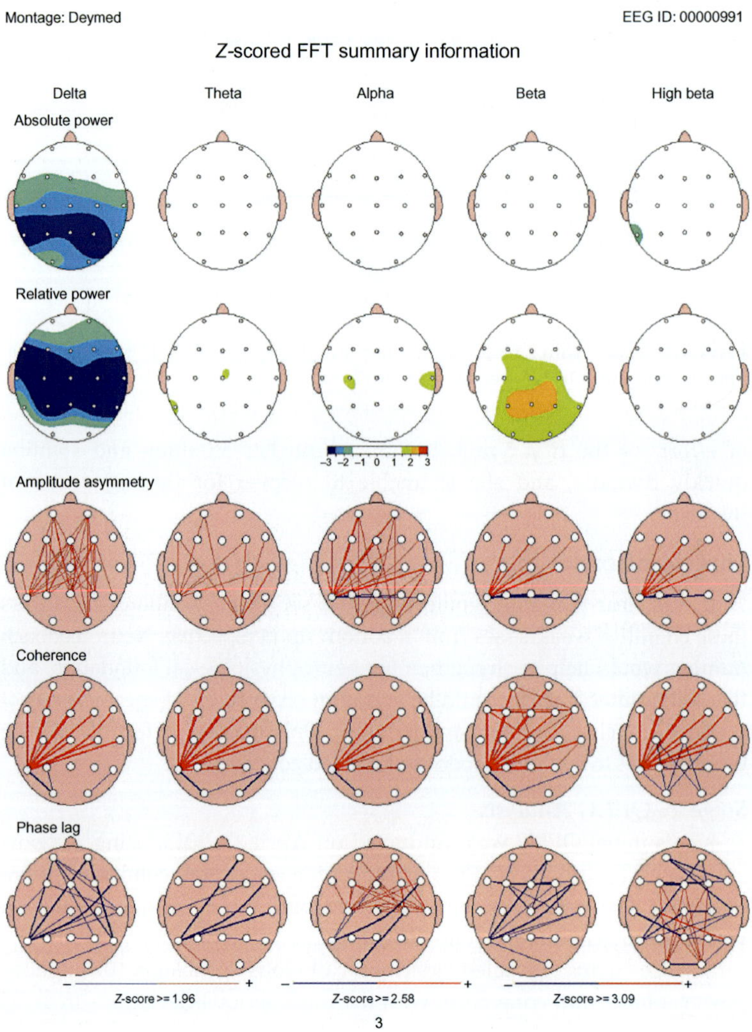

FIGURE 15.3 Kim's initial QEEG brain map, showing abnormalities throughout power and connectivity. The initial recording was taken April 17, 2013.

areas 13 (insular cortex) and 23 (cingulate cortex) were 1.94–3.25 standard deviations below the mean. Consistent with Kim's reported symptoms, these areas are heavily involved with lexical and semantic processing, two areas of weakness for Kim (Friederici, Rüschemeyer, Hahne, & Fiebach, 2003; Jessen et al., 1999).

Additionally, deviations in the 10 Hz band were both significant and pervasive in the left prefrontal cortex, auditory cortex, and posterior cingulate regions, as seen in Figure 15.4. Specific areas included Brodmann areas 8, 9, 44, 45, 46, 41, and 29, and showed excessive alpha activity well above 2 standard deviations from the mean. These areas are critical in Kim's symptomatology, as they include Broca's area, Heschl's gyrus in the auditory cortex, and prefrontal cortical areas, all of which comprise the networks involved in language generation, auditory processing, executive functions, and working memory (Heim, Eickhoff, & Amunts, 2008; Okuda, Fujii, & Yamadori, 2000;

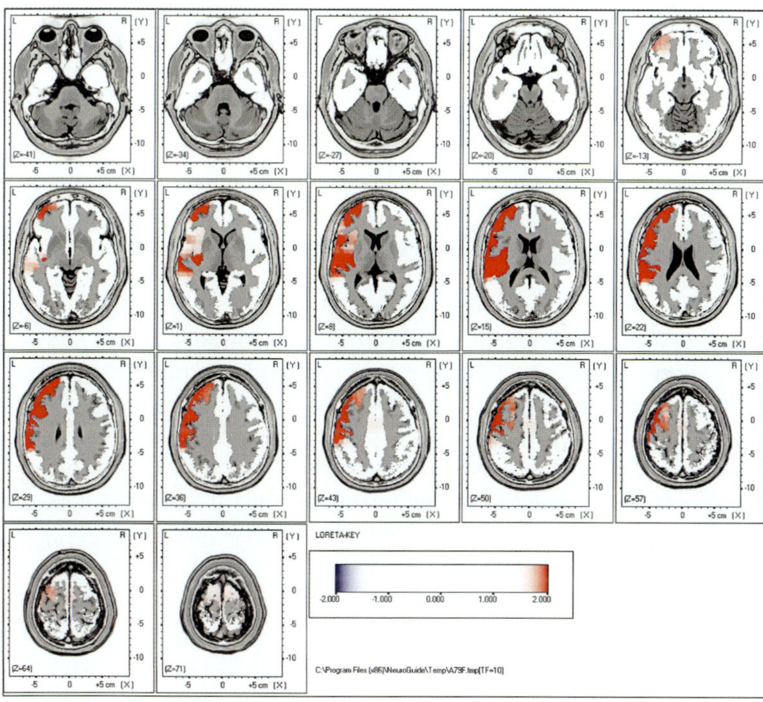

FIGURE 15.4 LORETA analysis of cortical slices showing increased activity at 10 Hz throughout the left prefrontal cortex and temporal regions, including Broca's area.

continued

CASE 1 *(cont'd)*

Rugg, Fletcher, Frith, Frackowiak, & Dolan, 1996), and all of which are related to Kim's challenges.

Phase 1: 2-Channel Z-Score Training

Kim completed several sessions of 2-channel Z-score training in order to resolve the focal discrepancies at T5, as well as increased connectivity between language areas and higher cortical information processing areas. Following the round of 2-channel training, Kim had resolved much of the power issues related to excess beta, as well as many of the hypercoherences seen in the initial mapping. Even more exciting was the report from Kim's mother of increased talkativeness, and a better overall use of vocabulary. Kim's mother felt that she was becoming much more fluid in her use of language, and was better able to articulate her thoughts, as opposed to giving up before being fully able to express what she wanted to say due to the frustration of having to piece it all together.

Phase 2: 19-Channel LORETA Z-Score Training

Although Kim had experienced some success with 2-channel neurofeedback training, it became clear that multiple nodes and networks were involved in her symptomatology, and that a more comprehensive approach would be needed. Kim then moved to 19-channel LORETA Z-score training, using Neuroguide software to generate selections for training.

Following analysis of a new updated QEEG, a Symptom Checklist was created from Kim's eyes open condition. One should note here the importance of building the Symptom Checklist from the eyes open condition, as Kim would be doing her training with her eyes open, and many of her symptoms involved processing visual data. This is not true for all individuals and presenting conditions, and it is at the discretion of the clinician to decide how to conduct training sessions and use the eyes open or eyes closed conditions accordingly.

Kim's updated QEEG, conducted approximately 4 months later, can be seen in Figure 15.5. Again, both eyes open and eyes closed conditions were conducted for comparison against her baseline QEEG. In the eyes open surface maps, deficiencies still exist in power in the lower frequencies, most specifically at 1 Hz. In looking at the updated map, we also begin to see areas of abnormal fast activity in the beta range which appear in areas associated with visual processing, language, and social cognition. It is important to note that Kim had recently returned to school at this point, which has been a consistent source of stress in

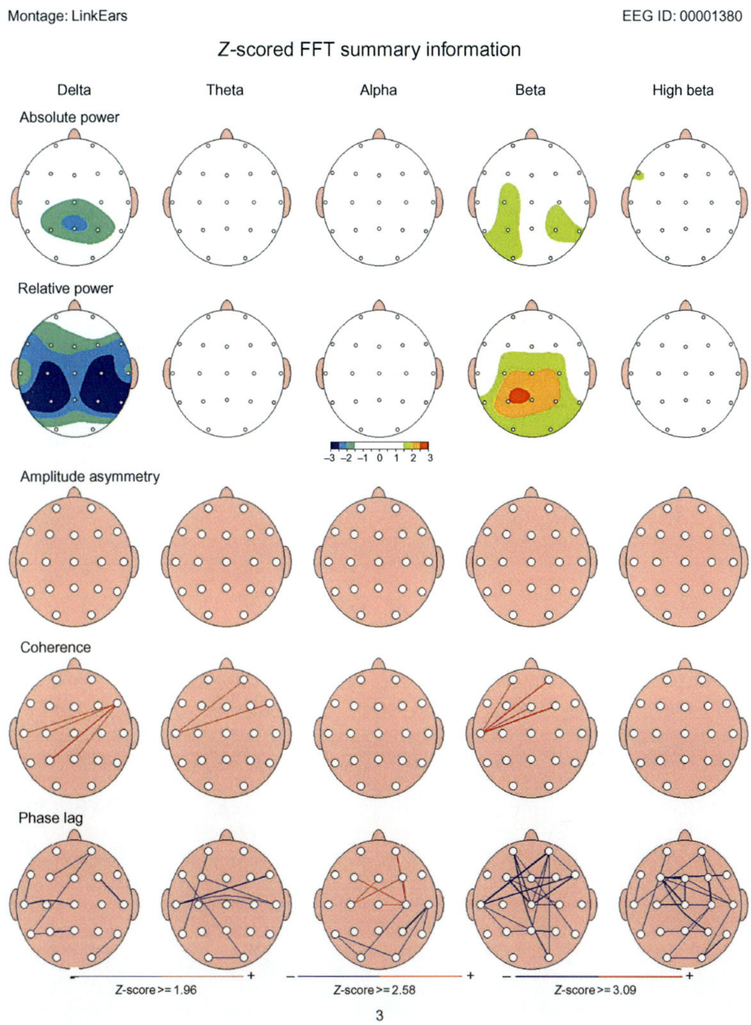

FIGURE 15.5 Kim's updated QEEG, taken August 6, 2013, showed dramatic improvements in connectivity, including resolution of the hypercoherence seen in the left temporal areas.

her life, and some of these deviancies, particularly the excessive beta activity in the anterior cingulate regions, may have been in part due to her anxiety about returning to school.

Significant improvements were made in measures of connectivity, as the hypercoherences associated with T5 had resolved completely.

continued

CASE 1 (*cont'd*)

In addition, abnormalities in amplitude asymmetry had normalized. LORETA analysis still showed unresolved power deficiencies in the 1–2 Hz bands, with localization in Brodmann area 7 bilaterally (superior parietal lobule, housing the association sensorimotor areas). This area was of particular interest, given its role in visuospatial information processing and working memory, as well as language comprehension (Yoo, Paralkar, & Panych, 2004) (Figure 15.6).

Some abnormal alpha activity remained present in the 10–11 Hz bands (seen in Figure 15.7), localized within the left and right temporal regions (Brodmann areas 41 and 43), although much of the activity originating from the left prefrontal cortex had resolved. However, the power abnormalities remaining continued to contribute to her difficulties processing and attending to spoken information, particularly in the classroom where sensory input is abundant.

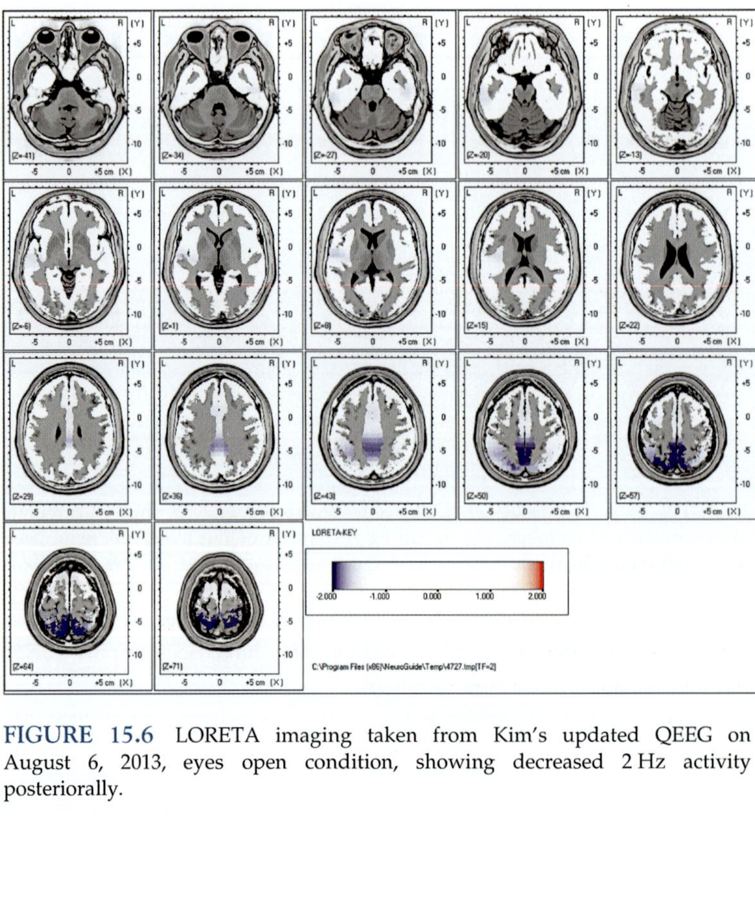

FIGURE 15.6 LORETA imaging taken from Kim's updated QEEG on August 6, 2013, eyes open condition, showing decreased 2 Hz activity posteriorally.

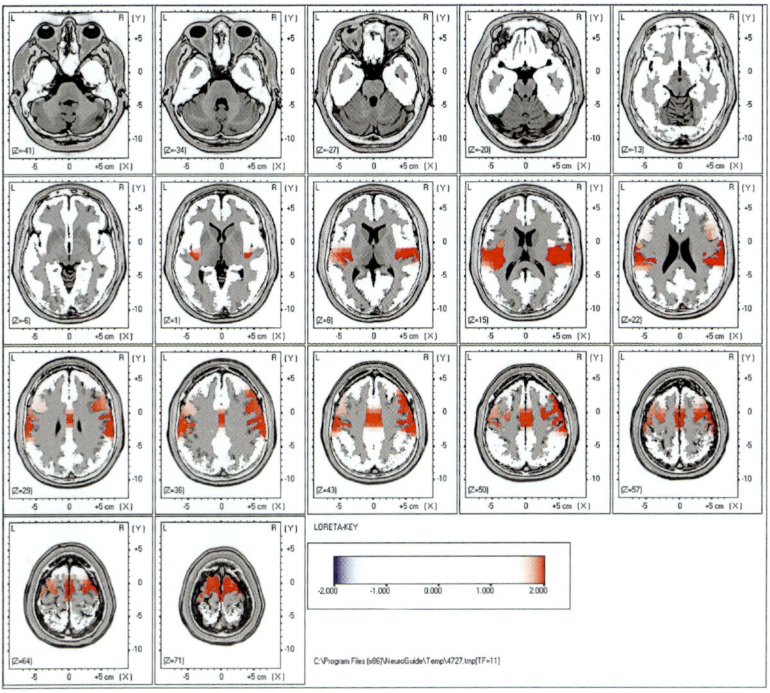

FIGURE 15.7 LORETA imaging showing increased activity in the 11 Hz band bilaterally. Taken from her QEEG recording on August 6, 2013.

Selections in the Symptom Checklist targeted symptom constellations. The decision was made to target-specific symptoms as opposed to networks due to more precise correlation between the symptom selections and the LORETA analysis. Symptoms chosen included *Slow Reader, Attention Deficits—Easily Distractible,* and *Anxiety.* Brodmann areas selected for training included areas 7, 13, 31, 40, 41, and 42, with metrics including power, absolute phase, and coherence. Selections were checked against the .tdt tables generated from LORETA Coherence and Phase in order to ensure that the protocol closely matched the deviant areas. Of importance to note here is that when choosing symptoms from the Symptom Checklist, there sometimes is no direct symptom listed for the presenting problem. For example, Kim may not be typically classified as a slow reader, as her challenge lies more within comprehension. However, upon examination of matched Brodmann areas, it is clear that *Slow Reader* brings in the appropriate areas of interest and thus should be selected.

continued

CASE 1 (*cont'd*)

Anxiety was selected because, although it does not directly relate to either information processing, attentional resources, or reading, it does have a circular relationship with all of these things. Anxiety is frequently observed in individuals with learning disorders, as they are often acutely aware of their difficulties as they relate to their peers. Not only is the anxiety caused by these root difficulties, but it further exacerbates them as well. Anyone who has felt a significant degree of anxiety well understands how difficult it is to pay attention or to try to piece together complex information when anxious thoughts are both intruding upon and overwhelming the cognitive processing systems. Therefore, it is often advisable to include the *Anxiety* symptom so as to capture the entire causal loop.

Conducting Training Sessions

Kim began training with 19-channel LORETA *Z*-score shortly following her second QEEG. She trained two times weekly, after school. Training sessions began with a check-in of symptoms and possible ab-reactions. Initially, Kim could tolerate no more than 12 min of training, with four sets of 3 min rounds. She would become easily fatigued, and in order to maintain her learning curve, we did not push her beyond her limits. After a period of time, however, she was able to work up to four sets of 4 min rounds, and sometimes even five sets. At times Kim was asked to hold the training parameters longer than the default 250 ms, and the time window was raised to 750 ms without detriment. Training was kept varied and interesting for her with the use of games, points, and the occasional reward. Kim was extremely self-motivated to work hard at her training, and so external rewards were less necessary than with other individuals who might not see the intrinsic value of neurofeedback. Indeed, Kim declined rewards offered at several points, making her the exception to the rule in that sense.

Periodic updated QEEGs were conducted, and new protocols subsequently made, ensuring that symptom constellations chosen continued to match the presenting symptoms, and incorporated Brodmann areas of interest as seen in LORETA analysis and .tdt files.

Phase 3: Introducing Complementary Interventions

Following a round of 20 sessions of LORETA *Z*-score training, Kim had begun to show significant improvements in her ability to learn and assimilate information. The holes in her cognitive foundation were being filled, and we felt that this would be a good time to begin to introduce complementary interventions which would build upon that foundation. We began by addressing her working memory, or the ability to hold and manipulate information in the mind. Working memory is imperative to any kind of problem solving, and in school children constantly need to use their working memory to solve math problems, take notes as they simultaneously listen to their teacher talk, and organize their essays in a coherent manner. Working memory is especially important in reading comprehension as well, especially for dyslexic readers who struggle so much with reading already. Cogmed Working Memory Training was a logical next step for Kim's treatment.

Cogmed is an intensive training program targeted at improving working memory and attention (Gray et al., 2012). Kim trained with the aid of a coach 5 days a week, for 30–40 min per day. Exercises were both visuospatial and auditory. She was still continuing with neurofeedback at the same time. After a week of this combined training, Kim's mother noticed that she was becoming easily fatigued and having trouble remaining awake and alert in school. For her, the dual approach of neurofeedback plus Cogmed was simply too much. She took a hiatus from neurofeedback to finish the remaining 20 days of the Cogmed program, which resolved the issue. She was then able to return to neurofeedback training without feeling strained and fatigued. She completed another 20 sessions before retesting her outcome measures.

Phase 4: Final Update and Outcomes

Kim took a break from training over the holiday season, and in February, 2014, returned for an updated QEEG and follow-up neuropsychological testing. The results were astonishing. Her parents reported a new-found confidence in herself, and a willingness to participate in school, whereas before she had been shy and withdrawn. Reading comprehension was significantly improved, as was her attention. Kim was again tested using the Quotient ADHD System, with remarkable improvement in her ability to sustain her cognitive effort and attention. Figure 15.8 shows her responses throughout the duration of the test, with fewer errors of omission and commission, thereby indicating decreased impulsivity and distractibility, as well as significantly less variability in her response time, indicating better attention overall.

In a breakdown of Kim's attention states taken over 30 s intervals (Figures 15.9 and 15.10), one can see the dramatic change in Kim's ability to maintain cognitive control, and it is easy to see how this would greatly improve her overall functioning in the classroom.

Kim's new QEEG looked similarly improved as well. As can be seen in Figure 15.11, deficiencies in the delta band had resolved, as well as

continued

CASE 1 (*cont'd*)

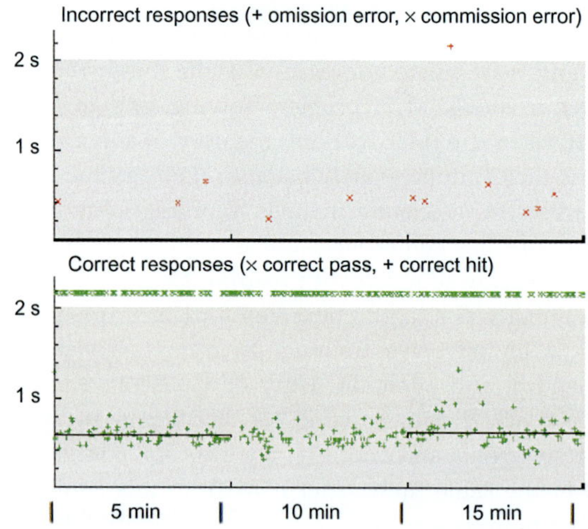

FIGURE 15.8 Kim's target and nontarget responses on the Quotient ADHD System showing improvement at the time of retesting, September 25, 2013.

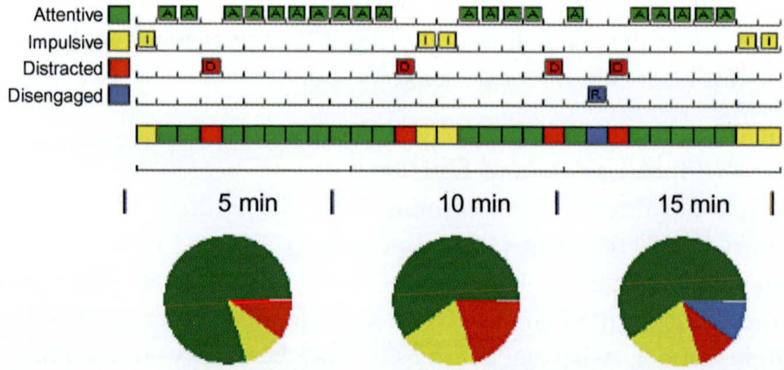

FIGURE 15.9 Kim's attention state analysis over 30 s intervals prior to training. Note that she spends a considerable amount of time responding impulsively, distractedly, and at one point, is completely disengaged from the task.

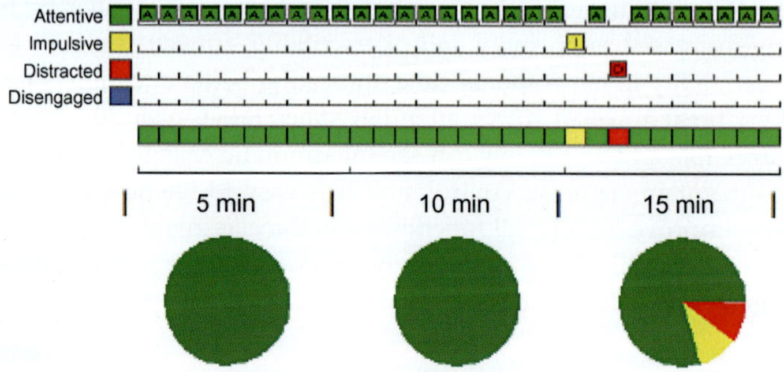

FIGURE 15.10 Kim's attention state analysis over 30 s intervals posttraining. She only has two intervals throughout the duration of the test where she is not completely on-task. Conducted September 25, 2013.

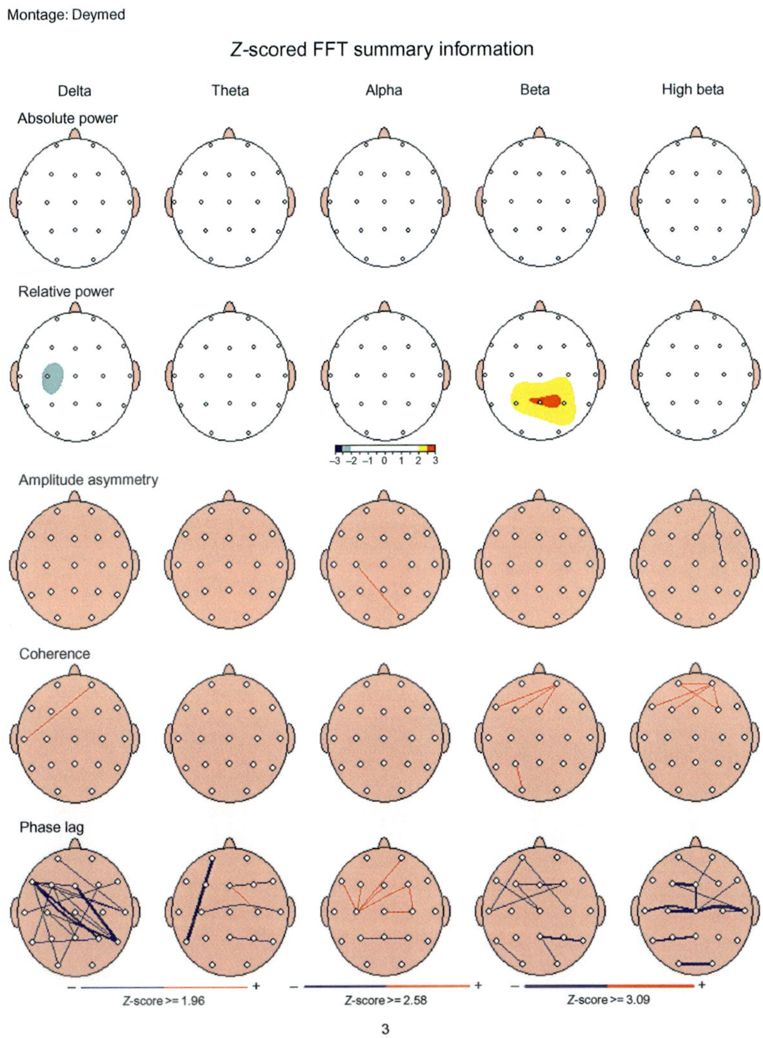

FIGURE 15.11 Surface maps taken from Kim's final QEEG taken February 26, 2014. Note the improvement in absolute power as compared to her baseline QEEG.

excess activity within the Alpha band. A few hypercoherences within the frontal regions still remained, as well as some abnormalities within absolute phase. Symptoms associated with executive skills had improved considerably. Kim was now able to organize her written and

continued

CASE 1 (*cont'd*)

spoken language much more precisely, as well as articulate the ideas which came into her head in a well-thought-out and cohesive manner. Her ability to hold and manipulate complex information in her head became much more pronounced, and subsequently her impoverished reading and mathematics skills became much less effortful, and on par with those of her peers. At this juncture, it was deemed unnecessary to continue training, instead moving the focus to more skill-based interventions.

Even more surprising than the improvements in the surface maps was the complete resolution of any deviant activity within the 10–11 Hz bands as seen in LORETA. Figure 15.12 shows the 11 Hz bins taken from her final QEEG on February 26, 2014, with no abnormalities in current density.

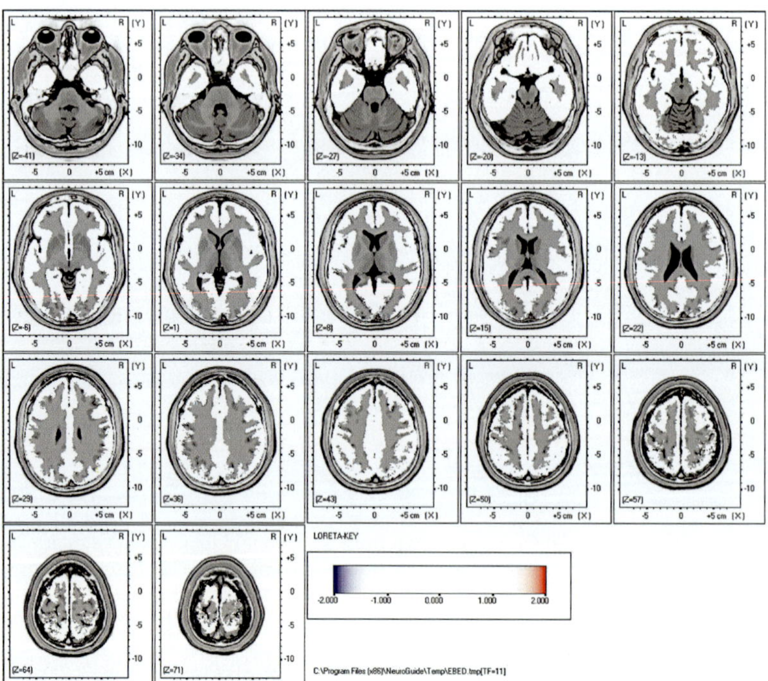

FIGURE 15.12 LORETA analysis detailing the normalized 11 Hz frequency band from Kim's final QEEG conducted February 26, 2014.

Conclusion

Kim's story is one of successful neurofeedback training, combined with complementary interventions and the use of neuropsychological testing in order to better understand her cognitive shortcomings. The use of 19-channel LORETA Z-score training enabled Kim to fully maximize her cognitive potential and gain cognitive resources that she never had before. This also paved the way for other focused interventions to be more effective. Kim continues to maintain her gains made via neurofeedback and Cogmed, and is now able to thrive in her classroom setting. Not only did she benefit academically, but emotionally as well, as she is now confident in her abilities to perform on par with her peers.

CASE 2

Symptom History

Sarah is a 10-year-old girl who came to our clinic following concerns in the classroom regarding her reading, writing, spelling, and mathematics skills. Sarah had been previously diagnosed with dyslexia and completed a 6-week intensive reading program, Linda-Mood Bell, following diagnosis. Although she made slight improvements following the program, she still had significant difficulty with reading fluency and comprehension. Sarah's parents sought a new assessment to receive updated information regarding possible diagnoses and to receive information about other available interventions.

In a clinical interview, Sarah's parents reported that she often skipped over words while reading and had difficulty comprehending information that she read. In addition to her reading challenges, Sarah's parents reported many difficulties with executive functioning; they addressed concerns regarding working memory, the ability to follow multistep directions, time-management, and task initiation. Sarah had trouble when asked how much time had passed or was remaining in regards to an event. For example, she was often unable to calculate the amount of time she had to get ready in the morning before school. Sarah's parents addressed concerns with her overall confidence as well and observed that she would often answer questions with a response of "I don't know," in order to avoid making a mistake.

continued

CASE 2 (*cont'd*)

Sarah attended a Montessori-based school, which typically provides a less structured classroom environment. Montessori schools differ from traditional schools in that they offer mixed-age classrooms, freedom to roam around and outside the classroom, and student-chosen activities. At the time Sarah entered our clinic, teachers were also noticing significant executive functioning difficulties in the classroom. Teachers reported that Sarah was distracted by her environment and often provided excuses to leave the classroom. In addition, she also had difficulty sitting down to begin her work. Although teachers provided Sarah with a list of work that she needed to do, she had trouble staying on task and often failed to complete assignments.

Assessment

Sarah completed a full neuropsychological assessment in our clinic. She completed a variety of measures, as well as an intelligence test against which her academic scores were compared. Similar to Kim, Sarah is a bright child, yet many of her scores on academic measures were severely discrepant from her overall abilities. Sarah presented as a friendly and outgoing child, but often had trouble maintaining appropriate effort during testing, especially when presented with a difficult task. Instead, Sarah would appear distracted or try to engage the examiner in irrelevant conversation. Sarah had a variety of strengths and weaknesses across all domains; however, her performance across measures of attention, reading, writing, and math was typically lower than would be expected when compared to her cognitive ability.

Figure 15.13 illustrates Sarah's overall intellectual functioning ability. Sarah demonstrated average verbal and nonverbal intellectual

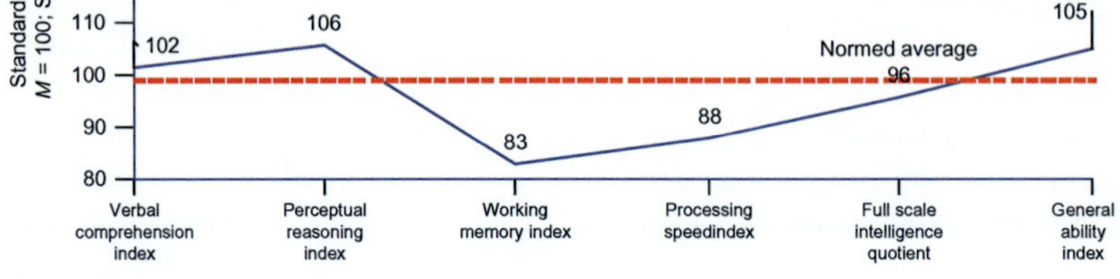

FIGURE 15.13 Sarah's intellectual profile compiled from composite scores on the Wechsler Intelligence Scale for Children—4th Edition, August 20, 2013.

abilities, and relative weaknesses in working memory and processing speed, consistent with parent and teacher reports.

In Figure 15.14, Sarah's performance on reading measures showed a relative weakness in reading accuracy and fluency compared to her cognitive ability. Her reading performance was slower and less accurate than expected, and she had a tendency to omit small words (e.g., "on," "now," "the"). Furthermore, as reading passages became more challenging, Sarah often inaccurately sounded out words and did not take the appropriate amount of time to recognize her mistake.

Figure 15.15 is an illustration of Sarah's attention states taken from the Quotient ADHD System, illustrating Sarah's inability to maintain

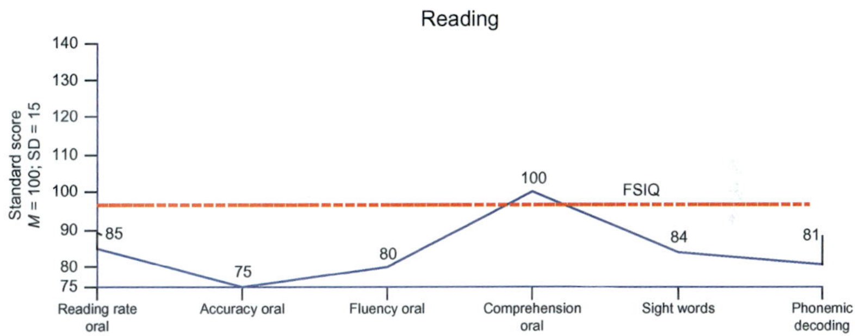

FIGURE 15.14 Sarah's intellectual profile compiled from composite scores on the Test of Word Reading Efficiency—2nd Edition, Form A (TOWRE-2) and Gray Oral Reading Test, 5th Edition, Form A (GORT-5), August 20, 2013.

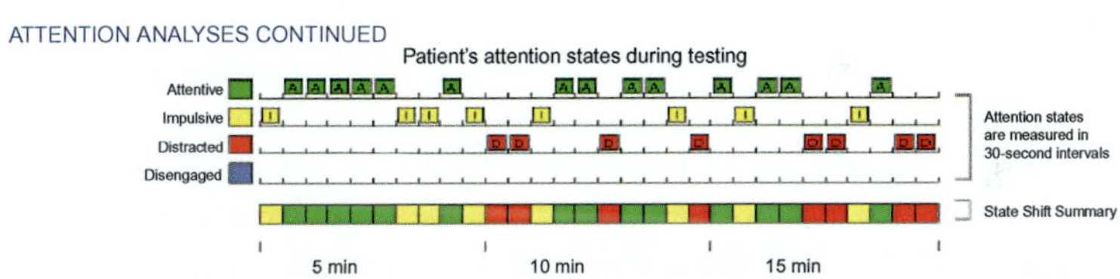

Attention State Results

Measure		Results	Reference Range (18-84 Percentile)	Age Percentile (t ≤ 16 Age Percentile)
Number of Shifts: *(number)* *A measure of how many times a change in behavioral states occurs over the course of a test.*		18	5 - 17	13 t
Attentive: *(percent)* *Percent of 30 second blocks in which subjects performed with very high level of accuracy.*		46.7	23.3 - 90.0	30
Impulsive: *(percent)* *Percent of blocks when subjects performed better than chance but made a significant number of commission errors.*		26.7	6.7 - 50.0	46
Distracted: *(percent)* *Percent of blocks when subjects performed better than chance but missed a significant number of targets.*		26.7	0.0 - 13.3	6 t
R.	**Random:** *(percent)* *Percent of blocks when subjects performed no better than predicted by random chance.*	0.0	0.0 - 6.7	99
M.	**Minimal:** *(percent)* *Percent of blocks when subjects performed no better than predicted by random chance and made few responses.*	0.0	0.0 - 0.0	99
C.	**Contrary** *(percent)* *Percent of blocks when subjects performed worse than predicted by random chance.*	0.0	0.0 - 0.0	99

FIGURE 15.15 Sarah's initial Quotient® ADHD System Continuous Performance Test: Attention States, August 26, 2013.

continued

CASE 2 *(cont'd)*

her attention over a 15 min period. Her attention states were broken down into 30 s intervals and graphed so as to better understand the percentage of time she spends actively engaged in a task. She struggled to maintain appropriate attention for the duration of the test, as reflected by an excessive number of errors of omission and commission, indicating relative weaknesses in distractibility and impulsivity over time. Sarah was often distracted or impulsive, and was attentive for less than half of the test.

Intervention

Since traditional measures were largely ineffective, we recommended that Sarah begin neurofeedback to address concerns regarding attention and executive functioning challenges. We also addressed areas associated with reading comprehension to assist with her reading difficulties.

Stage 1: QEEG Analysis

Sarah's initial QEEG was conducted on September 27, 2013, using a Nexus amplifier. Both eyes open and eyes closed conditions were obtained. The data was then artifacted and the eyes open condition was used to generate the following quantitative analyses.

Surface maps seen in Figure 15.16 yielded limited information. Apart from localized activity within the delta and beta ranges at FZ, maps also showed amplitude asymmetries generating from the right temporal regions, as well as deficiencies in absolute phase. It became clear that further analysis using LORETA would be needed to uncover the root of any further abnormal physiology.

LORETA current density analysis yielded a much clear picture, showing deficiencies in slow activity in delta 1–2 Hz ranging from −2.3 to −2.7 standard deviations in the areas of the cingulate cortex, bilateral parietal lobes, and insula (Figure 15.17) These areas are of particular significance in Sarah's case due to their heavy involvement in memory, sustained attention, and cognitive processing in general, all of which were of significant challenge to Sarah (Krause, Horwitz, & Taylor, 1999; Mencl, Pugh, & Shaywitz, 2000).

Moreover, there was excessive fast activity in the beta range (29–30 Hz) in the anterior cingulate and the superior and medial frontal gyri. Figure 15.18 shows the extent to which this excessive fast activity is present within Brodmann areas 6, 8, 9, 24, and 32. This activity may have been in part associated with Sarah's poor self-esteem and anxiety surrounding her perceived challenges, as well as her gross deficits in executive functioning (Burton, Noll, & Small, 2001; Fichtenholtz et al., 2004; Lane et al., 1998).

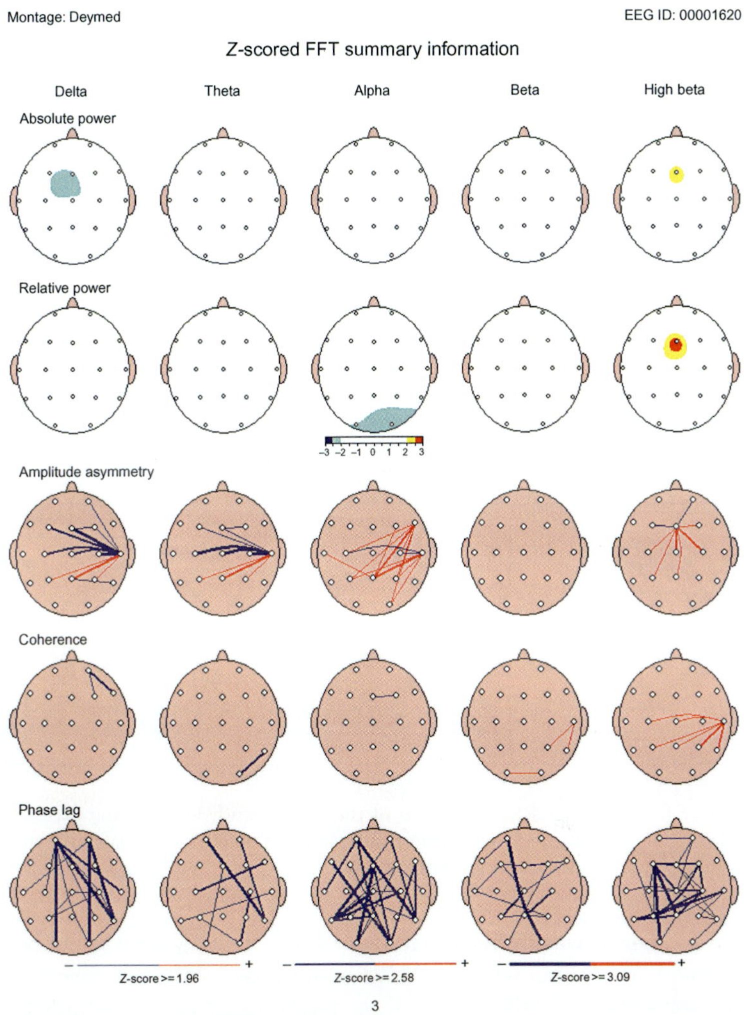

FIGURE 15.16 Sarah's surface maps taken from her initial QEEG on September 27, 2013. Localized absolute power abnormalities were noted surrounding FZ. However, the most concerning findings center around her short phase lag time across frequency bands.

Phase 1: 19-Channel Surface Z-Score Training

Following analysis of her first QEEG, areas of concern were selected using the Symptom Checklist in Neuroguide. Again, we cannot stress the importance of choosing constellations of symptoms which relate to

continued

CASE 2 (*cont'd*)

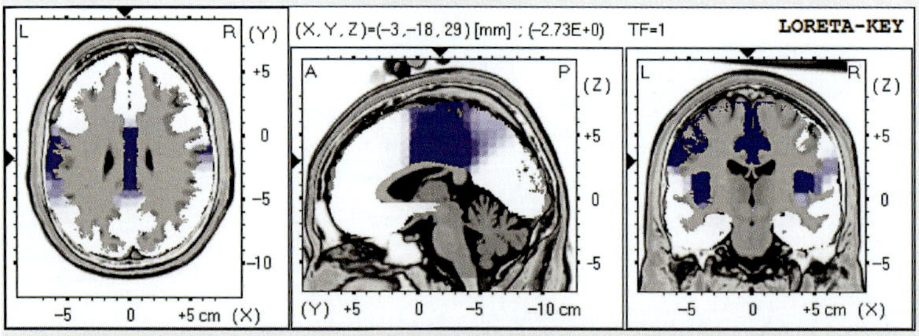

FIGURE 15.17 LORETA analysis of the 1 Hz band taken from Sarah's initial QEEG recording (condition: eyes open). Note that the deviant activity is nearly 3 standard deviations from the mean in the shaded areas.

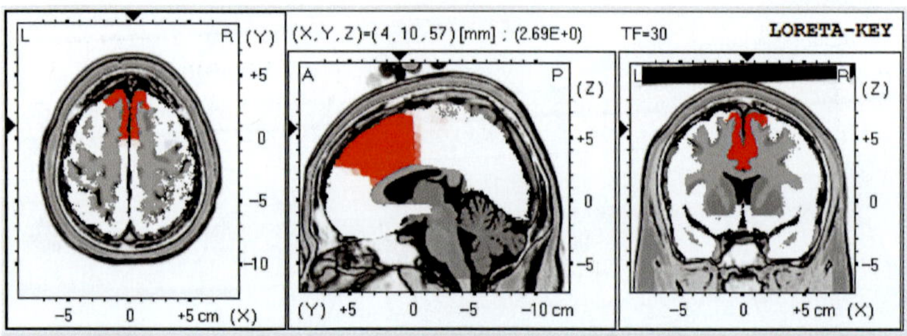

FIGURE 15.18 LORETA analysis of the 30 Hz band detailing the excessive beta activity within the frontal cortex, including the anterior cingulate and areas of the prefrontal cortex and premotor areas.

one another. It was decided that Sarah would initially train using NF1 to train surface EEG within coherence and phase shift and phase lock to resolve any anomalies within those measures. Selections included in Sarah's initial protocol were *Attention Deficits—Easily Distractible*, *Slow Reader*, and *Executive Function Problems*.

Conducting Neurofeedback Training Sessions

Sarah began neurofeedback sessions shortly after her first QEEG and came in before school twice a week. Initially, Sarah often failed to maintain an appropriate amount of effort for the duration of her neurofeedback session. She would have difficulty sitting still and would often stretch her arms, kick her legs, or attempt to initiate the therapist in conversation during her sessions. In addition, Sarah was unable to train longer than 12 min and often complained that she was tired. Sarah's parents and therapist worked together to create a reward system that encouraged her. Sarah earned prizes for the amount of points she earned while doing neurofeedback games, which appeared to ease her stress. For example, one prize which Sarah received was a pair of rollerblades once she reached 750 points earned during neurofeedback games.

Following session 14 (November, 27, 2013), Sarah's parents expressed concern that they had not seen any positive changes. They also spoke with her teachers, none of whom reported any changes regarding classroom behavior. An updated QEEG was completed to assess what changes had been made from neurofeedback so far. An analysis determined that while she had made significant improvements in the metrics included in her protocol (coherence, phase shift/lock), Sarah also experienced a significant decline in power.

Phase 2: 19-Channel LORETA Z-Score Training

Following a round of surface training, an updated QEEG analysis was conducted to examine Sarah's progress and to assess abnormalities within absolute power so as to better target those areas. Although coherence and phase discrepancies had largely resolved, there suddenly were a host of deficiencies across all frequency bands in LORETA current density. Sarah was exhibiting "blue brain." In Figure 15.19, one can see the pervasive deficiencies within the 30 Hz band, and how they have become exacerbated from her initial QEEG. This finding was consistent with nearly every frequency band, with Z-scores ranging to −3.64 standard deviations.

Beginning at session 15 (November, 29, 2013), Sarah began her training sessions on a new LORETA protocol, which again included the symptoms of *Attention Deficits—Easily Distractible, Slow Reader*, and *Executive Function Problems*. However, this time the focus was training absolute power. After Sarah completed five more sessions (December, 11, 2013) of neurofeedback on her new protocol, her therapist noticed that Sarah had been coming in more alert, energetic, and able to focus appropriately. Sarah's parents were also noticing some changes in her behavior at this time.

Sarah's parents emailed us (January, 16, 2013) following five more sessions and provided us with positive feedback expressed by Sarah's teachers. Sarah's teachers began to notice that she had been staying on task, finishing class assignments within the allotted time frame, and had also begun to self-correct errors.

continued

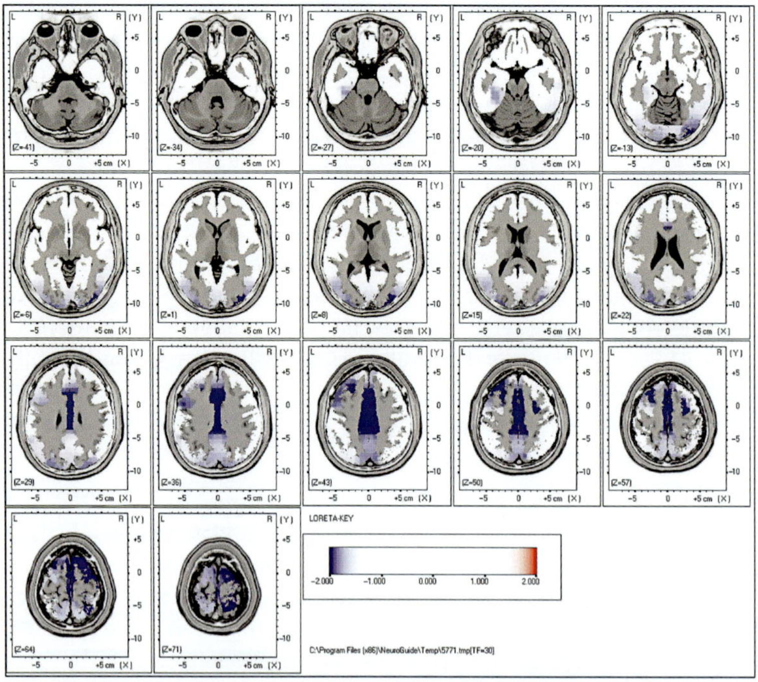

FIGURE 15.19 Cortical slices detailing deficiencies in the 30 Hz band throughout the brain. Taken from Sarah's updated QEEG on November 25, 2013.

After four more sessions, Sarah's parents and teachers had noticed observable changes in her behavior and work ethic. Sarah's teachers reported that her attention in class had significantly improved. They also had noticed she was no longer providing excuses to leave the classroom, and instead she was actively participating in the classroom by asking questions and helping other children. Furthermore, her teachers reported that although she was still having difficulty with some reading concepts, she had been taking the time to sound out words and self-correct mistakes.

In addition to these changes observed by her parents and teachers, we also noticed a significant shift in attitude when Sarah came in to our clinic for neurofeedback. During the first 2 months of neurofeedback, Sarah often complained and needed frequent rewards. She would fail to put forth an appropriate amount of effort and instead would stretch out in her chair, kick her legs, and attempt to engage in a conversation. Following approximately 25 sessions, it was noticeable that Sarah no longer needed frequent redirection. Instead, she was able to maintain focus and effort throughout the duration of her

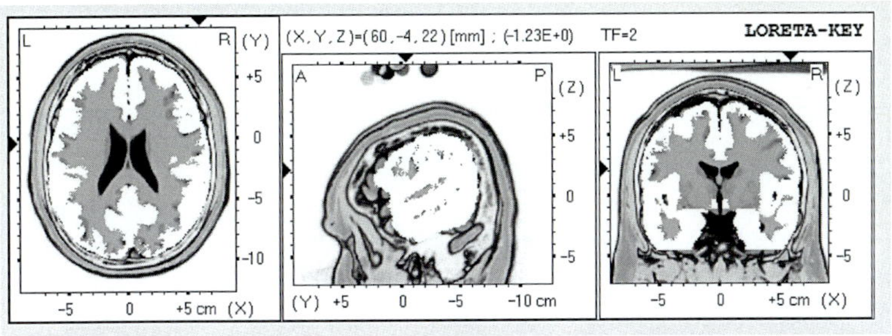

FIGURE 15.20 2 Hz bins showing complete resolution of abnormalities in current density, taken from Sarah's QEEG on March 26, 2013.

neurofeedback session. In addition, she enjoyed engaging in conversation at appropriate times and appeared to be much more confident when speaking.

Follow-Up

In an updated QEEG taken on March 26, 2013, Sarah showed remarkable improvements across frequency bands. In Figure 15.20, the resolution of deficiencies within the delta band can be seen.

Figure 15.21 shows the progress made within the beta range, specifically the 30 Hz band. If you will recall, the 30 Hz band was significantly deviant, with diffuse underactivity in the beta range. This is especially critical in the case of Sarah, as the lack of these faster organizing frequencies were contributing heavily to her symptoms of poor cognitive reserve.

Final Update and Outcomes

Sarah's neurofeedback treatments proved to be very successful. Following approximately 30 sessions, Sarah's parents e-mailed her neurofeedback therapist (January, 16, 2014) to provide astounding feedback; both parents and teachers had noticed significant changes in her behavior and work ethic.

Teachers had reported to Sarah's parents that the executive functioning difficulties observed at the beginning of the school year were no longer an issue. Sarah had been staying on task in the classroom and completing her assignments with ease. Previously, she required frequent monitoring and redirection in the classroom; however, teachers were now reporting that she was able to work from a checklist and manage classroom assignments on her own. Furthermore, teachers

continued

CASE 2 (*cont'd*)

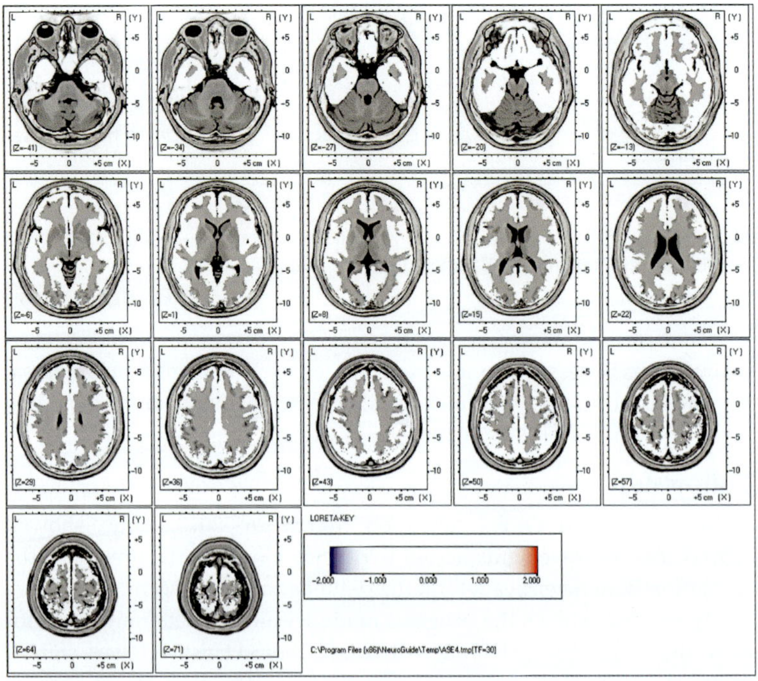

FIGURE 15.21 The 30 Hz band taken from Sarah's QEEG conducted on March 26, 2013, showing complete resolution within LORETA current density.

noticed that she was also checking her work for mistakes and self-correcting errors. They reported that her attention in class had significantly improved; she was no longer providing excuses to leave the classroom, and instead she was actively participating in the classroom by asking questions and helping other children stay on task. One teacher even mentioned that Sarah was "not the same kid that walked into the classroom at the beginning of the school year."

Additionally, her parents reported that Sarah had more confidence in herself and her abilities. She was now asking questions to clarify when something did not make sense to her and was able to maintain an appropriate amount of effort to learn and retain new material.

The success of 19-channel surface and LORETA neurofeedback training gave Sarah the ability to utilize her cognitive ability in both classroom and real-world settings. At the beginning of Sarah's neurofeedback treatment, she struggled with many executive functions and was often unable to put forth and maintain an appropriate amount of effort and focus. Following her neurofeedback training, those symptoms had been resolved. Sarah was no longer struggling at home or in class, and her teachers and parents with incredibly pleased her progress. Sarah's physiological changes due to neurofeedback made other facets of her academic work more enjoyable; she now had the mental stamina to approach new material, and the success she experienced with neurofeedback has dramatically improved her attitude and confidence in herself.

Conclusion

As seen in the illustrated cases, 19-channel LORETA Z-score training is a powerful tool in the treatment of learning disabilities and executive function deficits. It may be used in isolation, or in conjunction with other skill-based interventions to affect significant change in the physiology. Emphasis is placed on the importance of understanding the underlying symptoms in their entirety, and the cognitive processes which drive them via use of standardized measures and neuropsychological assessment. Although both Kim and Sarah were diagnosed with ADHD, they do not exhibit the classic signs of the disorder and conventional methods such as medication proved ineffective. Their attentional and executive function deficits, taken in conjunction with their learning disabilities, form a tangled web of symptoms which needed to be addressed in its entirety. Neurofeedback provided the physiological foundation upon which new connections could be built, paving the way for more skill-based interventions to be successful. This integrated model has proven successful with many other such cases at our clinic, and we continue to successfully treat many children and adults with similar profiles.

References

Burton, M. W., Noll, D. C., & Small, S. L. (2001). The anatomy of auditory word processing: Individual variability. *Brain Language, 77*(1), 119–131.

Fichtenholtz, H. M., Dean, H. L., Dillon, D. G., Yamasaki, H., McCarthy, G., & LaBar, K. S. (2004). *Cognitive Brain Research, 20*(1), 67–80.

Friederici, A. D., Rüschemeyer, S. A., Hahne, A., & Fiebach, C. J. (2003). The role of left inferior frontal and superior temporal cortex in sentence comprehension: Localizing syntactic and semantic processes. *Cerebral Cortex, 13*(2), 170–177.

Gray, S. A., Chaban, P., Martinussen, R., Goldberg, R., Gotlieb, H., Kronitz, R., et al. (2012). Effects of a computerized working memory training program on working memory, attention, and academics in adolescents with severe LD and comorbid ADHD: A randomized controlled trial. *Journal of Child Psychology and Psychiatry, 53*, 1277–1284.

Heim, S., Eickhoff, S. B., & Amunts, K. (2008). Specialisation in Broca's region for semantic, phonological, and syntactic fluency. *Neuroimage, 40*(3), 1362–1368.

Jessen, F., Erb, M., Klose, U., Lotze, M., Grodd, W., & Heun, R. (1999). Activation of human language processing brain regions after the presentation of random letter strings demonstrated with event-related functional magnetic resonance imaging. *Neuroscience Letters, 270*(1), 13–16.

Krause, B. J., Horwitz, B., Taylor, J. G., et al. (1999). Network analysis in episodic encoding and retrieval of word-pair associates: A PET study. *European Journal of Neuroscience, 11* (9), 3293–3301.

Lane, R. D., Reiman, E. M., Axelrod, B., Yun, L. S., Holmes, A., & Schwartz, G. E. (1998). Neural correlates of levels of emotional awareness. Evidence of an interaction between emotion and attention in the anterior cingulate cortex. *Journal of Cognitive Neuroscience, 10*(4), 525–535.

Mencl, W. E., Pugh, K. R., Shaywitz, S. E., et al. (2000). Network analysis of brain activations in working memory: Behavior and age relationships. *Microscopy Research and Technique, 51*(1), 64–74.

Okuda, J., Fujii, T., Yamadori, A., et al. (2000). Retention of words in long-term memory: A functional neuroanatomical study with PET. *Neuroreport, 11*(2), 323–328.

Rugg, M. D., Fletcher, P. C., Frith, C. D., Frackowiak, R. S., & Dolan, R. J. (1996). Differential activation of the prefrontal cortex in successful and unsuccessful memory retrieval. *Brain*(Pt 6), 2073–2083.

Yoo, S. S., Paralkar, G., & Panych, L. P. (2004). Neural substrates associated with the concurrent performance of dual working memory tasks. *International Journal of Neuroscience, 114*(6), 613–631.

Index

Note: Page numbers followed by "*b*," "*f*," and "*t*" refer to boxes, figures, and tables, respectively.

Edwards Brothers Malloy
Ann Arbor MI. USA
October 24, 2014